MANAGEMENT IN NURSING

An Experiential Approach That Makes Theory Work for You

Elaine L. La Monica, Ed.D., F.A.A.N., is Professor of Nursing Education at Teachers College, Columbia University, New York. Currently, she is Chair of the Department of Nursing Education. Her formal education includes a Doctor of Education degree in human relations and counseling from the School of Education, University of Massachusetts, Amherst; a Masters of Nursing in medical and surgical nursing administration from the College of Nursing, University of Florida, Gainesville; and a Bachelor of Science in nursing from Columbia Union College, Takoma Park, Maryland.

In addition to administrative and academic responsibilities at Teachers College, Dr. La Monica maintains a private consulting practice in management for health care organizations and other public and private industries throughout the United States and Canada. She also conducts training programs on organizational behavior both nationally and internationally.

Scholarly activities included serving as the Management Briefs Editor for *The Journal of Nursing Administration* and as a frequent author on management, empathy, and related topics in professional journals. Dr. La Monica's most recent books are *Nursing Leadership and Management: An Experiential Approach*, 1986, and *The Humanistic Nursing Process*, 1985; both are published by Jones and Bartlett, Boston, Massachusetts. *The La Monica Empathy Profile*, 1986, published by XICOM, Inc., Sterling Forest, Tuxedo, New York, is an instrument for measuring empathy in helpers—teachers, nurses, managers, and other caregivers.

Dr. La Monica maintains membership in the following professional organizations: American Academy of Nursing, American Nurses Association, American Psychological Association, Council of Nurse Researchers, New York State Nurses Association, and Sigma Theta Tau–Alpha Theta Chapter.

MANAGEMENT IN NURSING

An Experiential Approach That Makes Theory Work for You

Elaine Lynne La Monica,
Ed.D., F.A.A.N.

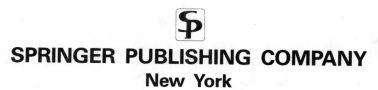

SPRINGER PUBLISHING COMPANY
New York

Copyright © 1990 by Springer Publishing Company, Inc.

Springer Publishing Company, Inc.
536 Broadway
New York, NY 10012

91 92 93 94 / 5 4 3 2

Library of Congress Cataloging-in-Publication Data

La Monica, Elaine Lynne, 1944-
    Management in nursing : an experiential approach that makes theory work for you / Elaine L. La Monica.
        p. cm.
    Includes bibliographical references.
    ISBN 0-8261-6580-X
    1. Nursing services—Administration. I. Title.
    [DNLM: 1. Leadership—nurses' instruction. 2. Nursing, Supervisory—organization & administration. WY 105 L234m]
RT89.L26 1990
362.1'73'068—dc20
DNLM/DLC
for Library of Congress   90-9455
                                                                  CIP

Printed in the United States of America

Dedicated to

My best friend,
Robert S. Rigolosi

For feeling without saying
And
For saying with feeling. . .

Always. . . .

Contents

PART III MANAGEMENT SKILLS

Preface

It is widely recognized that nurses must become effective managers and leaders in order to fulfill their responsibilities to themselves, to their clients, and to the nursing profession. Nurses' practice environments, roles, and educational programs are expanding. There is an actual and projected decline in the number of nurses entering the profession; there is an actual and projected need for increased professional nursing care services due to changing demographics of the population and crises emanating from disease states.

Other trends in health care include (a) changing emphases imposed by federal and state cost-containment regulations; (b) changing and alternative methods for health care delivery; (c) increasing focus on health maintenance–primary care–in addition to the ever-present foci on secondary care and tertiary care; and (d) greater quantities of data to support the mind/body relationship in health and disease, suggesting that not only is cure important, but altering behaviors is crucial so that the need to cure may be unnecessary or less frequent.

Wherever their placement in the health-care arena, nurses will be managers and leaders of themselves; of colleagues and peers in interdisciplinary clinical teams, of technicians and other health care providers; of colleagues in various management levels within formal health care organizations; of the public sector through media; of the individual clients, in city, state, national, and international political entities, and so forth. In these placements, nurses will be called upon for creative strategies, disciplined and cost-contained programs, and the abilities to research and analyze systems critically and chart growth—all in response to rapid health care changes. It is therefore mandatory that nurses perceive themselves in the roles of managers and leaders and increase their knowledge and application of theory and research in practice so that quality, comprehensive, efficient nursing care is provided to clients in any setting.

Leadership and management involve processes that are essential in making any nursing role, in any nursing environment, alive. Disciplines and professions such as organizational behavior, educational administration, and business have developed theories that assist managers in increasing the probability of achieving specified goals. Nurses must apply these theories into nursing leadership and management, and then extend them into nursing theory through research. Responsibility and authority granted by a state nurse practice act, an institution, an individual's unique experience and personality, and one's personal philosophy on the constituents of quality nursing care and effective management, must be integrated with knowledge and an ability to apply existing theories of management in nursing practice.

This book covers the processes of management and leadership in nursing practice. It evolves from my experience in teaching future nurse managers of health-care personnel in the delivery of nursing care. Content focuses on increasing organizational effectiveness in nursing service and practice. Theories and concepts from the professions of business, organizational psychology, and educational administration are applied to nursing topics in each chapter.

Sections of the book include simulations (for example, case presentations and multimedia activities) to provide practice experiences that illustrate the content of the chapters, as well as to expand the learner's range of experience. The simulations comprise the experiential approach; they provide learners with an opportunity to observe, experience, and carry out new behaviors in a safe, low risk practice environment. Careful explanations are provided for each simulation. The textbook and exercises are designed for use both in self-learning and classroom environments, in both individual and group learning experiences. It is suggested that study be weighted so that more time is devoted to the experiential elements, since enriched learning in management is derived more from actual and vicarious experiences than from reading and studying the printed word.

This book is written primarily for undergraduate nursing students in management and leadership courses. It is also intended as a resource for graduate administration nursing students, practicing nurses, learners in inservice and continuing education programs, and nursing faculty.

Acknowledgments

Even though the author first imagined and then created this book, the theory, exercises, and philosophy represented have been derived from many personal and professional resources. Some materials are original, and some are from established sources to whom credit is most gratefully given; others have evolved from an interchange with professionals and learners whose commitment has been to quality. I would like to particularly thank Donald Carew, Kenneth Blanchard, and Paul Hersey, whose teachings and writings were the foundation of my doctoral education and are the cornerstones of my current professional activities; Frederic Finch for sharing his knowledge; Phil Graf for his reinforcement and assistance—for believing many years ago that I had something to offer future nurse managers; and my colleagues in nursing education and practice for the constant interchange that has shaped today.

To all who have molded my beliefs, to all from whom I have received, I express my sincere gratitude.

Elaine Lynne La Monica

Introduction

Management and leadership in nursing involve an individual's efforts to influence the behavior of others in providing direct, individualized, professional nursing care. The basic premise of management is that managers set goals that represent some level of growth for a particular group in a particular environment. Managers then develop strategies for reaching these goals. Results are evaluated and altered or new directions are set. There is no value of good or bad to the actual state of the group, the group's goals, or the outcomes. Managers simply and constantly design strategies for moving groups of personnel to more efficient and more qualitative levels of functioning. The actual beginning points and the end points are of lesser importance than is the process of constantly developing strategies that result in identifiable, effective, and positive growth. In conducting these processes, nurse managers plan, organize, motivate, and control the work of other nurses and allied health-care personnel in the delivery of professional nursing care.

The processes of management and leadership are based on a scientific approach called the problem-solving method. The function of this scientific method is to increase the probability of success for a nurse manager's actions, given the particulars of a unique environment. In a typical nursing environment, there are staff members, clients, managers, situational variables such as policies and norms, and material resources; these are unique since it would be impossible to find this exact environment in another place or time. The goal of the nurse manager is to identify the environment's resources and put them to work as a whole system in accomplishing goals and facilitating growth. Use of the scientific method in management simply assists the manager in assessing many needs of the system and in choosing the priorities, identifying the people and situational elements that are important in carrying out specified goals, critically assessing the strengths of those people, and developing strategies that put those strengths to work.

A manager can be functional in the role without using the problem-solving method. This alternative, called "seat-of-the-pants" management, evolves from following only impulses and personal beliefs about self and others. Such management comes from involuntary behaviors that do not involve thinking about what a group needs from the manager in order to accomplish its goals. It is possible for seat-of-the-pants management to be successful. That is, by some stroke of luck, the impulses, beliefs, and behaviors of this manager are exactly what the system requires. Though possible, however, such success is unlikely.

Use of a scientific approach brings no guarantee of success; there is no way to predict the behavior of others with complete accuracy. An effective manager analyzes an environment and chooses the best strategy for achieving a specified goal, given the particular strengths and weaknesses of the employees who will be working to carry out that goal. There is always some unknown that cannot be controlled— the risk factor. Because all managers desire success, their goal in choosing the best strategy should be to identify the strategy that balances the lowest risk factor with the highest rate of return. This automatically increases the probability for success. A manager who uses seat-of-the-pants thinking will have a higher risk factor in every undertaking than will the manager who applies a scientific approach. The scientific management method forces the manager to plan, organize, motivate, and control logically and analytically. Further, it allows the manager to build contingency plans for all possible outcomes rather than to face problems unprepared.

Why does use of the scientific method offer so much? It is derived from methodologically sound research within the disciplines and professions of business, educational administration, and psychology—the purists in management. Given the numerous investigations that allow the label *theory* to be attached to a process or belief, the results suggest that this theory, applied in a particular way, produces these outcomes at least 95% of the time. A person who simply or randomly guesses in all decisions has an equal chance for being right or wrong. Managers, however, should not be satisfied with such a ratio—this is mediocrity. The use of intuition is appropriate and necessary only after the application of theory. It is the à la mode on homemade apple pie.

Parts I and II, "Conceptual Framework" and "Manager Responsibilities," present the process steps of nursing management and leadership. Each chapter has its own conceptual and theoretical discussions with nursing applications. In Chapter 7, the whole process of nursing management and leadership is presented through a case study. Part III, "Management Skills," takes a close look at the specific skills that managers must use to implement the management process effectively in a variety of nursing environments.

An experiential approach in learning management and leadership sets the book into motion for the learner. The simulations at the end of Parts II and III present specific ways to learn the chapter contents. These simulations are designed to provide experience in applying theory in a low-risk setting. It is known that as anxiety increases, perception decreases. When perception decreases, people most often do not think; they merely function intuitively. These intuitive behaviors are derived from practices and experiences earlier in life—from behaviors previously learned. It is also known that in a real management environment, a person's anxiety is generally greater than it is in a classroom or laboratory. This is due to tensions increasing when others are really looking to a person for guidance or are expecting something from that person. Because it takes time for learners to incorporate theory into practice, to think while doing instead of doing and then thinking, the use of simulations provides added experience so that the likelihood of a manager effectively applying theory while in any state of anxiety increases. This experiential model, the group dynamics laboratory, has been widely used in management training and this author has adapted it to nursing simulations.

The exercises in Part I of this book are ice-breaking, getting-acquainted activities. They are designed to help in the formation of effective groups and are most appropriately used at the beginning of study in a management and leadership course or program.

The ultimate goal of this book is identical to the ultimate goal of nursing: to assist the client to reach full health potential. In achieving this goal, an intermediate goal of assisting the nurse manager to achieve optimal effectiveness is emphasized. The educational process attends to the unique individual learner. A satisfied nurse manager has a high probability for having staff members who are also satisfied; satisfied staff members have a high probability for having satisfied clients; a satisfied client has a high probability for reaching full health potential.

A CONCEPTUAL FRAMEWORK

Part I provides a discussion of the theories and concepts on which management processes are based. These theories are derived from research in organizational psychology, business, and educational leadership; the theories are applied to a nursing environment.

Chapter 1 defines leadership and management, differentiating the roles of managers and leaders from the processes of managing and leading. The management process and the problem-solving method are the foci of this chapter.

Chapter 2 involves a discussion of the conceptual roots on which contemporary management practices are built—nonclassical organization theory. General system theory forms the basis for leader behavior, and the group dynamics laboratory is the mode used in this book for learning leadership and management content as well as process. The theory of motivation is then explained as it relates to management and leadership responsibilities.

The Management Process and the Problem-Solving Method

This chapter provides a definition of management and leadership and then discusses the general process of management. The management process frames all leader activities. Broad areas of management skills are then presented; the chapter concludes with a discussion of the problem-solving method, which is the scientific method for a leadership role. The content in this chapter forms the foundation for specific leadership responsibilities that are addressed in Part II of this book.

MANAGEMENT AND LEADERSHIP

Many definitions of management and leadership can be identified when surveying the literature (Brooten, Hayman, & Naylor, 1988; Koontz & O'Donnell, 1986; Lucio & McNeil, 1979; Marriner-Tomey, 1988; Newman & Warren, 1982; Sayles, 1979; Stevens, 1978). Themes, however, are evident. Hersey and Blanchard (1988) provided a comprehensive definition of management as "working with and through individuals and groups and other resources to accomplish organizational goals" (p. 3). Leadership also involves working through individuals and groups to accomplish goals, but these goals may be different from organizational goals, or they may involve one segment of the organizational goals. In a sense, the key difference between the concepts of management and leadership is the phrase "organizational goals." A manager works for an organization (for example, a Vice President for Nursing employed by a hospital) and carries the responsibility of accomplishing the organization's goals through specific professional services. Leadership is a much broader concept because all nurses are leaders. Anytime a person is a recognized authority and has followers who count on this person's expertise to carry out their objectives, the person is a leader. Furthermore, anyone who is responsible for giving assistance to others is also a leader. The staff nurse is a leader to clients; the student nurse also is a leader to clients; the head nurse is a leader to all team followers; and parents are leaders to children.

The organizational framework of a health-care agency is a clue to who is a leader as well as to whom the leader leads. Figure 1.1 presents a hypothetical organizational chart.

Moving from the bottom of the chart upward, the graduate nurse and student nurse are leaders in the direct care of clients. Primary nurses are responsible by position for all people beneath them; head nurses, supervisors, and directors follow the same pattern. It does not matter whether people are in top-, middle-, or lower-management positions; if someone relies on them, they are leaders.

It was necessary to define management and leadership in order to understand the differences between the roles of managers and leaders; to reiterate, the key difference is that managers are responsible for organizational goals while leaders may only be responsible for one segment of the overall goals. When management and leadership theory are applied to leader activities, however, the theory serves

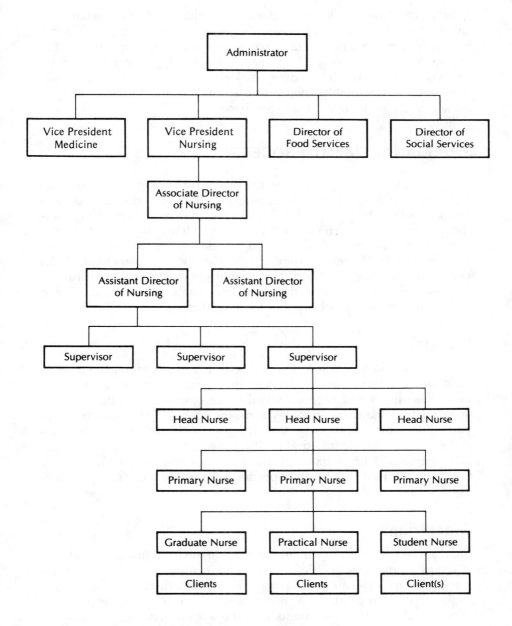

FIGURE 1.1 Hypothetical organizational chart

roles of both managers and leaders. What changes is the system that the leader influences. Obviously, the system that the primary nurse manages is much smaller than that of the supervisor or director. For clarity, therefore, there are both leader and manager roles in nursing. The theory that people in these roles apply, however, is called management and leadership theory and should be the foundation upon which all influencing activities are based.

THE MANAGEMENT PROCESS

The process of management is relevant to all people who seek to influence the behavior of others. Many authors who discuss management and leadership consider the process germane even though authors often differ semantically when identifying the process components (Brooten et al., 1988; Haynes, Massie, & Wallace, 1975; Longest, 1984; Marriner-Tomey, 1988). Hersey and Blanchard (1988) cited four managerial functions; planning, organizing, motivating, and controlling. Their definitions of these components are expanded here and combined with applications in nursing.

Planning

This involves identifying problems, setting and specifying both long-term and short-term goals, developing objectives, and then mapping how these goals and objectives will be accomplished. Longest (1984) asserted that planning involves a means to blend the actions of all participants in a system so that the group's members function together toward an identified goal. Planning greatly reduces the chance of being caught unprepared. Planning, according to Marriner-Tomey (1988), is the first and most important step of the management process.

Organizing

This part of the management process involves bringing all of the system's resources—people, capital, and equipment—into action toward goal accomplishment. Hersey and Blanchard (1988) discussed it as integrating resources. A nurse leader's desire is to include all people and situational elements into the system that will be carrying out a particular goal and to organize them so that the group is working together toward goal accomplishment.

Motivating

Motivation is a large factor in determining the performance level of employees and the quality of goal accomplishment (Hersey & Blanchard, 1988). William James of Harvard, conducting research on motivation, concluded that hourly employees could maintain their jobs by only working to 20 to 30% of their capacity. When properly motivated by their leader, however, they could work to 80 to 90% of their ability (Hersey & Blanchard, 1988). James felt that approximately 60% of employee performance can be affected by motivation. There is never a zero point or top level (100%) in employee performance because one should not say that people are at the maximum absolute level in their motivation to attain a goal. There are no limits on what human beings can accomplish, which is why Olympic records, for example, are broken. One must always strive to do a little bit better. Managers must always set goals that are higher than what employees had accomplished previously, based on the assessment that the goals are not beyond the capabilities of the people trying to attain them. That is the unidirectional process of growth.

Controlling

This last component in the management process involves setting up mechanisms for ongoing evaluation. Hersey and Blanchard (1988) said that controlling is obtaining feedback of results and periodically following up in order to compare results with plans. Adjustments in plans can be made accordingly. Quality-control systems, client-care audits, and client census and acuity information are examples of this aspect of the process.

Controlling is one aspect of management that is subject to myths and misinterpretations. This author often asks students to share the first adjective or emotion that comes to mind when the term *controlling* is presented. Responses include "manipulation," "rigid," "tight," "autocratic," and "oppressed." Controlling need not be any of these things; it is an essential aspect of managerial functions because a manager is ultimately responsible for followers' actions, given that a manager energizes the resources of a group to accomplish a goal. An effective nurse manager does not do everything. Rather, the manager leads the group to accomplish, and keeps track of what is happening at given points in time. Misinterpretations of controlling stem from the leader's verbal and nonverbal communications in the management process. It is possible to say, for example, that you as a manager would like to meet every week with your group in order to discuss progress and problems on a particular goal without being called autocratic, rigid, or tight. This is an area that should be role-played in a practice environment so that one's intent is perceived accurately.

Even though the four aspects of the management process are distinct, they are interrelated. When a leader plans, the plan also contains strategies for organizing, controlling, and motivating resources. Hence, all parts of the management process are connected. The case study in Chapter 7 illustrates this point further.

MANAGERIAL SKILLS

There are three general categories of skills that managers and leaders must possess: technical skills, human skills, and conceptual skills. Katz (1955) first classified these skills, and Hersey and Blanchard (1988) adapted them to the field of behavioral science.

> *Technical Skill*—Ability to use knowledge, methods, techniques, and equipment necessary for the performance of specific tasks acquired from experience, education, and training.
>
> *Human Skill*—Ability and judgment in working with and through people, including an understanding of motivation and an application of effective leadership.
>
> *Conceptual Skill*—Ability to understand the complexities of the overall organization and where one's own operation fits in the organization. This knowledge permits one to act according to the objectives of the total organization rather than only on the basis of the goals and needs of one's own immediate group (Hersey & Blanchard, 1988, p. 7).

For example, suppose a nurse leader has the goal of increasing the quality of nursing care. Technical skill is the leader's ability to perform the comprehensive individualized nursing care that is expected from staff nurses and from nursing practice standards. Human skill involves ability to influence others by teaching, role modeling, and so forth in order to accomplish the goal. Conceptual skill involves seeing how the goal that is being accomplished fits into

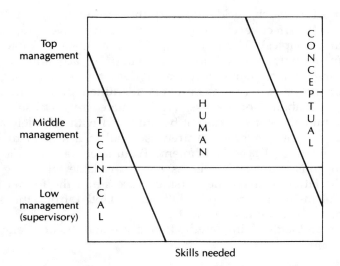

FIGURE 1.2 Management skills by levels of management.
Source: Reprinted by permission of the *Harvard Business Review.* From "Skills of an Effective Administrator," by R. Katz (January/February 1955). Copyright © 1955 by the President and Fellows of Harvard College; all rights reserved; and from Paul Hersey and Kenneth H. Blanchard, *Management of Organizational Behavior: Utilizing Human Resources*, 5th ed., © 1988, p. 8. Reprinted by permission of Prentice-Hall, Inc., Englewood Cliffs, NJ.

the overall organizational goals of client service in the agency—how it affects the entire health-care facility.

Research has shown that managers at different levels require varying amounts of technical and conceptual skills in order to carry out their responsibilities effectively. Human skills are a constant in all levels and occupy the greater part of the management function, as Figure 1.2 illustrates.

THE PROBLEM-SOLVING METHOD*

Effective management and leadership are not based on seat-of-the-pants thinking. The roles mandate methodical thinking that draws first from theory (what has been shown to be effective in a significant

---

*This section is an adaptation of the method presented by Hersey and Blanchard (1988) in their book and in their classes at the University of Massachusetts, 1973–1975.

number of research incidents) and then intuition (what has been shown to be effective in one's own experience, given application of research principles). The priority goal of a manager is to accomplish goals (commonly referred to as growing) by activating a system. Everything that a manager or leader does toward goal accomplishment should be based on a conscious, identified strategy that has the highest probability for success. Again, there are no absolute points because human behavior cannot be predicted with complete accuracy. Rather, the manager seeks awareness of all in a system to mobilize forces toward goal accomplishment. Fortunately, a scientific method for doing this is available, just as one is available for giving nursing care. The latter is called the nursing process and the former is called the problem-solving method. Both are adapted from the scientific method, as is evident in Table 1.1.

The problem-solving method is presented theoretically in this

TABLE 1.1 Comparison of the Problem-Solving Method, the Scientific Method, and the Nursing Process*

Problem-Solving Method	Scientific Method	The Nursing Process
		Problem Finding
1. Problem identification Point of view	1. Gathering information 2. Examining information 3. Interpreting information	Data collection Data processing
2. Problem definition and/or goal statement 3. Problem analysis	4. Identifying problem(s) 5. Stating the problem(s)	Nursing diagnosis
		Problem Solving
4. Alternative solutions 5. Recommended action	1. Developing alternatives 2. Making a decision 3. Deciding on a plan of action 4. Executing the plan of action 5. Evaluating the results 6. Redefining problem and change	Nursing orders Implementation Evaluation

*Source: La Monica, E. (1985). *The humanistic nursing process.* Boston: Jones and Bartlett.

chapter. It is the framework upon which all management practices are built. Part II of this book is devoted to the process of carrying out this method; examples for making the process alive are provided.

Problem Identification

This is the first step in the problem-solving method. A problem is identified by the difference between what is actually happening (the actual) in a situation and what one wishes to have occur (the optimal). Figure 1.3 illustrates this point. To determine a problem area, it is necessary to gather, examine, and interpret information from all sources available—primary and secondary—and to decide whether the problem area warrants attention. Primary sources are your followers, and secondary sources are all other people from whom information can be collected—clients, physicians, associates, superiors, and so forth. Data can be gathered from these sources on one-to-one or group bases. The manager's own point of view should be identified by being conscious of individual self-perceptions and beliefs. These data should be shared with members of the problem-solving group.

Problem Definition

After a situation has been assessed to determine a priority need area, to identify where a group is in relation to this need (the actual), and to identify where one wishes to go relative to this need (the optimal), then a problem can be stated. This procedure represents the difference between real and optimal and should be specific and tractable. Managers who identify problems may be comforted by the knowledge that problems are indicative of growth. A manager should al-

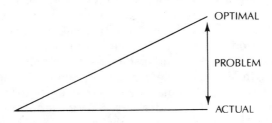

FIGURE 1.3 Identifying the problem.

ways be identifying problems—specifying where a group is and delineating where it can go. This is the process of growth. Once the optimal is attained, it becomes the actual or the real situation and the whole process of identifying problems should begin again.

Problems should be specific and tractable. For example, if performance is the focal point, it is necessary to determine the aspects of performance that one wishes to change. Is it that care plans are not routinely written? Or do employees spend too much time with administrative tasks? A clearly stated problem structures the whole problem-solving process because what has to be done to solve the problem and evaluate outcomes becomes apparent only when the problem statement is clear and specific. Further, Goode and Fowler (1949) demonstrated early that a clear statement of problems contributed to follower support in solving the problem because followers were aware of the focus of their efforts. Locke, Saari, Shaw, and Latham (1981) asserted that designating problems and setting goals "affect performance by directing attention, mobilizing effort, increasing persistence, and motivating strategy development" (p. 125).

A goal is simply a restated problem. Hence, goals flow from the problem statement. If a problem is that nursing-care plans are not written routinely, then the goal would be to have nursing-care plans written for all clients. A problem statement can be thought of as a negative statement—that is, something one wishes to eradicate or get rid of—and is similar to the nursing diagnosis. A goal is something one wishes to attain; it is a positive statement. Obviously, problems and goals comprise ends of the same continuum. It is individual choice whether a manager wishes to work with problems or goals or both. This author's preference is to always accentuate positive thinking by working with goals rather than problems.

The specification of the optimal can be a long-term or a short-term goal. Even though it is essential that a manager identify both types of goals, one should be aware that research in motivation suggests that people are more highly motivated at the beginning of task accomplishment and when the goal is almost accomplished (Atkinson, 1957). Since increased employee motivation usually results in an increase in productivity, with follower job-satisfaction as a byproduct, the manager should set goals with followers that can be accomplished in a reasonable amount of time. The success and rewards that follow goal achievement serve as both a reinforcement and a stimulus in further endeavors. Shorter-term goals may also be viewed by followers as more realistic and achievable. Livingston (1969) aptly stated that subordinates must consider goals as realistic in order to be motivated to reach high levels of productivity. For example, if care plans are never written for clients (the actual) and a leader desires that they be written for all clients (the optimal), an intermediate short-term goal might be to write care plans on clients who have chronic health problems. There are many rungs in the ladder toward accomplishment of the long-term goal. Each should be accomplished in stepwise progression toward a long-range goal.

Problem Analysis

After the problem is identified, it must be analyzed. Analysis entails four steps: (1) to determine why the problem exists; (2) to identify the unique group who will participate in solving the problem/achieving the goal; (3) to analyze the ability of a group to accomplish the goal (level of maturity); and (4) to specify an appropriate leader behavior style, indicated by the group's level of maturity, that is required in order to meet the needs of a group as it accomplishes the goal. It is in this fourth phase that leader behavior theories are brought into focus. By applying theory in each of these four steps, one increases the probability that analysis will be comprehensive and that the decision on the appropriate leader behavior style will be based on what works according to research findings.

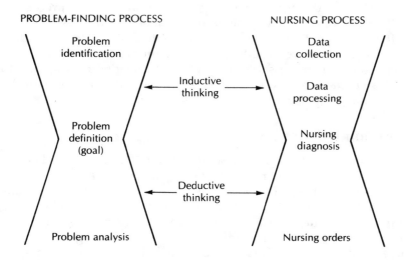

FIGURE 1.4 Comparison of the problem-finding process with the nursing process.

The problem-finding process that was previously discussed can be compared with the nursing process (La Monica, 1985), as portrayed in Figure 1.4. It is evident that vast information is boiled down in both methods to focus on a specific problem. Once the problem is specified, then analysis broadens in order to solve it. Problem identification and data collection and processing involve inductive thinking in order to make a conclusion about the problem; all information in these processes is used to identify a problem or a nursing diagnosis. Problem analysis and nursing orders, however, are examples of deductive reasoning; a focal area exists and all that follows relates to solving the problem or to getting rid of the nursing diagnosis.

Alternative Solutions

Based on analysis, the next step is to brainstorm various alternative solutions or strategies that have the potential to solve the problem or achieve the goal. Brainstorming, a step in the creative process (McNeil, 1973), can be used to foster creativity and to develop alternatives that reflect the individuality of a unique system—people, environment, and time. This process is a way to expand possibilities by answering the question. "If I could achieve this goal with this identified system, ideally doing anything I wished, reflecting my knowledge and experience, what would I want done and how should I get it done?" All ideas are important and during the process of brainstorming, no value judgments of good or bad operate.

After the ideas are listed, then each solution should be studied for anticipated positive results and anticipated negative results. In other words, it is necessary to play out behavior and attempt to predict reactions of followers; these reactions should include both the negative and the positive.

Recommended Action

Following analysis of alternative solutions, one strategy must be chosen. Unfortunately, it is rare when a strategy played out has no negative consequences. The recommended action, therefore, usually has the highest probability for reducing the discrepancy between real and optimal and the lowest probability for resulting in negative consequences, given that there are most often some negative consequences in all strategies. It should be noted that solution phases are too frequently hurried. A good analysis in these steps is important since it most often results in the recommended action becoming obvious.

SUMMARY

Management and leadership are different concepts when they are defined in terms of roles; managers are responsible for organizational goals while leaders are such because people look to them for guidance. In leader/manager activities, however, management and leadership theory is applied in both roles.

The management process contains four interrelated elements: planning, organizing, motivating, and controlling. Technical, human, and conceptual skills are required in order to carry out this process. Different levels of management require lesser or greater amounts of technical and conceptual skills; human skills are constant in all levels of management.

The problem-solving process is the manager's scientific method. It is the foundation on which all manager activity should be based. A problem must first be identified inductively, resulting in a specific problem statement. Deductive processes are then employed to analyze the problem and identify alternative solutions. A recommended action is the final outcome of the problem-solving method.

REFERENCES

Atkinson, J. (1957). Motivational determinants of risk-taking behavior. *Psychological Review, 64*, 365.

Brooten, D., Hayman, L., & Naylor, M. (1988). *Leadership for change: An action guide for nurses* (2nd ed.). Philadelphia: Lippincott.

Goode, W., & Fowler, I. (1949). Incentive factors in a low morale plant. *American Sociological Review, 14*, 618–624.

Haynes, W., Massie, J., & Wallace, M. Jr. (1975). *Management: Analysis, concepts, and cases.* Englewood Cliffs, NJ: Prentice-Hall.

Hersey, P., & Blanchard, K. (1988). *Management of organizational behavior: Utilizing human resources* (5th ed.). Englewood Cliffs, NJ: Prentice Hall.

Katz, R. (1955). Skills of an effective administrator. *Harvard Business Review, 33*, 33–42.

Koontz, H., & O'Donnell, C. (1986). *Essentials of management.* New York: McGraw-Hill.

La Monica, E., (1985). *The humanistic nursing process.* Boston: Jones and Bartlett.

Livingston, J. (1969). Pygmalion in management. *Harvard Business Review, 47*, 81–89.

Locke, E., Saari, L., Shaw, K., & Latham, G. (1981). Goal setting and task performance: 1969–1980. *Psychological Bulletin, 90*, 125–152.

Longest, B. (1984). *Management practices for health professionals* (3rd ed.). Norwalk, CT: Appleton-Lang.

Lucio, W., & McNeil, J. (1979). *Supervision in thought and action* (3rd ed.). New York: McGraw-Hill.

Marriner-Tomey, A. (1988). *Guide to nursing management* (3rd ed.). St. Louis: Mosby.

McNeil, J. (1973). The creative process. Unpublished paper, University of Massachusetts, Center for the Study of Aesthetics in Education, Amherst.

Newman, W., & Warren, E. (1982). *The process of management: Strategy, action, results* (5th ed.). Englewood Cliffs, NJ: Prentice-Hall.

Sayles, L. (1979). *Leadership: What effective managers really do . . . and how they do it.* New York: McGraw-Hill.

Stevens, W. (1978). *Management and leadership in nursing.* New York: McGraw-Hill.

Theory for Nursing Management and Leadership

The management process and the problem-solving method are the procedures for all management responsibilities. These procedures outline how managers should function. Chapter 2 discusses the concepts and theories explaining why managers function in particular ways. This chapter also provides the rationale for the educational design of the book, the intent of which is to enable learners to grow and therefore change; change is synonymous with growing or learning. The goal of this book parallels the goal of nurse managers and leaders, that leaders also facilitate change and growth in their personnel. The conceptual framework presented in this chapter applies to learning how to become a manager as well as to the role of being a manager. The conceptual framework, therefore, holds together the education of future leaders and managers as well as the process of management and leadership.

This chapter includes discussions of classical and nonclassical organization theory, general system theory, and the group dynamics laboratory as an educational mode. It concludes with the theory of motivation, which is an essential concept in understanding management and leadership processes.

CLASSICAL AND NONCLASSICAL ORGANIZATION THEORY

The literature reflects two categories of leadership: classical organization theory (COT) and nonclassical organization theory (NCOT). Prior to 1950, COT was the rule in organizations. NCOT, which has evolved from criticisms of COT, is the basis for contemporary management practices.

Classical Organization Theory

COT has a list of assumptions, delineated by McGregor (1966, 1960/ 1985), called Theory X assumptions about human nature. These are as follows:

1. People find work distasteful;
2. People are not ambitious and prefer direction;
3. People do not solve organizational problems creatively;
4. People are motivated only by physiologic and safety factors; and
5. People require close control and coercion to achieve goals.

Given these assumptions, organizations designed the leadership structure to counteract these traits of people so that organizational goals would be accomplished. The traditional organization therefore had centralized decision making and a pyramid form of superior-follower control. In essence, workers were told what to do and were not required to think. The leadership style used with the employees was autocratic (Davis & Newstrom, 1985; Hersey & Blanchard, 1988).

Severely criticizing classical organizations, which were built on Theory X assumptions, McGregor (1966, 1960/1985) asserted that people had those traits because the organization or past experience made them that way. When leaders treat workers as if workers have no thinking power or are robots, workers soon start behaving as if these traits are real. What motivation would one have to do otherwise?

Nonclassical Organization Theory

In contrast to Theory X assumptions about human nature, McGregor (1966, 1960/1985) further proposed the following Theory Y assumptions about people:

1. People regard work to be as natural as play, when conditions are favorable;
2. People are self-directed in achieving organizational goals;
3. People are creative in solving problems;
4. People are motivated at all levels of Maslow's (1970) hierarchy of needs—physiologic, safety, social, esteem, and self-actualization; and
5. People are self-controlled if properly motivated.

Nonclassical organizations, which have Theory Y assumptions about people, design the leadership structure so that workers will be able to grow within the organization; the aim is to have people fulfill the Theory Y assumptions.

Obviously, people are neither good nor bad, and it must be pointed out that McGregor had no intent of portraying them as good or bad when delineating Theory X and Theory Y. Theory Y assumptions allow managers in an organization to find out what motivates people and then give the appropriate leadership style that enables workers to grow within an organization. Some people may in fact need close control, for example; then the autocratic style of leadership is appropriate. Others may need support from the leaders and a democratic leader behavior style may be indicated. There may be those who are completely self-motivated and are committed to the growth of the organization. These people are usually best if left alone—the laissez-faire leadership style. Theory Y assumptions, therefore, permit the organization's leaders to respond to the needs of the people who make up the organization as these people work to achieve the organization's goals. Leader behavior reflects the needs of a group given a particular problem or goal. If the group changes or the goal changes, the appropriate leader behavior style must be reassessed and designated again.

GENERAL SYSTEM THEORY

All contemporary management practices are based on nonclassical organization theory. NCOT employs a situational approach to leadership. It assumes that all people can be helped and educated to achieve organizational goals, that people vary as to what motivates them, and that the styles of leadership used in organizations must respond to the needs of the organization's constituency (Argyris, 1971; Herzberg, 1966; Likert, 1967; McGregor, 1966, 1960/1985). The situational approach to leadership is based on an understanding of general system theory, which provides a construct for studying people within their environment and as builders of their environment.

General system theory is a model developed by von Bertalanffy (1968, 1975) and applied to nursing practice by Putt (1978). It mandates analysis of all the system's parts, the relationship between and among those parts, as well as the system's purposes, beliefs, and tasks. Yura and Walsh (1987) simplified general system theory by saying that it includes purpose, content, and process.

Von Bertalanffy (1968) designated two main types of systems, closed systems and open systems, as means of conceptualizing the world and the universe. Closed systems end when a quantity needed for fulfillment is obtained. Further, results are exactly predictable in closed systems. An example of a closed system is a chemical equation. If water (H_2O) is added to salt (NaCl), a chemist (or a nurse) can predict and quantify exactly what will occur—water plus the breakup of sodium and chloride ions. Hence, the balanced equation:

$$NaCl + H_2O = H_2O + Na^+ + Cl^-$$

Open systems have no designated quantity and are not exactly predictable. Human beings are open systems because even though one can spend great amounts of time finding out the properties, personality, wishes, and desires of people, there is and will always be the unknown. Open systems are the only concern for study, therefore, when general system theory is applied in management.

Von Bertalanffy (1968) identified four assumptions of open systems:

1. *A system is more than a sum of its parts.* In other words, a system is composed of all people and things within it, but the composite system contains more than its constituents. This composite has a character of its own, made up of the parts, but different from those parts. The system or group becomes the "I" or first person, not the individuals and things within the system.

Another example of the first assumption involves taking ten people in a group and giving each person an energy range that moves from 1 (lowest amount of energy) to 10 (highest amount of energy). If the assignment were given to one person in the group to use 10 units of energy and go out on an interstate highway and stop traffic in both directions from 8:00 A.M. to 8:30 A.M. one morning, would that person be successful? Maybe, but success is doubtful. Suppose the assignment were given to all ten people to do the same in the same spot but work independently. Then there would be 100 units of energy working on a goal. The ten people would have more chances of being successful than the single person. Give the same assignment to ten people, but instruct them jointly to plan a strategy for accomplishing the task—that is, to work together as a group on the goal. The chances of the group being successful would be far greater than the chances for success in either the single assignment or the task in which ten individuals worked alone.

Given a perfectly functioning group, the amount of energy contained within the group is not simply 10 times 10 or 100 units. The amount of energy is 10 to the tenth power (10^{10}) or 100,000,000,000 units of energy because the interaction between and among every combination of people in the group elicits energy toward goal accomplishment. So, a group of people working together toward a common goal is the manager's best bet, even though groups rarely function perfectly. The greater the amount of energy a group has working toward a goal, the higher the probability for effective goal completion. This is the principle behind collective bargaining units. The challenge for management, however, is to keep the groups working *for* the organization rather than against the organization.

2. *A system is ever-changing.* The absence of a member or part of a system or the inclusion of a new member or piece of equipment changes the system. On a smaller scale, the passage of time changes a system. Since humans are constantly learning from and therefore changing with the environment, people are different at every point in time. Even though a group may be composed of the same constituents, the group is always changing because the constituents are always changing. An effective leader must allow for the group's growth (or regression) to be reflected in the group's goals and the strategies that will best enable the goals to be attained. This process involves constant assessment of the group.

3. *A system has boundaries* that are defined by the system's purpose. A health-care agency can be considered as one system. All of the human and the material resources in this agency are part of the system. In fact, the community in which the facility is located can be conceptualized as the supra-system. The universe is our absolute outer system, given the limits of human knowledge. All that occurs in the world falls into subsystems. One system is always related to or is part of a larger whole. Figure 2.1 provides one example of how this principle works.

Problem solving requires that boundaries be designated. In increasing the quality of nursing care, for example, the subsystem of the community is important but not as important as the nursing care team. Boundaries are circumscribed by responding to the question: "What and who are the important components of the larger system that will have the most direct effect on solving a given problem?" The answer becomes the system for that problem. It follows that each system is unique for each problem, given the available human and material resources in a specified time and place. The system that has a goal of increasing the quality of nursing care in a given institution may not be the same system in another institution or at another time in the same institution. Part II will discuss designating systems in greater detail than is presented here.

4. *Systems are goal-directed.* This assumption flows directly from the previous one. Once the problem or goal is specified, the boundaries of a system can be specified. A system with no goal has no reason to exist, no motivation to function, and no drive to succeed. A system with no goals has nothing to evaluate because evaluation requires measurement points—a beginning point and an end point. Without goals, one can easily feel a lack of accomplishment and a feeling of "never getting anything done." Behaviorally, this can become a self-reinforcing negative cycle. Principles of time management, discussed in Chapter 17, are built on this goal-setting principle.

These four assumptions guide the manager to state problems/ goals, to designate the system that will be primarily responsible for goal attainment, and to understand how the group working as a

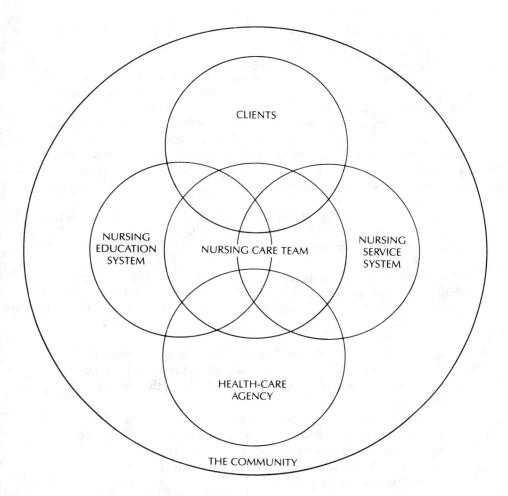

FIGURE 2.1 The nursing system viewed from a health-care service perspective.

single, integrated unit of one becomes foremost in effective goal accomplishment.

GROUP DYNAMICS LABORATORY

The group dynamics laboratory, the most widely used method for management training, has experiential learning as its focus (Fiedler, Chemers, & Mahar, 1984; Finch, Jones, & Litterer, 1976; Stogdill,

1974). Various group exercises form the laboratory experience: case studies, films, role playing, business games, and other media that involve group problem-solving projects.

The laboratory group is actually a microcosm of the real work world. Participants have an opportunity to apply and use the skills and behaviors that a manager must possess: how to lead, follow, draw out opinions, use power, resolve conflicts, be assertive, give and receive feedback, and so forth. Because the role of a manager always involves working with people in groups, the group dynamics laboratory serves to enable both learning the required content in management and leadership and the actual process of being a manager.

The group dynamics laboratory, developed by the National Training Laboratories in Bethel, Maine, grew from the sensitivity and T-group movement (Benne, 1969; Berne, 1978; Bradford, Gibb, & Benne, 1964; Perls, 1969; Schein & Bennis, 1965; Schutz, 1967). Several underlying assumptions about the learning process distinguish T-groups and the group dynamics laboratory from other modes of instruction. According to Seashore (1970, pp. 15–16), these assumptions are:

> *Learning Responsibility.* Participants are responsible for their own learning. What is learned depends upon style, readiness, and the relationships developed with other members of the group.
>
> *Staff Role.* The staff person's role is to facilitate the examination and understanding of the experiences in the group by helping participants to focus on the way the group is working, the style of an individual's participation, or the issues that are facing the group.
>
> *Experience and Conceptualization.* Most learning is a combination of experience and conceptualization. A major T-group aim is to provide a setting in which individuals are encouraged to examine their experiences together in enough detail so that valid generalizations can be drawn.
>
> *Authentic Relationships and Learning.* A person is most free to learn when authentic relationships are established with other people, thereby increasing one's sense of self-esteem and decreasing defensiveness. In authentic relationships, persons can be open, honest, and direct with one another so that they are communicating what they are actually feeling rather than masking their feelings.

Skill Acquisition and Values. The development of new skills in working with people is maximized as a person examines the basic values underlying behavior, as appropriate concepts and theory are acquired, and as one is able to practice new behavior and obtain feedback on the degree to which that behavior produces the intended impact.

The intent of the group dynamics laboratory is to accomplish one or more of the following changes in attitude or behavior on the part of the leader trainees (Stogdill, 1974, p. 182):

1. Greater sensitivity to follower needs and desires;
2. Greater openness and sharing of information;
3. Greater sharing of decision-making responsibilities with followers;
4. More intimate, friendly, and egalitarian interaction with followers; and
5. Less structuring, personal dominance, and pushing for productive output.

Studies by Gibb (1971), Harrison and Lubin (1965), Callahan and Wall (1987), Wright (1983), and Miles (1965) have all found the laboratory method to increase effective interpersonal communication among members; members can test and learn trust, risk-taking, openness, and interdependence. Further, outcome studies on the effects of the group dynamics laboratory approach in leadership training have been widespread and positive. Stogdill (1974) presented and discussed an extensive review of this body of literature.

Blumberg (1977, pp. 15–16) asserted that in order for training goals in laboratory education to be realized, certain conditions in the laboratory must be met. These are:

Presentation of Self. Until an individual has an opportunity to reveal the way one sees things and does things, there is little basis for improvement and change.

Feedback. Individuals do not learn from their experiences. They learn from bringing out the essential patterns of purposes, motives, and behavior in a situation where they can receive back clear and accurate information about the relevancy and effectiveness of their behavior. They need a feedback system which continuously operates so that they can change and correct what is inappropriate.

Atmosphere. An atmosphere of trust and nondefensiveness is necessary for people both to be willing to expose their behavior and purposes, and to accept feedback.

Cognitive Map. Knowledge from research, theory, and experience is important to enable the individual both to understand experiences and to generalize from them. But normally, information is most effective when it follows experience and feedback.

Experimentation. Unless there is opportunity to try out new patterns of thought and behavior, they never become a part of the individual. Without experimental efforts, relevant change is difficult to make.

Practice. Equally important is the need to practice new approaches so that the individual gains security in being different.

Application. Unless learning and change can be applied to back-home situations, they are not likely to be effective or lasting. Attention needs to be given to helping individuals plan application.

Relearning How to Learn. Because much of our academic experience has led us to believe that we learn from listening to authorities, there is frequently need to learn from presentation-feedback-experimentation.

Regarding the group mode of instruction in training, Carkhuff (1969) concluded that this model is goal- and action-directed in its work-oriented structure. Emphasis is on behavior one wishes to effect, leaving the trainee with tangible and usable skills. Longer retention of learned skills results because learning is an outcome of actual experience. Further, the nature of the systematic training involves steps that lead to measurable outcomes, thereby making evaluation explicit. "In summary, what can be accomplished individually can be accomplished in groups—and more!" (p. 184).

MOTIVATION

The theory of motivation is the last area to be discussed in the conceptual framework of management and leadership. Motivation, as stated in Chapter 1, comprises the largest area of a manager's responsibilities; its major importance in management activities remains constant regardless of one's management level.

In comparing motivated and unmotivated personnel generally, the more followers are motivated to accomplish a goal, the shorter time will be required to succeed. In addition, quality will increase, costs will decrease, and personnel will have a positive experience, which serves as a stimulus for motivating them to accomplish again. In short, as motivation increases, time and costs decrease while quality and satisfaction increase. Motivating personnel is the responsibility of managers. Theories are available that guide the leader to find out what motivates individuals and then to apply the appropriate leader behavior style that will increase the probability of motivating people to get the task done while enabling them to grow in their positions. Applications of these theories will be discussed and applied in Part II of this book. This section will present the theory of motivation, which is essential in understanding the applied motivation theory that is explained later.

Motivation Factors

The following definitions provide keys to understand motivation (Davis & Newstrom, 1985; Hersey & Blanchard, 1988):

> *Motives*—Needs, wants, drives, or impulses within an individual that prompt behavior; motives may be conscious or unconscious.
>
> *Motive Strength*—A means for categorizing the strength of a motive or need. Since people normally have a variety of motives all competing for fulfillment, the highest-strength motive is satisfied through behavior first. Once a need is satisfied, it decreases in motive strength and the need next in priority receives attention.
>
> *Goals*—"Hoped for" rewards, incentives, and external desires. Goals are outside an individual; they are what one wishes to attain.
>
> *Behavior*—What a person does and what others perceive. Behavior is observable, measurable action.

Figure 2.2 diagrams how these concepts work. If a need is present within an individual, the need (internal) is attached to a goal in the environment (external) and causes the individual to work toward attaining that goal, thereby satisfying the need. Davis and Newstrom (1985) discussed external goals as intrinsic and extrinsic factors. Intrinsic factors occur at the time work is performed, an example of

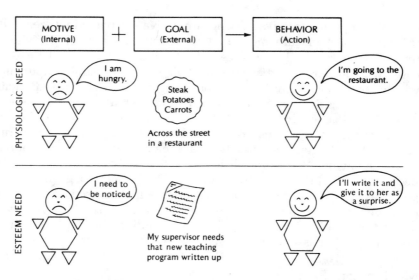

FIGURE 2.2 Motivation factors.

which is positive reinforcement from a supervisor immediately following task completion. Extrinsic factors occur away from work, for example, fringe benefits and days off.

People work on satisfying needs in an orderly fashion. Those

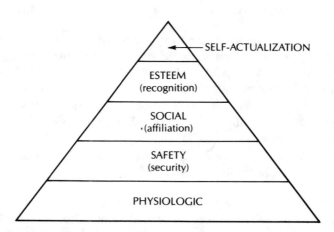

FIGURE 2.3 Maslow's hierarchy of needs.

Source: "Hierarchy of Needs" from *Motivation and Personality*, 2nd ed., by Abraham H. Maslow. Copyright 1954 by Harper & Row Publishers, Inc. Copyright ©
1970 by Abraham H. Maslow. Reprinted by permission of the publisher.

needs that have the highest motive strength receive attention first. Maslow (1970) presented a theory that designates categories of needs and their strength when unsatisfied. The theory is called Maslow's hierarchy of needs and is shown in Figure 2.3. According to Maslow's widely accepted theory of motivation, the physiologic needs (shown at the bottom of the pyramid in Figure 2.3) are top priority in motive strength when unsatisfied. Physiologic needs have the highest priority until satisfied. Once physiologic needs become less important or are in balance, safety needs take priority. This format follows as the pyramid climbs to self-actualization, which is a priority only when the other four needs are satisfied. It must be noted that all needs are present within an individual; the priority of the needs, however,

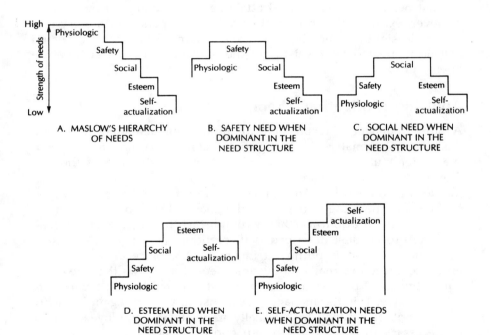

FIGURE 2.4 Movement of Maslow's hierarchy of needs.

Source: Paul Hersey & Kenneth H. Blanchard, *Management of Organizational Behavior: Utilizing Human Resources,* 5th ed., pp. 33–35, © 1988. Reprinted by permission of Prentice Hall, Inc., Englewood Cliffs, NJ. "Hierarchy of Needs" from *Motivation and Personality*, 2nd ed., by Abraham H. Maslow. Copyright 1954 by Harper & Row Publishers, Inc. Copyright © 1970 by Abraham H. Maslow. Reprinted by permission of the publisher.

shifts. A person may be functioning at a physiological level at 12:00 noon and then be at an esteem level after lunch. Hersey and Blanchard (1988) diagrammed this movement as shown in Figure 2.4. Theorists such as Argyris (1971), Herzberg (1966), Hersey and Blanchard (1988), and McGregor (1966) presented variations on motivation factors. These theories are discussed and compared in Part II of this book.

In order to understand motivation fully, another concept requires discussion. This concept involves the difference between internal and external motivation. Internal motivation comes from within a person; external motivation is outside a person. The old saying, "You can lead a horse to water but you cannot make it drink," is true. A leader cannot make someone behave in a certain way. If someone has an internal need, the sight of an external goal increases the probability that behavior aimed at goal attainment will follow; no guarantee, however, exists. Going back to Figure 2.2, if a person is hungry and food is in sight at a nearby restaurant, it is probable that the person will be motivated to travel to get the food but one cannot be absolutely sure.

Applying Motivation Theory

A nurse manager is responsible for motivating personnel to accomplish organizational goals. Using motivation theory toward this end, the leader must first assess the highest motive strength of the employee and then designate a goal having a reward that directly meets the need of the worker. The leader uses intrinsic and extrinsic factors in the goal. The route to obtaining the goal and thereby satisfying the need is through a journey that accomplishes the organizational goal.

The process just described is theoretically how people are externally motivated; it is portrayed in Figure 2.5. Since a manager can only attempt to externally motivate someone, it follows that the external motivational process may not work; it may fail to lead a person to act or behave. It is the manager's responsibility to try again by delineating another strategy to externally motivate the employee. It may be necessary to reassess or to rediagnose the needs of the follower. Obviously, if the first assessment was not on target, the chances increase that the external motivational strategy will not work. Also, different things work for different people. In a sense, being a manager or leader is a commitment to struggle—to constantly develop ways of motivating people to get the work done. If a strategy for accomplishing an immediate organizational goal does not work, an-

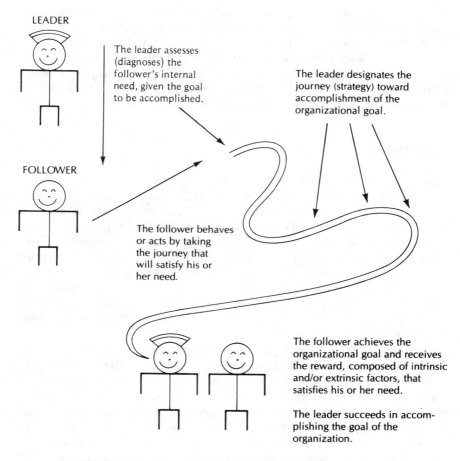

LEADER

The leader assesses (diagnoses) the follower's internal need, given the goal to be accomplished.

The leader designates the journey (strategy) toward accomplishment of the organizational goal.

FOLLOWER

The follower behaves or acts by taking the journey that will satisfy his or her need.

The follower achieves the organizational goal and receives the reward, composed of intrinsic and/or extrinsic factors, that satisfies his or her need.

The leader succeeds in accomplishing the goal of the organization.

FIGURE 2.5 Motivation process for manager activities.

other strategy must be developed or the goal may be adjusted. Once the immediate goal is attained, another goal should be designated and new strategies must then be built on the needs of workers at that particular point in time.

The motivation process previously described was applied to motivating one person. Since a nurse leader is most often trying to motivate a group to accomplish a task, motivation theory is applied to individual people in the group first. Individual needs are assessed and then the need that is the group mode is used by the leader in planning a strategy for externally motivating the group to accomplish an organizational goal. It is logical to conclude that the strategy may not be best for all people in the group; however, it should be best for the majority of people in the group. A leader may not be all things to everyone. A leader should be on target for the majority (mode) of people in a group and then try to work on a person-to-person basis with those individuals who are not directly satisfied. Application of the theory of motivation is extended in Chapter 4.

SUMMARY

Two categories of leadership styles are discussed in this chapter: classical organization theory and nonclassical organization theory. NCOT forms the basis of contemporary leadership models and assumes that people must be motivated to fulfill themselves within the organization. Because people are different, leaders must diagnose what people need and then provide the appropriate leader behavior style that will enable a goal to be accomplished and enable workers to grow while in their positions. NCOT employs a situational approach to leadership and sees an organization as a system that is composed of human and material resources working as one unit toward goal accomplishment.

Von Bertalanffy's (1968, 1975) general system theory is the framework that explains how systems work. The group dynamics laboratory is the educational mode that enables experiential learning of management and leadership content. The group dynamics laboratory enables future leaders to experience the process of being a manager through an application of theory. A manager's primary responsibility is externally motivating followers to achieve organizational goals. This is accomplished by diagnosing the internal need of a person, specifying an external goal and reward, using intrinsic and extrinsic factors that fulfill the follower's need, and setting a path through which the follower can attain the goal and reward through behavior that accomplishes the particular goal of the organization at a given point in time.

REFERENCES

Argyris, C. (1971). *Management and organizational development: The path from XA to YB*. New York: McGraw-Hill.
Benne, K. (1969, January). The self, the group or the task: Differences among growth groups. Paper presented at the Ninth Annual Conference on

Personality Theory and Counseling Practice, University of Florida, Gainesville.

Berne, E. (1978). *Games people play.* New York: Ballantine.

Blumberg, A. (1977). Laboratory education and sensitivity training. In R. Golembiewski, & A. Blumberg (Eds). *Sensitivity training and the laboratory approach: Readings about concepts and applications.* Itasca, IL: Peacock.

Bradford, L., Gibb, J., & Benne, K. (Eds.). (1964). *T-Group theory and laboratory methods: An innovation in re-education.* New York: Wiley.

Callahan, C., & Wall, L. (1987). Participative management: A contingency approach. *Journal of Nursing Administration, 17*(9), 9–15.

Carkhuff, R. (1969). *Helping and human relations: A primer for lay and professional helpers* (Vol. 2). Amherst, MA: Human Resource Development Press.

Davis, K., & Newstrom, J. (1985). *Human behavior at work: Organizational behavior* (7th ed.). New York: McGraw-Hill.

Fiedler, F., Chemers, M., & Mahar, L. (1984). *Improving leader effectiveness: The leader match concept.* New York: Wiley.

Finch, F., Jones, H., & Litterer, J. (1976). *Managing for organizational effectiveness: An experiential approach.* New York: McGraw-Hill.

Gibb, J. (1971). The effects of human relations training. In A. Bergin, & S. Garfield (Eds.). *Handbook of psychotherapy and behavior change.* New York: Wiley.

Harrison, R., & Lubin, B. (1965). Personal style, group composition and learning. *Journal of Applied Behavioral Science, 3,* 286–301.

Hersey, P., & Blanchard, K. (1988). *Management of organizational behavior: Utilizing human resources* (5th ed.). Englewood Cliffs, NJ: Prentice-Hall.

Herzberg, F. (1966). *Work and the nature of man.* Cleveland: World Publishing.

Likert, R. (1967). *The human organization.* New York: McGraw-Hill.

McGregor, D. (1966). *Leadership and motivation.* Boston: MIT Press.

McGregor, D. (1985). *The human side of enterprise: 25th anniversary printing.* (Original work published 1960). New York: McGraw-Hill.

Maslow, A. (1970). *Motivation and Personality* (2nd ed.). New York: Harper & Row.

Miles, M. (1965). Changes during and following laboratory training: A clinical experimental study. *Journal of Applied Behavioral Science, 1,* 215–242.

Perls, F. (1969). *Gestalt therapy verbatim.* Lafayette, CA: Real People Press.

Putt, A. (1978). *General system theory applied to nursing.* Boston: Little, Brown.

Schein, E., & Bennis, W. (Eds.). (1965). *Personal and organizational change through group methods: The laboratory approach.* New York: Wiley.

Schutz, W. (1967). *Expanding human awareness.* New York: Grove Press.

Seashore, C. (1970). What is sensitivity training? In R. Golembiewski, & A. Blumberg (Eds.). *Sensitivity training and the laboratory approach: Readings about concepts and applications.* Itasca, IL: Peacock.

Stogdill, R. (1974). *Handbook of leadership.* New York: Free Press.

von Bertalanffy, L. (1968). *General system theory.* New York: Braziller.

von Bertalanffy, L. (1975). *Perspectives on general system theory: Scientific-philosophical studies.* New York: Braziller.

Wright, M. (1983). The humanistic side of management. *Nursing & Health Care, 4,* 178–180.

Yura, H., & Walsh, M. (1987). *The nursing process* (5th ed.). Norwalk, CT: Appleton-Lang.

Part I

Ice-Breaking and Getting Acquainted: Experiential Exercises

EXERCISE 1　　Group Formation

Purposes

1. To divide the group into subgroups of six to eight members.

2. To increase group members' awareness of their self-perceptions concerning the roles assumed in group activities.

Facility

Large comfortable room in which participants can mill around.

Materials

Magic markers or crayons, 5" × 7" index cards, scotch tape, paper, and pencils.

Time Required

Thirty to 45 minutes.

Group Size

Unlimited.

Design

1. Participants should choose one word from each of the following three pairs of words. The word chosen should describe what they believe their behavior is when they are working on a group activity.

   A. Leader/follower

   B. Obsessive/carefree

   C. Rigid/flexible

2. Have members use a magic marker or a crayon to write their three chosen words in large print on the index card.

3. Tape the index card to their clothes, back or front.

4. Instruct members to mill around the room, talk with each other, and form into groups of six to eight people. These small groups will stay the same throughout the course and will work as one unit on all small-group exercises. Explain that a group should be com-

posed of all kinds of people—leaders, followers, obsessive, carefree, rigid, and flexible—in order for the group to be balanced. Balance plays a large part in the effective outcomes of group activities (15 to 30 minutes).

5. When groups have been formed, ask that each group record the names, addresses, and phone numbers of the members. These records should be duplicated and given to every member of the smaller group.

Discussion The formation of groups early in a class is necessary to encourage a group identity to begin. The groups will further develop throughout the course as they do the experiential exercises that require small groups. If possible, do not add any members to the groups once they have been formed.

Variation The word pairs can be expanded to include other areas that might be important. Examples are: smoker/nonsmoker; likes to write/hates to write; enjoys presenting to a large group/ hates presenting to a large group; and needs to talk/ needs to listen. The longer the list of word pairs, the longer time is required to decide on group membership. Having more than seven word pairs should be avoided because arriving at a balance in the group is too complicated and time-consuming.

EXERCISE 2   Member Introductions

Purposes
1. To introduce members of the small group to each other.
2. To begin formation of the team.
3. To establish an atmosphere that is conducive to experiential learning.

Facility
Large room with tables so that the members of the small group can sit facing one another.

Materials
None.

Time Required
Thirty minutes.

Group Size
Six to eight.

Design
1. Have small group members form into pairs or triads (if there is an odd number in the group).
2. Request that each pair (triad) share information about themselves—thoughts, experiences, backgrounds, goals, hobbies, likes, dislikes, and so forth (15 minutes). Discussion should avoid labels such as age, class level, and marital status. Labels do not tell others about the true self—what is inside.
3. Form into a group of the whole, which is composed of the six to eight members.
4. Ask each member of the pair (triad) to introduce the other(s) to the rest of the group.

Discussion
This exercise should be done after the small groups have been formed in Exercise 1. It does not matter if members of the pairs or triads know one another. If they do, instruct them to introduce themselves by telling their partner(s) something they know is unknown to the partner(s).

Variations

1. Have members wear name tags on which they have only drawn a picture. Then proceed with the design and have them relate to the picture in introducing themselves.

2. Use adjectives or animals in the above variation instead of a picture.

EXERCISE 3   **Self—My Management Shield***

Purposes

1. To look at the thoughts, feelings, and experiences that develop one's desire to become a nurse manager.

2. To become aware of one's personal values or philosophy of nursing management.

3. To explore one's desires and beliefs about ideal nursing management practice.

4. To probe into the ways one actually practices while in a management position.

5. To identify personal goals in nursing management.

Facility

Large room with tables so that the members of the small group can sit facing one another.

Materials

Construction paper and felt-tipped pens or crayons.

Time Required

One hour.

Group Size

Six to eight.

Design

1. Working individually, have participants draw a large shield on construction paper and divide it into six parts as shown.

2. Have them place their names at the top of the shield. Explain that this is their personal management shield, symbolizing various aspects of themselves as nurse managers.

3. Request that the areas in the shield be lettered from 1 to 6, as shown.

4. Ask that members draw in each designated area a picture or symbol that answers one of the following six questions:

---

*This exercise is based on the PELLEM Pentagram, a model of self developed by Elaine L. La Monica and Eunice M. Parisi. It is an adaptation of an exercise published in: La Monica, E. (1985). *The humanistic nursing process.* Boston: Jones and Bartlett.

NAME

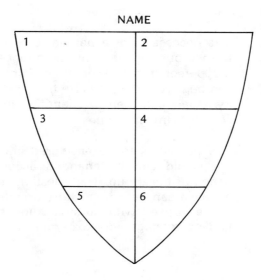

A. What or who has been significant to me in developing a desire to become a nurse manager?

B. What describes the "best" nurse manager I have known?

C. What do I believe the essence of nursing management to be?

D. What signifies my personal practice in nursing management?

E. How do I feel as a nurse manager?

F. In five years, if all were ideal, how would I be as a nurse manager?

5. After completing the shield, ask the small group members to discuss their shields with each other. Suggest that they explore the reasons, thoughts, and feelings that went into each picture or symbol.

6. Discuss the experience.

(continued)

EXERCISE 3 *(continued)*

Discussion   It is necessary for a person to explore globally
                         the various feelings and experiences that form
                         the person today. From this point, the person
                         can begin to conceptualize the ideal versus real-
                         ity. Goals can then be identified and strategies
                         set up to meet them.

Variation   The questions to be answered and pictured in
                         the shield can be changed according to the
                         needs of the group. The questions stated in the
                         exercise can be made future-oriented if the ex-
                         ercise is used with nursing students who have
                         had no management experience.

EXERCISE 4   Beginnings

Purposes
1. To begin formation and group interchange.

2. To assist with group introductions.

3. To assist participants to identify personal goals relative to the experience.

Facility
Large room with tables so that the members of the small groups can sit facing one another.

Materials
Worksheet A, pencils or pens, a blackboard, and chalk.

Time Required
Thirty to 45 minutes

Group Size
Six to eight

Design
1. Each participant should sit alone and complete the questions on Worksheet A. This should take approximately 15 minutes.

2. After participants complete the questions on Worksheet A independently, they should share their responses with each other in the small groups. Someone should record the list of major goals that the participants in the small group identified for the course/experience/workshop.

3. In the large group, the facilitator should list the major goals from all of the groups on the blackboard and themes should be identified. These themes can be woven into the course content or can be achieved in course assignments or extra activities.

Discussion
Participants should have the opportunity to see that they can achieve their personal objectives by moving through an organized experience. By combining a participant's needs with the course objectives, motivation can be increased.

(continued)

EXERCISE 4 (*continued*)
WORKSHEET A

1. What is your name, where do you attend school/work, and what do you do?

2. What is your major goal while attending this course/workshop/experience?

3. What do you like most about your current educational program/position?

4. What is the most difficult aspect of your current program/position?

5. What is the easiest aspect of your current program/position?

6. Describe one of your recent achievements.

7. Write some words you would use to describe yourself.

Part II

MANAGER RESPONSIBILITIES

Part II contains a discussion of a manager's responsibilities in motivating followers to accomplish goals. Motivating followers is the most important aspect of management and leadership. As has already been discussed, properly motivated employees, in comparison with unmotivated employees, accomplish tasks more quickly, thereby costing the organization less money. Also, quality of outcomes increases and employees have a greater chance for being satisfied. Employee satisfaction is a built-in positive reinforcer for accomplishing again.

Chapter 1 emphasized that effective management and leadership begins with the identification of a problem/goal. The system must then be filled in with material and human resources that are important in carrying out the goal or solving the problem. People and things that are essential and/or helpful in order to get the task done should be included in a system. Every system, therefore, is unique given the particular problem. System boundaries should be methodically identified so that important parts are not omitted, and nonessential parts are not included. One wishes to create a group that contains as much energy as possible working toward goal accomplishment. Nonessential parts of a system tend to detract from the group because energy can shift elsewhere. Remember that a group working together is affected by all parts of the group so you want to build a system that has as much positive energy as is possible.

It is helpful to consider the followers' human and material resources when identifying a system for a particular problem:

1. *Superiors*—those above the leader in the organizational chart. If a problem is not delegated to the manager to solve in any way deemed appropriate, superiors maintain varying amounts of control in how a problem is solved. Therefore, they may have to be included in the planning process.

2. *Associates*—those on the same level as the manager in the organizational chart. If associates have roles in the problem, they must be part of the system. If associates do not have roles in the problem but have had positive experiences in solving a similar problem, they should be included in the system if they are willing to participate.

3. *Followers*—those below the manager in the organizational chart. Followers usually comprise the largest part of the system.

4. *Situational Variables*—time demands, budget allocations, and the nature of the task.

5. *Material Resources*—technical equipment and other things that are available for use in solving a problem.

After the problem and the system for solving the problem have been designated, members of the system must be effectively motivated and educated to solve the problem and accomplish the goal. The manager behaves with the goal of influencing and motivating others. Leader behavior thereby responds to the needs of the environment and can be expressed in the following equation:

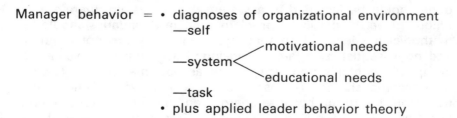

Manager behavior = • diagnoses of organizational environment
—self
—system
—motivational needs
—educational needs
—task
• plus applied leader behavior theory

The manager behavior that results from following this equation becomes the pivot on which alternative solutions and the ultimate recommended action for solving a problem through the system are based. The appropriate manager behavior can be thought of as an umbrella, guiding leaders in the strategy for goal accomplishment with ways that have the highest probability for success, given a unique problem and a unique system.

This equation forms the focus of Part II. Chapter 3 provides a discussion of how to diagnose self. Diagnosing the system is explained in Chapter 4. Given the system diagnosis, an appropriate leader behavior is identified in Chapter 5. Chapter 6 discusses how to diagnose the task, Chapter 7 applies the theories and processes by presenting and discussing a case study, and Chapter 8 contains a discussion of a foundation for management—ethics. Experiential exercises conclude Part II.

Diagnosing Self

CONCEPTUAL FRAMEWORK
POINT OF VIEW
  Stereotyping
  Halo-Horn Effect
  Implicit Personality Theory
LEADER BEHAVIOR STYLE
SUMMARY

Chapter 3 focuses on diagnosing self since the manager is an important part of the environment, and diagnosing self is the first step of the equation for diagnosing the organizational environment. This diagnosis involves identifying the manager's view of the problem/goal and of the unique environment, a viewpoint that will be influenced by the manager's values and perceptions. The manager must also diagnose the behavior style that is part of his or her leader personality—how the manager behaves involuntarily without cognitively thinking about actions. A discussion of the conceptual framework for diagnosing self begins this chapter.

CONCEPTUAL FRAMEWORK

The PELLEM Pentagram (named for its originators, Elaine L. La Monica and Eunice M. Parisi) is a model of self, comprised of five interrelated yet separate parts (La Monica, 1985):

- ■ Thoughts, feelings
- ■ Philosophy, values
- ■ Desires
- ■ Behaviors
- ■ Experiences

Figure 3.1 depicts the five-pointed star. While each point of the star represents one aspect of self, the aspects merge in the center to form the total self. The body is represented by a circular line running through each point. It is symbolized in this way because the body affects how and what one experiences, feels, and thinks, as well as how one behaves.

The points of the model represent what theorists believe to be operating within a person's total experience. The body is the vehicle for self-expression—it is one's language—and therefore crosses all facets of the pentagram. Self, portrayed in the center of the model, is the blending of all.

The influence of psychic powers and mystical phenomena that may have a part in total experience is absent from the model. These energies are neither denied nor claimed as fact even though their influence is undetermined and looked upon by pure scientists as based on superstition or at least unknown.

The PELLEM Pentagram provides a way to study self holistically. The interplay of all parts produces the unique individual. It is all of the components acting in unison that determine experience at any given moment. Denying the significance of any one part denies an important aspect of being. This model provides one simple though comprehensive way to view the complexities of a person. It stems

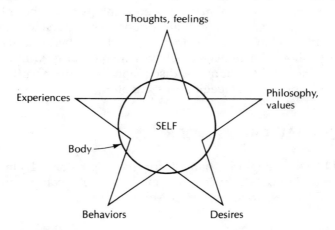

Figure 3.1 PELLEM Pentagram.

Source: Based on the PELLEM Pentagram, a model of self developed by Elaine L. La Monica and Eunice M. Parisi. La Monica, E. (1985). *The Nursing Humanistic Process*. Boston: Jones and Bartlett.

from personal and professional struggles to know and understand self, to direct self.

The areas of the PELLEM Pentagram should be explored in analyzing why problems and goals are considered important, why people are perceived in certain positions, and why self and others behave in certain ways. Self-exploration will provide the manager with insight, thereby raising self-awareness so that the environment being studied is looked at as objectively as is possible. Finch, Jones, and Litterer (1976) asserted that "accurate self-perception increases the likelihood of accurate interpersonal perception, and realistic perceptions of others are key elements in our ability to communicate, engage in joint problem-solving, and otherwise work with others" (p. 167).

POINT OF VIEW

Identifying the leader's point of view means starting honestly with one's perceptions of the problem/goal, feelings about followers in the system, past experiences relating to the problem/goal, personal desires, and so forth. Frieze and Bar-Tal (1979) and Kelley (1967) studied attribution theory, which is concerned with understanding perceptions of the causes of an event. They explain that people first form an idea about something or somebody and then collect data to support that idea. Krech, Crutchfield, and Ballachey (1962) posited that the first step in responding to another is to form an impression. This impression influences the interpersonal behavior in the event; it steers reactions.

Based on the previously cited theories, therefore, leaders' and managers' points of view affect the outcomes of a problem-solving process. Hersey and Blanchard (1988), Livingston (1969), and Likert (1961) discussed this concept in terms of an effective cycle and an ineffective cycle. In an effective cycle, people respond to a manager's high expectations with high performance. In an ineffective cycle, a manager's low expectations of employees generally result in low performance. Even though it is human nature to form impressions, a manager can reduce the impact his or her own perceptions may have on others by being conscious of them and then controlling them. A manager cannot control impressions if not aware of them. Cognitively thinking about personal perceptions increases the probability that the manager will not behave solely on the basis of those perceptions—at the very least not to the same degree that one would behave given no consciousness of the perceptions.

It is also important to note that even though high expectations generally result in high performance, set goals should be within the reach (with some stretching) of the people who are to be involved in accomplishing the goal. Setting expectations or goals that are unattainable results in high follower anxiety that becomes counterproductive and results in decreased motivation and maybe even "giving up" (Livingston, 1969). Managers should always examine goals carefully and then set reasonable expectations that can incrementally move a group to a much better level of performance over a period of time. Major change can then be charted and visualized by looking backward and adding all of the smaller accomplishments that were made. Figure 3.2 portrays this principle.

Finch, Jones, and Litterer (1976) and Krech, Crutchfield, and Ballachey (1962) have documented three persistent human tendencies that influence a manager's point of view: stereotyping, the halo-horn effect, and implicit personality theory.

Stereotyping

Stereotyping occurs when an individual attributes characteristics to someone that are assumed, given the individual's past experience, to typify a particular group (Finch, Jones, & Litterer, 1976). Racial, ethnic, and sexual stereotyping are most common, but stereotyping is

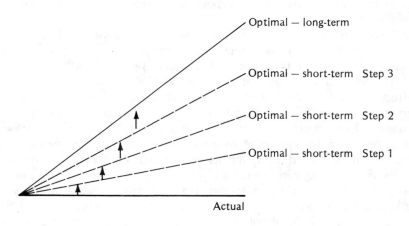

Figure 3.2 Progressive setting of attainable goals.

seen in other areas as well. There are stereotypes about nurse educators, physicians, nurse executives, hospital administrators, nurses who have been in the same position for 40 years, and so forth. These stereotypes can blind a nurse manager to the unique characteristics of an individual filling any of these roles. Further, stereotypes can cause the manager to respond inappropriately to another person based on past values and assumptions about people in those roles. It does not matter whether the stereotypes are negative or positive; behavior based on a stereotype has a high chance of being inappropriate.

Halo-Horn Effect

The halo-horn effect is another human tendency that must be checked. The halo effect refers to a favorable impression of one characteristic in an individual that the manager sees as important. This favorable impression becomes generalized to all of that individual's traits or characteristics. The horn effect is the same principle applied to an unfavorable impression of a characteristic the manager deems important. For example, if a nurse is efficient in organizing responsibilities, and the evaluating manager loves organized people, then the manager assumes the nurse must be good in carrying out all of those responsibilities. Conversely, if a nurse cannot organize work properly, the chances of being perceived as a good bedside nurse are slim. Such thinking is not discriminating; rather, it is biased and generally results in ineffective management.

Implicit Personality Theory

Implicit personality theory refers to grouping personality traits together (Finch, Jones, & Litterer, 1976). If a person is observed to be inflexible, is that person also demanding, cold, and hostile? Maybe and maybe not. Managers should always try to separate traits from one another in order to diagnose each unique individual objectively. Otherwise, misperceptions, misunderstandings, and inaccurate communication may result.

Informal group discussions with associates and superiors are effective means for uncovering biases such as those presented. Exploring why a problem is considered personally important and why one reacts negatively and/or positively to certain people and traits is an excellent consciousness-raising activity that reaps rewards in management and leadership. A trusting relationship among those discussing is essential for positive outcomes to this process.

LEADER BEHAVIOR STYLE

A nurse manager behaves first as a human being with unique personality characteristics and second in the role of nurse manager. Some managers enjoy working with people who are unskilled, training the unskilled worker every step of the way. Other managers most enjoy working with skilled people who are socially inclined—those who work together and also socialize together. Still other managers are inclined to lead people who need little on-site direction and reinforcement. All such inclinations are normal and expected given the humanness of an individual.

If a manager's system for solving a problem requires the behavior style that is the leader's forte, leading that system toward accomplishing a goal will be natural and will require only moderate cognitive thinking about leader actions. A perfect match is not often the case, however, especially in every problem situation. Since the system is always changing and the manager's goal is to facilitate growth so that followers are both willing and able to carry out their responsibilities, using only one leader behavior style is rarely enough. A manager must be able to function appropriately using different leader behavior styles.

Since all the styles of leadership are seldom the forte of the nurse leader, the manager must know one's inclinations (that which comes involuntarily) and then cognitively think about how to behave in order to meet the requirements of followers for other leader behavior styles. This requires diagnosing one's personal leader behavior style. The experiential exercises at the end of Part II contain an instrument that is valid for this purpose—the Leader Behavior (Self) Questionnaire, developed by staff members of the Ohio State Leadership Studies, Center for Business and Economic Research (see Exercise 1: Worksheet A).

SUMMARY

Identifying the manager's view of a problem/goal, as well as the unique environment, are aspects of diagnosing self. The PELLEM Pentagram (La Monica, 1985), a model of self, is the conceptual basis for the process of diagnosing self. A manager must be aware of personal beliefs such as stereotypes, halo-horn effects, and implicit personality groupings. Only with such insight can the manager reduce the impact of self-perceptions on others. This is necessary in

management so that leader behavior responds to the unique characteristics of people and things in a system rather than to the effects of
past experience, which may not be present reality. A manager must
also be aware of personal inclinations toward a specific leader behavior style. Because followers require all styles of leadership at different
points in time, the manager must know his or her own inclination
and then plan to meet the follower's needs for other leader behavior
styles.

REFERENCES

Finch, F., Jones, H., & Litterer, J. (1976). *Managing for organizational effective-
ness: An experiential approach.* New York: McGraw-Hill.
Frieze, I., & Bar-Tal, D. (1979). Attribution theory: Past and present. In I.
Freize, D. Bar-Tal, & J. Carroll, (Eds.). *New approaches to social problems:
Applications of attribution theory.* San Francisco: Jossey-Bass.
Hersey, P., & Blanchard, K. (1988). *Management of organizational behavior: Uti-
lizing human resources* (5th ed.). Englewood Cliffs, NJ: Prentice-Hall.
Kelley, M. (1967). Attribution theory in social psychology. In D. Levine (Ed.).
Nebraska Symposium on Motivation (Vol. 15). Lincoln: University of Ne-
braska Press.
Krech, D., Crutchfield, R., & Ballachey, E. (1962) *The individual in society.*
New York: McGraw-Hill.
La Monica, E. (1985). *The humanistic nursing process.* Boston: Jones and
Bartlett.
Likert, R. (1961). *New patterns of management.* New York: McGraw-Hill.
Livingston, J. (1969). Pygmalion in management. *Harvard Business Review, 47,*
81–89.

CHAPTER 4

Diagnosing the System

MASLOW'S HIERARCHY OF NEEDS
  Physiological Needs
  Safety Needs
  Social Needs
  Esteem Needs
  Self-Actualization Needs
HERSEY AND BLANCHARD'S LEVELS OF READINESS
McGREGOR'S THEORY X AND THEORY Y
ARGYRIS'S IMMATURITY–MATURITY
  CONTINUUM
HERZBERG'S MOTIVATION-HYGIENE THEORY
SUMMARY

The introduction to Part II contained a discussion of the human and material resources that must be considered when designating the system that will carry out a goal or solve a problem. Once a system is identified, it must be diagnosed. This system diagnosis is part of the equation that was introduced in Part II:

Manager behavior = • diagnoses of organizational environment
              —self

                         motivational needs
              —system<
                         educational needs

              —task
           • plus applied leader behavior theory

Five theories that can be used to diagnose a system are presented, discussed, and applied in this chapter. These theories are: Maslow's (1970) hierarchy of needs, Hersey and Blanchard's (1988) levels of readiness, McGregor's (1966, 1960/1985) Theory X and Theory Y, Argyris's (1971) maturity-immaturity continuum, and Herz-berg's (1966) motivation-hygiene theory.* Maslow's theory can best be used to diagnose the motivational needs of the system, as previously introduced in Chapter 2, while the balance of theories are best used to diagnose the educational needs of the system. Building a strategy for goal accomplishment therefore involves a focus on (a) what the system needs in order to be motivated and willing to achieve and (b) what the system needs in order to be educated and able to achieve, thereby accomplishing the stated goal within an acceptable range of that identified as optimal. The strategy is implemented by the man-ager using the most appropriate leader behavior indicated, given the maturity level of the majority of people in the unique system.

The general purpose of diagnosing a system is to determine the maturity level of the system regarding the system's ability to carry out the goal or to solve the problem; this is commonly referred to as diagnosing the maturity of the system. Maturity has nothing to do with chronologic years. Rather, its only concern is discriminating the system's ability to solve a problem or accomplish a goal. Leader behavior rests predominantly on this diagnosis. The system's diagno-sis, therefore, is the most important assessment that managers make. Accurate assessment results in appropriate leader behavior, which increases the probability for success in solving the problem. Unfortu-nately, the converse—that inaccurate assessment results in inappro-priate leader behavior and a decreased probability for success—is also true. The case called Urban City Hospital at the end of Part II is designed to enable learners to sharpen their diagnostic skills.

The theories provide various clues to managers concerning differ-ent behaviors and/or concepts that may be studied in the system. Each theory offers a different perspective, and the assessor should choose a theory or a combination of theories that best fits the system and seems most appropriate in a particular situation. The leader first assesses the individual parts of a system and then combines data on the system to determine the level of maturity of the system as a whole. Because leader behavior must respond to the majority in the group, the group mode (majority) of maturity is then used to deter-mine the appropriate leader behavior style for solving a specific prob-lem. If only one individual is in the system, then the manager can base leader behavior specifically on the individual's level of maturity.

---

*The integration of theories into maturity levels and their comparisons is an adaptation of that presented by Hersey and Blanchard (1988).

It is also essential to point out that leader behavior varies according to the needs of the system in solving a particular problem. Even though the leader may be the same person for two systems and even though the systems may be the same for two problems, the level of maturity of the system may be different as that system is diagnosed for its ability to solve different problems. Diagnosis is always done in response to a unique system's needs regarding a specified goal/ problem.

MASLOW'S HIERARCHY OF NEEDS

The first theory to be discussed in diagnosing a system belongs to Maslow (1970), who developed a hierarchy of human needs that contains five categories. In order of priority, these needs are: physiological, safety, social, esteem, and self-actualization. All of these needs are vital parts of a person's system but physiological needs are top priority when unsatisfied. When physiological needs are satisfied or are in balance, then safety needs become top priority. This ladder effect follows to self-actualization, which is top priority only when all other needs are satisfied. All needs are present within an individual, but the priority shifts according to the time, the place, and the activity of an individual. Maslow's (1970) hierarchy of needs is diagrammed and discussed in Chapter 2. The nurse manager can use Maslow's theory to diagnose the system's level of maturity, specifically their motivational needs, for accomplishing a particular problem. How the theory is applied for this purpose is discussed in the next section of this chapter; how this assessment leads to the decision of the appropriate leader behavior style that should be used to get the problem solved is the focus of Chapter 5. Remember, in order to diagnose a system, diagnose the individual parts of the system first and then decide the group's (system's) modal level of maturity.

Physiological Needs

Physiological needs are those that sustain life. They are biological and personal in nature and include air, water, food, clothing, and shelter. Assurance of income in order to meet physiological needs is an essential aspect in this area. Since most people can always use more money, assurance of income only becomes a need priority when basic needs are threatened or when a lower standard of living would occur due to decreased income.

Adults are usually able to satisfy their own physiological needs when these are a priority. A wise manager, however, tries to make easy fulfillment of these needs possible. For example, if a leader plans a 9 A.M. meeting and the system contains coffee drinkers, provide coffee for the group at the beginning of the meeting. Do not expect that people will be so dedicated to hearing about the agenda that they will forget about their physiological needs or that the people will bring their own coffee—these chances are risky. Rather, most people during the meeting will start thinking about how nice it would be to have a cup of coffee. This means that participants will not be thinking about business.

Another example is that nurses are often accused of spending much of their time at the nurses' station or in the conference room eating and/or smoking. If a leader knows that such behavior is prevalent in a group, to say that these nurses are remiss or not dedicated is foolish; it will only make the nurses resentful of authority and increase the need, which will in turn decrease the amount and the quality of time spent with clients. Rather, keep the coffee pot going, set up a system so that munchies are easily available, and tell the members of the system that even though they are on the unit to give nursing care, it is recognized that they need frequent breaks—give people what they need. At the same time, tell followers that management's hopes are that frequent breaks will increase the quality of nursing care provided because the nurses will be more satisfied. By giving system members what they need, thereby satisfying their need, a manager moves them to the next need level. Ideally the manager wishes to move the system to esteem and self-actualization levels because motivation to solve a problem is highest at these levels. Physiological needs are also the easiest to satisfy.

Safety Needs

Hersey and Blanchard (1988) defined safety needs as involved with self-preservation. Protection from physical injury in the environment is a safety need. Douglass (1988) further included stability and predictability in life, freedom from constant stressful situations, familiar surroundings, and provision for job security.

A leader can conclude that a member of a system is at a safety level of maturity when the physical environment is potentially harmful, when the member's position or status quo is threatened, when someone is new in a position, or when the problem involves a noticeable change from normal service. Suppose that new cardiac monitors were installed in the Intensive Care Unit (ICU). The goal is to orient the ICU staff to these new monitors. Even though the ICU staff members were mature in ICU nursing care, they would be at a safety level regarding the new monitors until they become proficient in running the new equipment.

A new graduate beginning a first position is at a safety level of maturity; so is a 20-year veteran taking a position in a new agency. Given the goal of orienting new staff, the new graduate is most probably in a stressful state, not knowing the environment, the expectations others will have for the role, and whether the ability to fulfill the role is present. The 20-year nurse veteran will most likely be concerned with the new environment and the expectations of others. Because the veteran has a library of experience, however, this person may move out of the safety level of maturity more quickly than will the new graduate. Nevertheless, at the outset, both can be diagnosed as at a safety level of maturity.

Social Needs

Hersey and Blanchard (1988) cogently expressed social needs as meaningful interpersonal relationships. Social needs involve a concern for others in the environment with focus of attention moving from self to others. Since the client should be the primary focus in health-care agencies, health-care personnel ideally should be at the social need level at the minimum whenever they are interacting with clients. If not, personnel will be more concerned with self—this is not the intent of any helping relationship. Even though the ideal just stated is not always possible, the manager should work toward this goal.

Examples of people who are functioning at a social level are those who enjoy working together in groups or in teams, sharing warm relationships, viewing the work environment as a social situation (Douglass, 1988), encouraging people to feel a part of the work group, and generally expressing concern for others in the environment. People who come to work primarily because they need the stimulation from and affiliation with others are at a social level of maturity. Social needs are a priority only when safety and physiological needs are in balance or are satisfied.

Esteem Needs

Maslow (1970) identified two types of esteem needs: (1) the desire for achievement, competency, and mastery of one's personal and professional activities and (2) the desire for prestige, status, importance, and recognition.

People who have esteem needs seek fulfillment by overtly and covertly asking to be noticed. They may want to be told that they are super nurses, that they always follow through on their responsibilities, that they are accountable, and so forth.

Overt esteem needs of people are obvious because a person asks for what is wanted—"What is your reaction to my ability?" Covert esteem needs must be diagnosed. For example, if a person comes back after having been asked to do something and shares that it was necessary to shorten lunch in order to get the task done, take this as a covert request for praise. Tell this person how much you appreciate what was done and how good it is to be so accountable and dependable. Maslow (1970) cautioned against being superficial when giving praise and reinforcement because a person motivated at the esteem level wants respect, not phoniness. Therefore, be clear about your own positive feelings about what was done and then share those feelings.

Self-Actualization Needs

This need structure is of the highest order, becoming prominent when all other needs are satisfied. It involves one's desire to reach fullest potential (Hersey & Blanchard, 1988). Furthermore, this potential is reality-based on awareness of one's own strengths and weaknesses.

Douglass (1988) characterized self-actualized employees as those finding meaning and personal growth in work; they actively seek new responsibilities, and work becomes play. Further, these people reinforce self (intrinsic reinforcement) rather than seeking reinforcement from others (extrinsic reinforcement). Extrinsic reinforcement characterizes people at the esteem level. Self-actualized people will accomplish, tell the manager what is required, and then go on with responsibilities. They are dependent, interdependent, and independent according to their own direction and as the situation demands. A nurse at this level strives to help self and others in the environment without being told to do so.

HERSEY AND BLANCHARD'S LEVELS OF READINESS

The second theory that is considered to be appropriate in diagnosing nursing environments is Hersey and Blanchard's (1988) levels of readiness, which has two major components: ability and willingness. The first component involves one's ability to solve a problem, including knowledge and experience. The second component refers to one's willingness to carry out a task with self-confidence, commitment, and self-respect (Hersey & Blanchard, 1988).

Using the variables ability, willingness, and confidence, Hersey and Blanchard (1988, p. 176) designated four benchmarks in readiness levels:

Readiness level:	*Follower is:*
R1—Low maturity	Unwilling and unable or insecure
R2—Moderate maturity	Unable but willing or confident
R3—Moderate maturity	Able but unwilling or insecure
R4—High maturity	Able and willing or confident

Suppose that the middle managers in an acute-care hospital decided to change from team nursing to primary nursing as the nursing-care delivery model. Further assume that one nursing unit was chosen as the pilot group for this goal. All of the registered nurses for all shifts on this unit, plus the head nurse, supervisor, and assistant director in charge of the unit, became the system. The assistant director was the manager for solving the problem. This director was involved as a middle manager in making the decision to change from team nursing to primary nursing.

The system would be at the Rl (unwilling and unable) level of readiness if the majority of its members neither knew about the primary-nursing concept nor had experience with primary nursing and if the members verbally and nonverbally expressed no desire for change. If the members were excited about the change, wanting to gain the knowledge even though primary nursing was new, the system would be diagnosed as R2 (unable but willing or confident). Using the same hypothetical example, the system would be at the R3 level of readiness (able but not willing or confident) if the majority of the system's members had knowledge of primary nursing and had previously experienced it but did not have a positive experience with the model and felt that team nursing was what they wanted. If the majority of members had knowledge about and experience with primary nursing, liked it, and were eager to put it to work on their unit, this system would be at the R4 level of readiness (able and willing).

This hypothetical example illustrates how to diagnose a system using all of the levels in Hersey and Blanchard's (1988) theory of readiness. If the problem of the example were real, a manager would choose the unit with the highest readiness level as the target for the pilot project. This unit would provide the best chance for initial success, which is especially important when attempting a major change.

Another factor to remember when applying this theory is that a person is either willing or unwilling and able or not able. There are no gray areas. For example, if a person is willing to try something even though doubting its usefulness, then for the purpose of applying the theory, consider the person to be unwilling. People are able only when able to be left completely on their own—when they have the knowledge, the experience, and they understand the job requirements. People are willing or confident when they are willing to take responsibility, when they are secure in their abilities to perform effectively and when they need to achieve.

McGREGOR'S THEORY X AND THEORY Y

The third theory that can be used to diagnose a system is McGregor's (1966, 1960/1985) Theory X and Theory Y. It was introduced in Chapter 2 in a discussion of classical and nonclassical organization theory. Although McGregor's theory was intended for the purpose used in Chapter 2, it can be used appropriately for diagnosing the system. Table 4.1 lists the assumptions about human nature that underlie McGregor's theory.

Table 4.1 lists five traits and opposite statements for each trait.

TABLE 4.1 Assumptions About Human Nature That Underlie McGregor's (1966, 1960/1985) Theory X and Theory Y

Theory X Immature	Trait	Theory Y Mature
1. People find work distasteful	Work attitude	1. People regard work as natural as play, given favorable conditions.
2. People are not ambitious and prefer direction.	Ambition	2. People are self-directed in achieving organizational goals.
3. People do not solve organizational problems creatively.	Creativity	3. People are creative in solving problems.
4. People are motivated only by physiological and safety factors.	Motivation	4. People are motivated at all levels of Maslow's (1970) hierarchy of needs.
5. People require close control and coercion to achieve goals.	Control	5. People are self-controlled if properly motivated.

TABLE 4.2 McGregor's (1966, 1960/1985) Theory X and Theory Y: A Continuum for Diagnosing a System

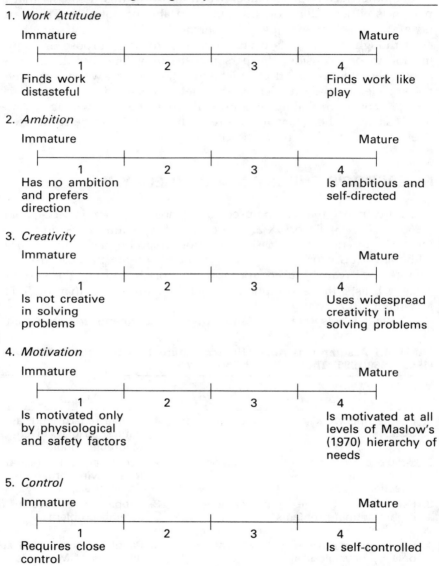

1. *Work Attitude*

   Immature   Mature

   ├────────1────────┼────2────┼────3────┼────4────────┤

   Finds work   Finds work like
   distasteful   play

2. *Ambition*

   Immature   Mature

   ├────────1────────┼────2────┼────3────┼────4────────┤

   Has no ambition   Is ambitious and
   and prefers   self-directed
   direction

3. *Creativity*

   Immature   Mature

   ├────────1────────┼────2────┼────3────┼────4────────┤

   Is not creative   Uses widespread
   in solving   creativity in
   problems   solving problems

4. *Motivation*

   Immature   Mature

   ├────────1────────┼────2────┼────3────┼────4────────┤

   Is motivated only   Is motivated at all
   by physiological   levels of Maslow's
   and safety factors   (1970) hierarchy of
                                                 needs

5. *Control*

   Immature   Mature

   ├────────1────────┼────2────┼────3────┼────4────────┤

   Requires close   Is self-controlled
   control

The statements are explicit descriptions of how the traits can be observed in people. Since most people, however, may not fit totally into an either/or category, the nurse manager should use McGregor's (1966, 1960/1985) theory as a continuum for diagnosing a system. Table 4.2 is one example of how this continuum can be established. The manager can indicate on Table 4.2 an assessment of where a system member is for each particular trait. These individual assessments can then be tallied according to the number of people in each category of the trait. The category with the highest number of people (the modal category) should be used to determine the appropriate leader behavior style. The reader is cautioned against averaging the assessments because the average (or mean) is affected by extremes and is not a purely representative figure of the majority of people. A manager should base leader behavior on the modal level of maturity.

ARGYRIS'S IMMATURITY—MATURITY CONTINUUM

The fourth theory that can be used to diagnose a system, developed by Argyris (1971), is called the immaturity-maturity continuum. Argyris depicted seven changes that take place in the personality of healthy people as they develop from immaturity to maturity.

First, people move from a passive state to a state of activity. Second, people are dependent on others and grow to an independent

TABLE 4.3 Argyris's (1971) Immaturity—Maturity Continuum

Immature	Trait	Mature
1. Passive	Work attitude	1. Active
2. Dependent	Dependence	2. Independent
3. Behaves in a few ways	Behavior	3. Behaves in many ways
4. Erratic, shallow interests	Interests	4. Deep, strong interests
5. Short time perspective	Concern	5. Long time perspective (past and future)
6. Subordinate position	Position	6. Equal or superordinate position
7. Lack of self-awareness	Self-awareness	7. Awareness and self-control

state. Third, immature people possess few behaviors, but when mature they can behave in many ways. Fourth, immature people have erratic and shallow interests while mature people have deep and intense interests. Fifth, people move from a concern only for the here and now (a short time perspective) to a concern for the past, present, and future (a long time perspective). Sixth, people move from a subordinate position to an equal or superordinate position. Seventh, a lack of self-awareness characterizes the immature whereas awareness and control over self characterizes the mature. Table 4.3 lists these changes. Like McGregor's (1966, 1960/1985) Theory X and The-

TABLE 4.4 Argyris's (1971) Immaturity-Maturity Continuum: A Continuum for Diagnosing a System

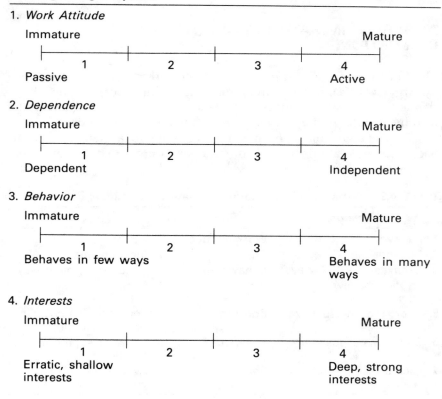

1. *Work Attitude*

Immature — Mature

| 1 | 2 | 3 | 4 |

Passive — Active

2. *Dependence*

Immature — Mature

| 1 | 2 | 3 | 4 |

Dependent — Independent

3. *Behavior*

Immature — Mature

| 1 | 2 | 3 | 4 |

Behaves in few ways — Behaves in many ways

4. *Interests*

Immature — Mature

| 1 | 2 | 3 | 4 |

Erratic, shallow interests — Deep, strong interests

TABLE 4.4 (continued)

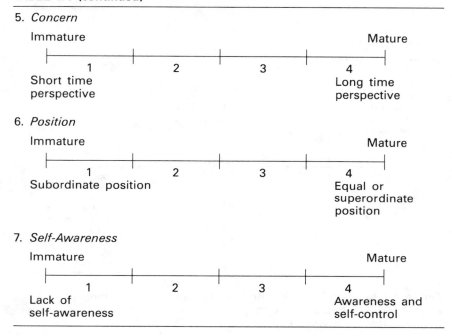

5. *Concern*

Immature   Mature

```
|-------------+-------------+-------------+-------------|
      1             2             3             4
```
Short time   Long time
perspective   perspective

6. *Position*

Immature   Mature

```
|-------------+-------------+-------------+-------------|
      1             2             3             4
```
Subordinate position   Equal or
                                                    superordinate
                                                    position

7. *Self-Awareness*

Immature   Mature

```
|-------------+-------------+-------------+-------------|
      1             2             3             4
```
Lack of   Awareness and
self-awareness   self-control

ory Y, Argyris's (1971) immaturity—maturity continuum (Table 4.4) can be used to assess individual people in a system.

HERZBERG'S MOTIVATION–HYGIENE THEORY

The last theory to be discussed for diagnosing a system is Herzberg's (1966) motivation-hygiene theory, commonly referred to as his two-factor theory. Herzberg identified higher-order needs relating to job content that can raise performance and increase one's total work output—motivators, such as achievement, recognition, challenging work, responsibility, advancement, and growth. Herzberg also delineated lower-order needs that referred to the job environment and context—hygiene factors, such as organizational policies, working conditions, interpersonal relations, money, status, security, and personal life. Herzberg found that employees who were dissatisfied with

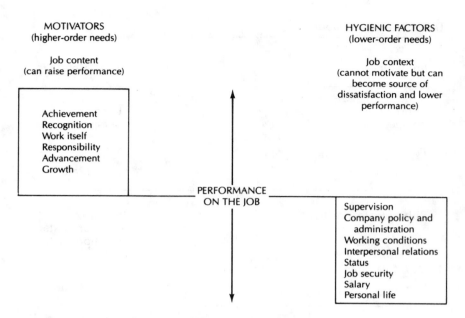

Figure 4.1 Herzberg's motivation-hygiene (maintenance) theory.
Source: Herzberg F., Mausner B., & Snyderman B. (1959). *The Motivation to Work* (2nd ed.). New York: Wiley. Reproduced by permission.

hygiene factors had lower performance. Claus and Bailey (1977) conceptualized this theory, as shown in Figure 4.1 (Herzberg, Mausner, & Snyderman, 1959)

Herzberg's theory is useful for the nurse manager in identifying insights to the goals and incentives that may satisfy needs according to Maslow's (1970) hierarchy. For this purpose, Davis and Newstrom (1985) compared Maslow's need-priority model with Herzberg's (1966) motivation-hygiene model, as shown in Table 4.5. Herzberg's theory, therefore, can be used to amplify the diagnosis made using Maslow's theory and to provide greater insight into the reasons for the diagnosis and strategies for motivating.

Herzberg (1966) is often credited with the concept of job enrichment—the Herzberg Solution. According to Herzberg, the way to enrich a job is to enlarge the responsibility, scope, and the challenge in the position. In this way, the motivators of achievement, recognition, responsibility, and advancement would be amplified, thereby giving employees what they value in the position.

TABLE 4.5 Parallels Between Maslow's Hierarchy of Needs and Herzberg's Motivation-Hygiene (Maintenance) Theory

Maslow's *Need-Priority Model*		*Herzberg's* *Motivation-Maintenance Model*
Self-actualization and fulfillment	*Motivational factors*	Work itself Achievement Possibility of growth Responsibility
Esteem and status		Advancement Recognition
Belonging and social needs	*Maintenance factors*	Status Relations with supervisors Peer relations Relations with subordinates Quality of supervision
Safety and security		Company policy and administration Job security Working conditions
Physiological needs		Pay

Source: Davis, K., & Newstrom, J. (1985). *Human Behavior at Work: Organizational Behavior* (7th ed.) New York: McGraw-Hill. p. 77. Reproduced by permission.

SUMMARY

Diagnosing the maturity level of a system in terms of the system's ability to solve a problem is the most important aspect of the environmental diagnosis. Leader behavior is based on the system's diagnosis. A manager diagnoses the individuals in a system first and then uses the modal level of maturity to determine leader behavior. This leader behavior is then used to begin implementation of the strategy for goal accomplishment.

Five theories for diagnosing a system were presented and discussed in this chapter. The manager may use one or more theories to diagnose a system, depending on what seems to be appropriate in a given context. Table 4.6 provides a concise summary and comparison of the theories presented.

TABLE 4.6 A Comparison of Five Theories for Diagnosing a System

I M M A T U R I T Y   *Maslow's (1970) Hierarchy of Needs*   M A T U R I T Y

M1	M2	M3	M4
Physiological Safety	Social	Esteem	Self-actualization

Herzberg's (1966) Motivation-Hygiene Theory

Hygiene (maintenance) factors   Motivational factors

M1	M2	M3	M4
Salary; Working conditions; Job security; Company policy and administration	Supervision; Interpersonal relations	Status; Advancement; Recognition	Work itself; Achievement; Growth opportunities; Responsibilities

Hersey and Blanchard's (1988) Levels of Readiness

R1	R2	R3	R4
Unwilling and unable or insecure	Unable but willing or confident	Able but unwilling or insecure	Able and willing or confident

McGregor's (1966, 1960/1985) Theory X and Theory Y

Theory X   *Theory Y*

M1	M2	M3	M4

1. Finds work distasteful
2. No ambition; prefers direction
3. No creativity
4. Motivated by physiological and safety factors
5. Requires close control

1. Finds work pleasant
2. Ambitious and self-directed
3. Widespread creativity
4. Motivated at all levels of Maslow's hierarchy
5. Self-controlled

TABLE 4.6 (continued)

Argyris's (1971) Immaturity-Maturity Continuum

M1   M2   M3   M4

1. Passive	1. Active
2. Dependent	2. Independent
3. Behaves in a few ways	3. Behaves in many ways
4. Erratic, shallow interests	4. Deep, strong interests
5. Short time perspective	5. Long time perspective
6. Subordinate position	6. Equal or superordinate position
7. Lacks self-awareness	7. Awareness and self-control

REFERENCES

Argyris, C. (1971). *Management and organizational development: The path from XA to YB.* New York: McGraw-Hill.

Claus, K., & Bailey, J. (1977). *Power and influence in health care.* St. Louis: Mosby.

Davis, K., & Newstrom, J. (1985). *Human behavior at work: Organizational behavior* (7th ed.). New York: McGraw-Hill.

Douglass, L. (1988). *The effective nurse: Leader and manager* (3rd ed.). St. Louis: Mosby.

Hersey, P., & Blanchard, K. (1988). *Management of organizational behavior: Utilizing human resources* (5th ed.). Englewood Cliffs, NJ: Prentice-Hall.

Herzberg, F. (1966). *Work and the nature of man.* Cleveland: World Publishing.

Herzberg, F., Mausner, B., & Snyderman, B. (1959). *The motivation to work* (2nd ed.). New York: Wiley.

Maslow, A. (1970). *Motivation and Personality* (2nd ed.). New York: Harper & Row.

McGregor, D. (1966). *Leadership and motivation.* Boston: MIT Press.

McGregor, D. (1985). *The human side of enterprise: 25th anniversary printing.* New York: McGraw-Hill. (Original work published 1960).

Leader Behavior

This chapter contains a discussion of leader behavior theory with an application of theory to the system diagnosis in order to determine the appropriate leader behavior for a unique system that will achieve a goal.

Leader behavior will be defined, followed by a discussion of the common leader behavior styles. Theoretical components of leader behavior and leadership styles will then be discussed. A leader behavior model will be applied in determining the appropriate leader behavior style, given a system's diagnosis. An examination of the components of leader effectiveness concludes this chapter.

DEFINITION OF LEADERSHIP

Stogdill (1974) aptly noted that "there are almost as many different definitions of leadership as there are persons who have attempted to define the concept" (p. 7). He does, however, provide a rough scheme of classification and a thorough review of the literature in this area. Highlights of Stogdill's discussion are presented in the following paragraph.

In early literature (Cooley, 1902; Knickerbocker, 1948), leadership was thought of as a focus of group processes. The idea that leadership was a personality trait also appealed to early theorists (Bingham, 1927/1973; Kilbourne, 1935). Allport (1924) and Bennis (1959) viewed leadership as the art of inducing compliance, and Shartle (1951) and Tannenbaum, Weschler, and Massarik (1961) similarly saw it as the exercise of influence. Fiedler (1967) suggested that leadership was an act or a behavior, and Koontz and O'Donnell (1986) regarded it as a form of persuasion. Numerous theorists have suggested that leaders are instruments of goal achievement (Cattell, 1951; Urwick, 1953). Other organizational behaviorists have viewed leadership as an interactive effect (Merton, 1969), a differentiated role (Sherif & Sherif, 1956), and the initiation of structure (Homans, 1950).

The definitions of leadership developed by Fleishman (1973) and Hersey and Blanchard (1988) will be combined. For the purpose of this book, leadership is using communication processes to influence the activities of an individual or of a group toward the attainment of a goal or goals in a unique and given situation; leader behavior is how a manager acts toward members of the system. Fleishman (1973) pointed out that leadership always involves attempts to influence; further, he stated that all interpersonal relationships can involve elements of leadership. This latter remark affirms the statement, which was made in Chapter 1, that all people in the health-care system who influence others are leaders.

COMMON LEADER BEHAVIOR STYLES

There are three common labels for leader behavior: autocratic, democratic, and laissez-faire. Autocratic leaders are often described as authoritarian, firm leaders who make unilateral decisions, whereas democratic leaders involve the group in decision making, giving responsibilities to followers. Laissez-faire leaders generally maintain loose control over their followers.

An informal survey of leaders' and followers' opinions of the best leader behavior style usually results in the democratic style obtaining the most votes. But imagine the following scene:

> You are in a car with two of your associates driving home on a country road after work. The car in front of you is sideswiped; you and your associates are the only people at the scene. The driver in the accident has a severely lacerated hand and is semiconscious. You must do something. The bleeding must be stopped, and an ambulance must be called.
>
> Being a democratic leader, you say to your associates, "Listen, the bleeding must be stopped, and someone has to walk through the woods to a house in order to call an ambulance. It does not matter who does what . . . both of you jointly decide and let me know your decision."

The beauty of the democratic style is that participants have choice, but is choice appropriate in the situation just described? No! An autocratic statement is quickly needed to tell your associates what each must do. It is important to point out that autocratic statements are frequently perceived as hostile, mean, and unfriendly. Remember that any statement can be hostile or warm, depending on the verbal and nonverbal communication patterns that are used by the speaker.

Changing the scene slightly, suppose that you and your associates were emergency room nurses and had worked together for five years. Would it be necessary for anyone to say what should be done? No! In this example, laissez-faire leader behavior would be appropriate.

Each leader behavior style can be appropriate, depending on the situation. Determining the appropriate leader behavior style is often more complex than in the previously cited example. For this reason, theorists have broken leader behavior into components and then used models to determine scientifically the appropriate behavior for a specific situation.

COMPONENTS OF LEADER BEHAVIOR

Management theorists designate two basic components of leader behavior, even though the theorists name the components differently. One component deals with getting the job done, and the other is

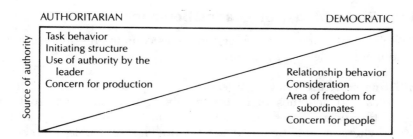

Figure 5.1 The balance of leader behavior components.

Source: Adapted and reprinted by permission of the *Harvard Business Review.* An exhibit from "How to Choose a Leadership Pattern" by Robert Tannenbaum and Warren H. Schmidt (March/April, 1958). Copyright © 1958 by the President and Fellows of Harvard College; all rights reserved.

concerned with interpersonal behavior. Hersey and Blanchard (1988) referred to *task behavior* and *relationship behavior.* The Ohio State Leadership Studies staff call the components *initiating structure* and *consideration* (Kerr & Schriesheim, 1974). Tannenbaum and Schmidt (1958) labeled the components as *use of authority by the leader* and *area of freedom for subordinates* and Blake and Mouton (1964, 1978, 1984) said it is *concern for production* and *concern for people.*

A leader's behavior style is never one component or the other. Rather, one's leader behavior is a composite of both components with the weight of each varying, given the whole. Figure 5.1 portrays this balance.

In the figure, leader behavior is conceptualized as filling the rectangle. As task behavior decreases, relationship behavior increases. There is always an element of job-related behavior and relationship behavior in any style.

LEADERSHIP MODELS

There are several theories that delineate leadership styles. Authors differ on the style labels, as with the components of leader behavior, even though the framework and meaning of the models remain the same. Three prominent leader behavior models will be discussed and compared. The Ohio State model has been used to diagnose leaders' personal behavior styles in Chapter 3 and will be used predominantly in later sections of this chapter and in Chapter 7.

Ohio State Model of Leader Behavior

The Ohio State model for leadership styles contains the following two components of leader behavior:

Initiating structure refers to a leader's attempt to organize and define the roles and activities of group members. It is stating a goal and delineating what is to be done, how it will be done, when it will be done, where it will be done, and who is responsible for specific tasks. Structure involves one-way communication; the leader tells followers what to do in order to accomplish a goal.

Consideration involves two-way communication, responding to the group's needs by requesting opinions, beliefs, desires, and so forth. Group activities and discussions are consideration interventions. Further, consideration refers to establishing mutual trust between and among group members, showing respect and warmth. Establishing effective interpersonal relationships is part of consideration.

The Ohio State model can be seen in Figure 5.2 (Stogdill &

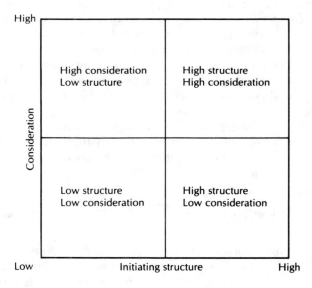

Figure 5.2 Ohio State model of leadership.
Source: Paul Hersey and Kenneth H. Blanchard, *Management of Organizational Behavior: Utilizing Human Resources* (5th ed), © 1988, p. 92. Reprinted by permission of Prentice Hall, Inc., Englewood Cliffs, N.J.

Coons, 1957). When the two components of leadership are placed on separate axes and the window boxes are filled in, four leader behavior styles result.

Situational Leadership Theory

Situational leadership theory (Hersey & Blanchard, 1988) grew out of the Ohio State model and can be seen in Figure 5.3. This theory looks exactly like the Ohio State model except that the names of the leader behavior components are different. Task parallels structure, and relationship parallels consideration.

The four quadrants in the Ohio State model and in situational leadership theory can be explained as follows:

1. *High structure/task and low consideration/relationship.* A leader primarily defines the task, explains to the group each person's responsibility, and states when tasks should be done. One-way communication characterizes the leader's behavior even though the low relationship behavior should be observable.

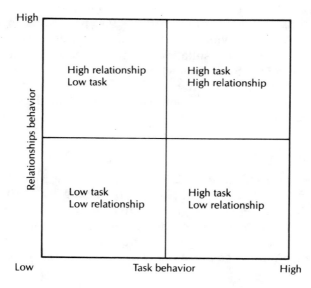

Figure 5.3 Situational Leadership Theory.

Source: Paul Hersey and Kenneth H. Blanchard, *Management of Organizational Behavior: Utilizing Human Resources* (5th ed.), © 1988, p. 117. Reprinted by permission of Prentice Hall, Inc., Englewood Cliffs, N.J.

The low relationship behavior is simply respect and warmth toward another and positive reinforcement after a goal is completed. No group decision making is included in this style.

2. *High structure/task and high consideration/relationship.* A leader balances concern for the intricacies of getting a task accomplished with a concern for the beliefs, desires, and needs of the group. The leader might define a goal, designate what needs to be done and who has specific responsibilities, and invite questions or reactions. The leader's original plan might be altered given the followers' reactions. In this style of leadership, the leader is still in full control but group interaction is begun.

3. *High consideration/relationship and low structure/task.* In this style, the leader's primary concern is not the task and its various intricacies. Rather, concern is for the process, for getting the group to work together effectively to accomplish the task. The leader still has some control over how the group accomplishes the task. In this style, for example, a leader might define the problem and ask the group members to make further decisions about how they will work together to accomplish the task.

4. *Low structure/task and low consideration/relationship.* The leader maintains a low profile in this style, permitting followers to function within previously defined limits. At times, the leader may be available for consultation, to give direction, or for positive reinforcement. Such interaction is not planned on a regular basis but rather occurs as the need arises. This leader behavior style is delegation because control is shifted from the leader to the follower(s).

Managerial Grid®

Blake and Moutin (1964, 1978, 1984) developed the Managerial Grid (see Figure 5.4) and recently applied it to nursing leadership (Blake, Mouton, & Tapper, 1981). The grid has five styles of leadership based on a combination of concern for production and concern for people. The scale for each component moves from one (low) to nine (high). The five leadership styles are described as follows (Blake & Mouton, 1964):

Authority-Obedience (Task) (9,1). The leader assumes a position of power by arranging work conditions efficiently and in such a way that human elements interfere minimally.

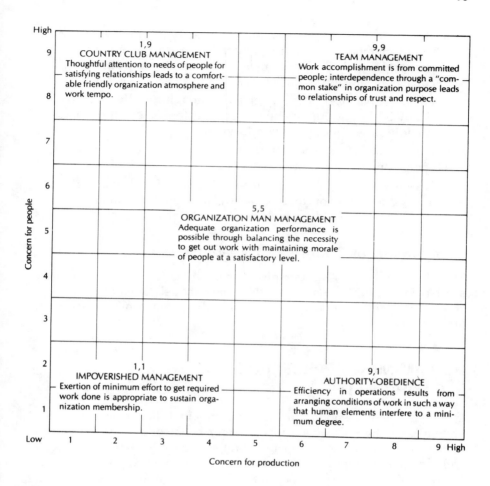

Figure 5.4 The Managerial Grid®.

Source: The Managerial Grid figure from *The New Managerial Grid III: The Key to Leadership Excellence*, by Robert R. Blake and Jane Srygley Mouton. Houston: Gulf Publishing Company, copyright © 1985, p. 12. Reproduced by permission.

Team (9,9).* People are committed to accomplishing a task; group members are interdependent, and everyone holds a "common stake." Relationships of trust, respect, and equality characterize the work climate.

Country Club (1,9). The leader pays thoughtful attention to the needs of group members and fosters a comfortable, friendly atmosphere and work tempo.

Impoverished (1,1). The leader extends minimal effort in accomplishing the required work.

Organization Man (Middle-of-the-Road) (5,5). The leader balances the behavior that is task-related while maintaining the morale of group members at a satisfactory level.

Comparison of Theories of Leadership

The three models of leadership discussed earlier are conceptually similar. Figure 5.5 merges the Ohio State model, Situational Leadership Theory, the Managerial Grid, and the three common styles of leadership.

DETERMINING APPROPRIATE LEADER BEHAVIOR STYLE**

Leader behavior responds to the environmental diagnosis of self, the system, and the task plus applied leader behavior theory. Diagnoses of the task will be discussed in Chapter 6. In this chapter, a bridge will join the diagnosis of the system and the appropriate leader behavior style. This bridge becomes the most important element in determining leader behavior. Self-diagnosis, which was discussed in Chapter 3, is information for the leader concerning what needs to be done and/or thought about so that one can actually behave according to the theory-specified leader behavior style in a given situation.

The leader behavior that will be used in this section is the Ohio State model, shown in Figure 5.2. Chapter 4 contained a discussion of five theories that can be used to diagnose a system (see Table 4.6). These theories are combined in Figure 5.6.

---

*Recent research by Blake and Mouton (1981) determined that managers prefer the team (9,9) style.

**This section grew from the work of Hersey and Blanchard (1988).

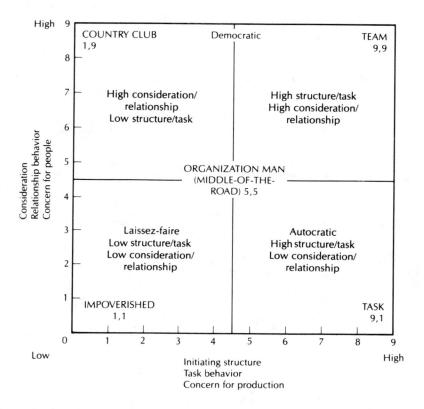

Figure 5.5 Theories of leadership: Ohio State model, Situational Leadership Theory, Managerial Grid®, and common leader behavior styles. Adapted from Hershey & Blanchard, 1988.

The theories used to diagnose the system read in progression from right to left in Figure 5.6. In other words, the lowest level of development is on the right side and the highest level of development is on the left side. Also, leader behavior numbers (LB1, LB2, LB3, and LB4) are placed in the four leader behavior quadrants, moving counterclockwise from least to most mature.

In order to determine the appropriate leader behavior style given a system's diagnosis, the bottom part of Figure 5.6 (system diagnosis) must be bridged to the top part of the figure (leader behavior). Suppose that the task is to change from team nursing to primary nursing as the model of nursing care delivery on one nursing unit. The leader uses Hersey and Blanchard's (1988) theory for diagnosing the maturity of the people in a system regarding their readiness to

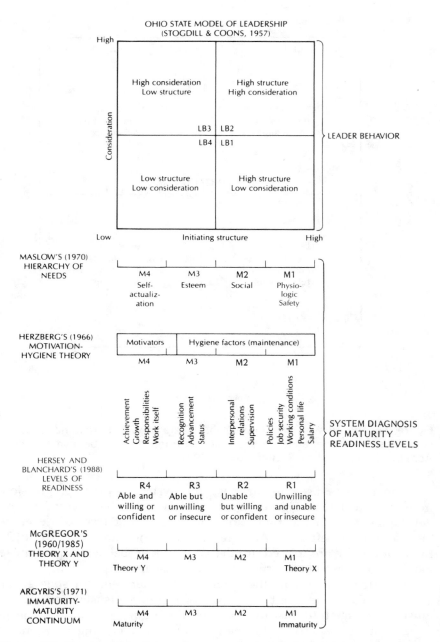

Figure 5.6 Theories for diagnosing a system and determining appropriate leader behavior. Adapted from Hershey & Blanchard, 1988.

accomplish a goal. Suppose the readiness level is designated as R1. The group, therefore, is predominantly unwilling or insecure and unable to carry out the task. The numbers in the theories to diagnose the system and the numbers in the leadership model should be paired. Therefore, R1 level of readiness corresponds directly to LB1. In order to accomplish the task, therefore, the leader's best bet is to begin goal accomplishment by behaving according to LB1, high structure and low consideration. This leader behavior style is the pivot on which alternate solutions and the ultimate recommended action are based. In the example given, task behavior from the leader becomes paramount at this point in time. The leader must develop a strategy that gives people knowledge about primary nursing and lets people know their responsibilities. In other words, the leader must take full responsibility for getting this task accomplished at this point in time.

The diagnosis and designation of a leader behavior style gives the leader a place to start—a place that, according to research, has the highest probability for success. Once a start has been made, the changing maturity of the system should be reflected in the leader's behavior, either moving forward one quadrant (growth) or backward one quadrant (regression). Recalling the example, if a leader started in LB1 and found that the group was becoming more receptive to primary nursing, then the leader should gradually change from LB1 to LB2, high structure and high consideration. In LB2, group interaction is started, but the leader still maintains control of task accomplishment. If a leader is in LB2 and finds that the group is regressing in maturity, that is, becoming less willing to carry responsibility for the task, then a leader would have to move back to LB1. The stepwise move from LB1 to LB4 represents a gradual decrease in leader control concerning how the group accomplishes the goal and a gradual increase in follower control concerning the process of goal accomplishment. The opposite stepwise move, LB4 to LB1, represents increased leader control and decreased follower control.

Determination of the appropriate leader behavior style is necessary before the leader develops solutions to a problem. Once in the leader behavior model, move forward one quadrant or backward one quadrant in response to the growth or the regression of the system in relation to accomplishing the task. The speed with which leader behavior movement occurs is variable, depending solely on the system. The goal of the leader is to move the system to requiring LB4, low structure and consideration. The right side of Figure 5.6 represents immaturity, and the left side represents maturity. When a system is mature, it can monitor itself and accomplish the task. The leader can then delegate to the system and be free to work toward getting another task accomplished. Delegation occurs only in LB4.

One simple example has been used to show how to bridge the system diagnosis with the leader behavior that should be used as the pivot for solutions to a problem. The steps in the example were:

1. *Determine the system diagnosis* using one or more theories, depending on preference and ease in application.

2. *Pair the maturity/readiness number with the same leader behavior number* to determine where leader behavior should begin.

3. *Move one leader behavior style forward or one leader behavior style backward* depending on the growth or regression of the system in relation to task accomplishment. The leader's goal is ultimately to have the system require LB4.

Now that the basics for determining the appropriate leader behavior style have been presented, examples from each theory or combination of theories will be discussed. A case study in Chapter 7 will amplify this discussion, and Urban City Hospital, an experiential exercise at the end of Part II, can be used for practice in applying the presented content.

It is most unlikely that a person or group can be diagnosed as mature using one theory and immature using another theory, given the same task. A leader makes a decision based on an individual's predominant need. If a nurse is predominantly motivated to achieve (Maslow's theory), then it is most unlikely that she or he would be able but unwilling (Hersey and Blanchard's theory), primarily concerned with working conditions (Herzberg's theory), or passive and dependent (Argyris's theory). The variety of theories that can be used to diagnose offer different aspects or descriptions of the same process—the development of a person from immaturity to maturity. For this reason they can all be applied toward the same purpose. Each theory should offer information that can be helpful in building a specific strategy for goal accomplishment that *motivates* and *educates* people to accomplish a goal.

Maslow's Hierarchy of Needs

Suppose that a new nurse with the title "coordinator" joins a home health care agency. After six months, the coordinator wishes to streamline the charting system, eradicating any routine nurses' notes. This need is based on feedback from the staff. The system is composed of the entire staff—ten registered nurses. After individually diagnosing each nurse on ability to accomplish the task, the modal level of maturity is at the esteem level on Maslow's (1970) hierarchy. Data suggest that the nurses are diligent, independent, motivated to achieve, and like to be noticed for quality and quantity of work done.

Esteem is M3; the corresponding leader behavior style is high consideration and low structure, LB3. Strategies for accomplishing the task, therefore, should focus on getting the group working together on the problem. The leader, for example, could convene the group, broadly state the issue based on comments received from the group, and facilitate the group's work in further specifying the problem and developing solutions.

Maslow's theory is predominantly used to diagnose motivational needs and is best used in combination with another diagnostic theory in order to diagnose educational needs.

Herzberg's Motivation-Hygiene Theory

An acute care hospital unit admits approximately three newly diagnosed clients with diabetes per week. No diabetic teaching program has been formalized. The manager has been on the unit two years; the unit has registered nurses, licensed practical nurses, and orderlies on staff. The goal, therefore, is to develop a diabetic teaching program. The system involves the registered nurses.

The manager assesses the system's ability to carry out the task and finds that members are often talking together about the idea, seem enthused about it, and have some knowledge about diabetic teaching; all want to be leaders in the process. Furthermore, they are pushing to plan the program over dinners and after working hours. The system can be diagnosed as M2, because the focus is on interpersonal relations and supervision. The leader should start behavior in LB2, high structure and high consideration, and be alert to the ability of the group to control how to accomplish the goal. If the leader believes that the group is able, then a gradual move into LB3 is appropriate, providing reinforcement for the group's work and some structure as needed. The manager could then function simply as a group member, letting the group establish its own informal leader and structure itself. The manager provides predominantly support and reinforcement in this quadrant.

Hersey and Blanchard's Levels of Readiness

Nursing care plans are not being done on clients and accreditation from the Joint Commission on Accreditation of Hospitals (JCAH) is six months away. Care plans are supposed to be written and updated by the team leaders on all shifts; the team leaders on the evening shift should take a nursing history on new clients and begin the process. The manager decides to start toward goal accomplishment with the three evening team leaders. The system is diagnosed as able but unwilling—R3. Rationale for this decision is that the team leaders have each worked on the unit a minimum of three years, they all have had formal education that taught the nursing process, and they have previously written excellent care plans.

High consideration and low structure, LB3, is the appropriate style to use for an R3 system diagnosis. Since the team leaders know what they are supposed to do, telling them in a high-structure style will probably only make them more defensive. It is necessary first to find out why they are unwilling to do the nursing care plans and then work from there. This involves two-way communication, which is high consideration. Once a manager knows why the team leaders are unwilling, solutions to these causes must be sought. Once the unwillingness is relieved, then the team leaders should be able and willing.

McGregor's Theory X and Theory Y

Suppose a director of in-service for nursing must set up an orientation program for six new baccalaureate graduate nurses who have just graduated and will take their boards in eight weeks. They were hired as staff nurses. The director must plan the program without having met the graduates.

What would be safe to assume about the maturity level of the graduates using cues from McGregor's Theory X and Theory Y? It would be helpful for the director to think back to how he or she felt in the situation. This is likely to be a high stress state promoting unsafe feelings and a need for direction—definitely on the Theory X side at an M1 level. The director should therefore be high in structure and low in consideration—LB1. A detailed plan of activities should provide knowledge of the environment, practical experience with supervision, and clear expectations of the graduates. The director should be warm and caring but be the guide and leader in satisfying the graduates' needs for structure. At the same time, the director must be acutely alert for signs of growth from the new graduates; when evident, a gradual move to LB2 is indicated.

Argyris's Immaturity—Maturity Continuum

The director of nursing needs three nurses from the intensive care unit to revise the emergency resuscitation plan for the hospital. The head nurse of the unit posts a notice on the desk asking each shift to nominate a fulltime nurse who would be willing to serve.

The head nurse's behavior is low structure and low consideration—LB4. This choice was based on the following data about the nurses: they (a) are all equal in ability, (b) have worked on the unit a minimum of three years, (c) are flexible and effectively meet the demands of a situation, (d) are all able to assume the role of charge nurse, and (e) are insightful. Given these data, the director can assume the nurses are at a mature point on Argyris's continuum—M4.

DISCUSSION OF APPLIED
LEADER BEHAVIOR THEORIES

The initial determination for the appropriate leader behavior style is the leader's best bet at the start of goal accomplishment (Fiedler, 1987; Hammer & Turk, 1987; Vecchio, 1987; Zenger, 1985). It has the highest probability for motivating people to accomplish the task. How one operates within the style, given that it can be interpreted broadly, depends on the particular needs of the group that were identified during the diagnosis. These particulars are then used in the alternate solutions and recommended action. The umbrella leader behavior style remains constant unless the system matures or regresses. Then movement is only one quadrant forward or backward—in systematic, gradual stepwise progression or regression.

A leader never jumps from LB1 to LB3, for example. Why? Because the leader behavior model is designed from learning theory, which says that reinforcing behavior increases the probability that the behavior will continue. Because the task is the most important concern for the leader, it is primary in LB1. It is reinforced in LB2 but consideration for the individual employee/group becomes equal in importance. If the task is not getting accomplished, the manager must move back to LB1. Should LB1 be successful, reinforcement of the task behavior would not occur if one jumped to LB3. Another example would be an employee to whom you have always delegated responsibilities (LB4). Noticing that quality in outcome is slipping, the manager should move to LB3 and use high consideration in order to discover why quality is slipping. Jumping back to any other style would be inappropriate at this time because the leader is aware that the employee knows what to do; high structure therefore would not be the leader's best bet unless LB3 failed to work and minimum quality standards were in jeopardy. Then the leader would need to become firmer and more structured, gradually moving back to LB2 and then to LB1.

The leader is advised that if any serious doubt exists concerning the system's readiness/maturity, then it is better to hold on to control until data are observed suggesting that followers are mature enough to carry effectively the responsibility that comes with control. A manager's move from LB2 to LB3, for example, is usually interpreted as a positive, rewarding change. Should a manager relinquish control too quickly and then have to take it back, such as a quick move from LB3 to LB2, this is often interpreted as punishment or leader dishonesty. Both interpretations are negative forces that may make goal accomplishment difficult because of the defensiveness that they engender in participants.

Another issue that is often raised concerns feelings that leader behavior must be consistent. Leader behavior responds to the context and system of resources; leader behavior, therefore, changes as indicated from diagnoses. Experience has shown that employees respond negatively to changes in a leader's affect and tone but not to caring and respectful changes in how one carries out leader responsibilities. By using a situational approach, a manager essentially is giving employees what they need. Moodiness, however, is not what employees need—so self-diagnose before you act.

A leader behavior application that is worthy of understanding is Ouchi's (1981a, 1981b) Theory Z. This is a term that represents management behavior in successful Japanese organizations. Smith, Reinow, and Reid (1984) contrasted typical Theory Z Japanese management practices with those routinely used in the United States. Japanese concepts involve permanent employment, few evaluations and promotions, nonspecialized career options, implicit managerial control, collective decision making (quality circles), work group responsibilities, and holistic concern for employees. Management practices in the United States seem dissimilar. For example, the emphasis in the United States is on specialization, accelerated evaluation and promotion, explicit organization control, individual accountability, and delegation of authority to individuals.

While much has been written applying Theory Z practices in the United States, it is not considered to be the answer in all managerial problems, even though some adaptations may be beneficial (Adair & Nygard, 1982; Smith, Reinow, & Reid, 1984; Younger, 1983). Theory Z practices predominantly incorporate democratic approaches to leadership—leader behavior styles 2 and 3—high relationships/ consideration and high task/structure. Use of only these two styles assumes that followers are all at moderate levels of maturity/readiness and that followers should be kept at that level of maturity/readiness. This author does not believe that those assumptions about followers hold in the United States; however, they obviously must be appropriate in Eastern cultures. Techniques that are used from Theory Z should therefore be carefully evaluated so that leader behavior matches the needs of the majority of followers.

LEADER EFFECTIVENESS

A leader's behavior or influence over an individual or group can be either successful or unsuccessful. If the desired goal is reached (approximately or exactly), then the specific leader behavior used by the manager can be called successful. Conversely, if the desired goal is not reached within an acceptable range, then the leader behavior can be called unsuccessful (Hersey & Blanchard, 1988). When leader behavior fails to influence an individual or a group to achieve a specified goal, then the manager must evaluate what occurred using the steps of the management process and redesign the strategy for goal accomplishment.

When leader behavior is successful, success can range from very ineffective to very effective depending on how followers feel about the leader's behavior (Hersey & Blanchard, 1988). For example, if the leader used personal power to influence followers, thereby making goal accomplishment a personally rewarding experience for the followers, then the leader's behavior is both successful (the goal was accomplished) and very effective (the followers feel terrific about accomplishing).

On the other hand, followers can be coerced to accomplish by a manager who uses position power, close supervision, and the use of rewards and punishments. Even though the leader's behavior was successful, the leaders behavior is also very ineffective if the followers were unhappy and carrying negative feelings toward the leader. Generally, when leader behavior is successful and effective, the followers are self-motivated to accomplish the goal even when the manager is not present. When leader behavior is successful and ineffective, followers often relax the drive to accomplish when the manager is absent (Hersey & Blanchard, 1988).

ORGANIZATIONAL EFFECTIVENESS

The effectiveness of a leader's behavior should be determined on the basis of its relationship to the growth of an organization during a specified period of time (Hersey & Blanchard, 1988). Likert (1967) identified three sets of variables: causal variables, intervening variables, and output variables. Hersey and Blanchard (1988) also looked at short-term and long-term goals. Organizational effectiveness should be a result of evaluating all four sets of variables in order to decrease the halo-horn effect, which was discussed in Chapter 3. Even though subjectivity is an element in any evaluation, looking at separate variables usually decreases the amount of subjectivity that will bias the incident. The following variables are used to evaluate the effectiveness of the organization over time.

Causal Variables

Causal variables have influence on the developments within an organization, including results or accomplishments (Hersey & Blanchard, 1988). These variables are under management control; they can be changed or altered.

Causal variables refer to the following:

1. Appropriateness of leader behavior to the system's level of maturity;
2. Accuracy of the system's diagnosis;
3. Appropriate involvement of the system in decision making;
4. Effectiveness of the organization's philosophy and objectives in guiding its constituents; and
5. Use of available technology in a particular organization.

Intervening Variables

Intervening variables refer to the resources (people) within an organization. Likert (1961) asserted that they represent the internal state of the organization. Intervening variables refer to employees' commitment, motivation, morale, and skills in leadership, communication, and conflict resolution (Hersey & Blanchard, 1988).

Output Variables

Output variables represent the achievements of the organization. Output variables are quantifiable and include production (output or services), costs, earnings, turnover, management-union relations, and so forth.

Long-Term Goals and Short-Term Goals

This aspect involves long-term and short-term planning. Long-term goals refer to the future development of the organization. A short-term perspective refers to immediate output (Hersey & Blanchard, 1988). An effective management team in an organization must balance both.

SUMMARY

Leadership has many definitions, all of which converge on several points. Leadership involves using communication processes to influence the activities of an individual or of a group toward the attainment of a goal in a unique situation. Democratic, autocratic, and laissez-faire are common labels for leader behavior styles. Even though democracy is often connoted as a best style, each style is appropriate, depending on the unique situation.

Management theorists have designated two major components of leader behavior: one refers to getting the task accomplished and the other is concerned with interpersonal behavior. Theorists have different labels for these components. The Ohio State model of leadership has structure and consideration as its components. Structure refers to a leader's attempt to organize and define the roles and activities of group members. Consideration involves two-way communication—establishing trust, openness, respect, warmth, and effective interpersonal relationships between and among group members.

Several leadership models were presented, discussed, and compared. All of the models are appropriate to apply in nursing systems. The Ohio State model was applied in this chapter. The appropriate leader behavior style for a given system is determined by diagnosing the system's level of maturity readiness and then pairing the maturity/readiness level with the parallel leader behavior. This results in a place for the leader to start and represents the pivot upon which solutions for solving the problem are based. A leader then changes from one style to another, depending upon the growth or regression of the system. The ultimate goal of the leader should be to facilitate (1) getting the tasks accomplished and (2) moving the group members to the highest level of maturity and then delegating to them.

Leader behavior can move on a range from successful or unsuccessful. If successful it can further range from very ineffective to very effective. The effectiveness of an organization over time should be evaluated on the stimuli (causal variables) that act upon an organism (intervening variables) to create responses (output) (Hersey & Blanchard, 1988). Long-term goals and short-term goals must also be considered.

REFERENCES

Adair, M., & Nygard, N. (1982). Theory Z management: Can it work for nursing? *Nursing & Health Care, 4,* 489–491.

Allport, F. (1924). *Social Psychology.* Boston: Houghton Mifflin.

Argyris, C. (1971). *Management and organizational development: The path from XA to YB.* New York: McGraw-Hill.

Bennis, W. (1959). Leadership theory and administrative behavior: The problems of authority. *Administrative Science Quarterly, 4,* 259–301.

Bingham, W. (1927). In H.C. Metcalf. *The psychological foundations of management.* New York: Shaw.

Bingham, W. (1973). In H.C. Metcalf. *The psychological foundations of management.* Easton, PA: Hive. (Original work published 1965)

Blake, R., & Mouton, J. (1964). *The Managerial Grid.* Houston, TX: Gulf Publishing.

Blake, R., & Mouton, J. (1978). *The new Managerial Grid.* Houston, TX: Gulf Publishing.

Blake, R., & Mouton, J. (1981). Management by Grid principles or situationalism: Which? *Group and Organization Studies, 6,* 439–455.

Blake, R., & Mouton, J. (1984). *The Managerial Grid III* (3rd ed.). Houston, TX: Gulf Publishing.

Blake, R., Mouton, J., & Tapper, M. (1981). *Grid approaches for managerial leadership in nursing.* St. Louis: Mosby.

Cattell, R. (1951). New concepts for measuring leadership in terms of group syntality. *Human Relations, 4,* 161–184.

Cooley, C. (1902). *Human nature and social order.* New York: Scribner.

Fiedler, F. (1967). *A theory of leadership effectiveness.* New York: McGraw-Hill.

Fiedler, F. (1987). When to lead, when to stand back. *Psychology Today, 21*(9), 26–27.

Fleishman, E. (1973). Twenty years of consideration and structure. In E. Fleishman, & J. G. Hunt (Eds.). *Current developments in the study of leadership.* Carbondale: Southern Illinois University Press.

Hammer, T., & Turk, J. (1987). Organizational determinants of leader behavior and authority. *Journal of Applied Psychology, 72*(4), 674–682.

Hersey, P., & Blanchard, K. (1988). *Management of organizational behavior: Utilizing human resources* (5th ed.). Englewood Cliffs, NJ: Prentice-Hall.

Herzberg, F. (1966). *Work and the nature of man.* Cleveland: World Publishing.

Homans, G. (1950). *The human group.* New York: Harcourt Brace Jovanovich.

Kerr, S., & Schriesheim, C. (1974). Consideration, initiating structure, and organizational criteria—an update of Korman's 1966 review. *Personnel Psychology, 27,* 555–568.

Kilbourne, C. (1935). The elements of leadership. *Journal of Coast Artillery, 78,* 437–439.

Knickerbocker, I. (1948). Leadership: A conception and some implications. *Journal of Social Issues, 4,* 23–40.

Koontz, H., & O'Donnell, C. (1986). *Essentials of management* (4th ed.). New York: McGraw-Hill.

Likert, R. (1961). *New patterns of management.* New York: McGraw-Hill.

Likert, R. (1967). *The human organization.* New York: McGraw-Hill.

McGregor, D. (1960). *The human side of enterprise.* New York: McGraw-Hill.

McGregor, D. (1985). *The human side of enterprise: 25th anniversary printing.* New York: McGraw-Hill. (Original work published 1960)

Maslow, A. (1970). *Motivation and personality* (2nd ed.). New York: Harper & Row.

Merton, R. (1969). The social nature of leadership. *American Journal of Nursing, 69,* 2614–2618.

Ouchi, W. (1981a). *Theory Z.* Reading, MA: Addison-Wesley.

Ouchi, W. (1981b). Organizational paradigms: A commentary on Japanese management and Theory Z organizations. *Organizational Dynamics, 9,* 36–43.

Shartle, C. (1951). Leader behavior in jobs. *Occupations, 30,* 164–166.

Sherif, M., & Sherif, C. (1956). *An outline of social psychology.* New York: Harper & Row.

Smith, H., Reinow, F., & Reid, R. (1984). Japanese management: Implications for nursing administration. *Journal of Nursing Administration, 14*(9), 33–39.

Stogdill, R. (1974). *Handbook of leadership.* New York: Free Press.

Stogdill, R., & Coons, A. (Eds.). (1957). *Leader behavior: Its description and measurement* (Research Monograph No. 88). Columbus: Bureau of Business Research, Ohio State University.

Tannenbaum, R., & Schmidt, W. (1958). How to choose a leadership pattern. *Harvard Business Review, 37,* 95–102.

Tannenbaum, R., Weschler, I., & Massarik, F. (1961). *Leadership and organization: A behavioral science approach.* New York: McGraw-Hill.

Urwick, L. (1953). *Leadership and morale.* Columbus: College of Commerce and Administration, Ohio State University.

Vecchio, R. (1987). Situational leadership theory: An examination of a prescriptive theory. *Journal of Applied Psychology, 72*(3), 444–451.

Younger, J. (1983). Theory Z management and health care organizations. *Nursing Economics, 1,* 40–45, 69.

Zenger, J. (1985). Leadership: Management's better half. *Training, 22*(12), 44–53.

CHAPTER 6

Diagnosing the Task

THE VROOM AND YETTON MANAGERIAL
  DECISION-MAKING MODEL
APPLICATION OF THE DECISION MODEL
DISCUSSION OF THE MODEL
SUMMARY

Part II of this book is devoted to identifying the appropriate leader behavior for motivating people in a system to accomplish a goal. This process involves diagnosing the environment—self, system, and task—and applying leader behavior theory.

Diagnosing self, presented in Chapter 3, is necessary in identifying the leader's personal point of view on the problem/ goal and on the environment. Further, diagnosing one's personal leader behavior style is helpful in order to approximate more closely behavioral intent with others' perceptions of behaviors. Diagnosing self is a consciousness-raising experience with an intent of reducing leader bias.

Chapter 4 contained a discussion of theories that can be used to diagnose a system. Once a diagnosis is made, leader behavior theory is applied in order to determine the leader behavior style that has the highest probability for motivating people to accomplish a task. This leader behavior style is the umbrella or pivot upon which problem solutions are based.

Diagnosing the task is the last segment of leader responsibilities and completes the equation that forms the basis for this part of the book:

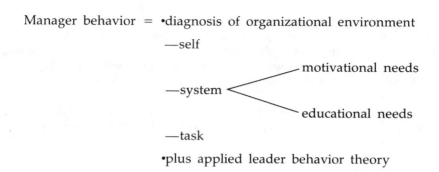

Manager behavior = •diagnosis of organizational environment

—self

—system — motivational needs

— educational needs

—task

•plus applied leader behavior theory

THE VROOM AND YETTON MANAGERIAL DECISION-MAKING MODEL

The conceptual framework for diagnosing the task is the Vroom and Yetton managerial decision-making model (Vroom, 1973; Vroom & Jago, 1974, 1978, 1988; Vroom & Yetton, 1973). This decision-making model is another theory destroying the myth that managers who use democratic styles are "good" and those who do not are "bad." The decision process used by the manager in a situation should depend on the nature of the unique situation. The model, therefore, provides a means to diagnose situations (tasks) in determining the most appropriate problem-solving technique for the manager to use in getting something accomplished. While diagnosing the nature of the task should be only one of three determinants of leader behavior, the Vroom and Yetton decision-making model is a powerful one that reports validity for its purpose (Field, 1982; Vroom & Jago, 1978).

A general guide for diagnosing the task can be depicted by the following equation (La Monica & Finch, 1977):

Effective decisions =
function of (quality + acceptance + time)

Quality refers to whether there are a number of possible solutions to the problem and some alternatives could result in better outcomes than others—a qualitative judgment on the best solution must be made. *Acceptance* is concerned with whether staff members must accept the problem's solution in order for the problem to be eliminated—must the staff do anything? *Time* relates to how much time is available to work on the problem. The Vroom and Yetton managerial decision-making model integrates answers to these three variables and suggests a decision-making style that has the highest probability for effectiveness. These results will be combined with other diagnoses from previous chapters in determining leader behavior.

Table 6.1 contains five different managerial decision styles. Read each and then study the case in Box 6.1. Select the decision-making

TABLE 6.1 Management Decision Styles

Type	Description
AI	You solve the problem or make the decision yourself, using information available to you at that time.
AII	You obtain the necessary information from your subordinates(s), then decide on the solution to the problem yourself. You may or may not tell your subordinates what the problem is in getting the information from them. The role played by your subordinates in making the decision is clearly one of providing the necessary information to you, rather than generating or evaluating alternative solutions.
CI	You share the problem with relevant subordinates individually, getting their ideas and suggestions without bringing them together as a group. Then you make the decision that may or may not reflect your subordinates' influence.
CII	You share the problem with your subordinates as a group, collectively obtaining their ideas and suggestions. Then you make the decision that may or may not reflect your subordinates' influence.
GII	You share a problem with your subordinates as a group. Together you generate and evaluate alternatives and attempt to reach agreement (consensus) on a solution. Your role is much like that of chairman. You do not try to influence the group to adopt "your" solution, and you are willing to accept and implement any solution that has the support of the entire group.
DI	You delegate the problem to your subordinate(s), providing him [them] with any relevant information that you possess, but giving him [them] responsibility for solving the problem . . . you may or may not request him [the group] to tell you what solution . . . [has been] reached.

Source: AI-GII—Reprinted by permission of the publisher, from "A New Look at Managerial Decision Making," by Victor H. Vroom, *Organizational Dynamics*, Spring, 1973, © 1973. American Management Association, New York. All rights reserved.

DI—Vroom, V., Yetton, P., 1973. *Leadership and Decision Making*, p. 13.

BOX 6.1 Case Example

You are an assistant director of nursing in a large city hospital. The management has recently put into effect, at your request and consultation, the unit manager system on two floors. This was expected to relieve the nurses of administrative responsibility, increase their abilities to provide quality care to clients, ensure that health assessments and care plans could be accomplished for every client, and lower the nursing budget. Quality health care and nursing care plans reflected the suggestions made by the hospital accreditors. To the surprise of everyone, yourself included, little of the above has been realized. In fact, nurses are sitting in the conference room more, quality has maintained a status quo, and employees and patients are complaining more than ever.

You do not believe that there is anything wrong with the new system. You have had reports from other hospitals using it and they confirm this opinion. You have also had representatives from institutions using the system talk with your nursing personnel, and the representatives report that your nurses have full knowledge of the system and their altered responsibilities.

You suspect that a few people may be responsible for the situation, but this view is not widely shared among your two supervisors and four head nurses. The failure has been variously attributed to poor training of the unit managers, lack of financial incentives, and poor morale. Clearly, this is an issue about which there is considerable depth of feeling within individuals and potential disagreement among your subordinates.

This morning you received a phone call from the nursing director. She had just talked with the hospital administrator and was calling to express her deep concern. She indicated that the problem was yours to solve in any way you think best, but she would like to know within a week what steps you plan to take.

You share your director's concern and know that the personnel involved are equally concerned. The problem is to decide what steps to take to rectify the situation.

Decision style you would use: _____

Source: La Monica, E., & Finch, F. (1977). Managerial decision-making. *Journal of Nursing Administration 5*, 21. Reproduced by permission. This case was adapted into nursing from a business example. The original material is presented by Vroom, 1973, pp. 72–73.

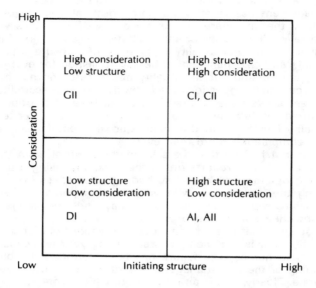

Figure 6.1 Vroom and Yetton's decision styles and the Ohio State model of leadership.

style that you would use if you were the manager in the case. Write your response in the space provided after the case.

As you have probably noted, the five managerial decision styles can be considered as a continuum. AI and AII are autocratic styles, CI and CII are consultative styles, and GII is a group decision-making style. Delegation (DI) has been discussed by Vroom and Yetton (1973) and Vroom and Jago (1988) as one in a two-person superior/follower relationship; delegation is at the opposite end of the continuum from AI. These decision styles can be paralleled with the Ohio State model of leadership, as shown in Figure 6.1. As a manager moves from AI to GII, the amount of time involved in solving the problem increases.

APPLICATION OF THE DECISION MODEL

Now that a decision-making style has been chosen for the case example, the Vroom and Yetton (1973) model should be applied in diagnosing the task. Vroom (1973) developed the decision model using a tree format; it is commonly referred to as the decision-making tree, shown in Figure 6.2.

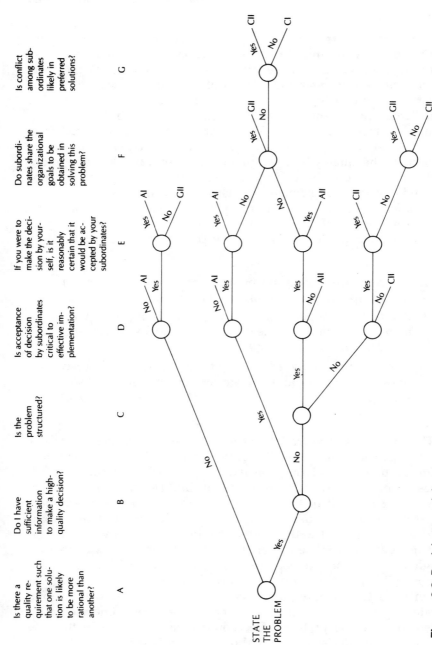

Figure 6.2 Decision model.

Source: Reprinted by permission of the publisher, from "A New Look at Managerial Decision Making," by Victor H. Vroom, *Organizational Dynamics*, Spring, 1973, © 1973. American Management Associations, New York. All rights reserved.

Notice that there are seven questions across the top of Figure 6.2. Questions A, B, and C refer to the variable of quality and questions D through G refer to the variable of acceptance. Referring to a case, it is necessary to start at the left of the model, question A, and answer the question in a yes-no format. If the answer to question A is "no," then follow the "no" line to the next node and answer the question on top of the node. Follow this format until the tree ends with a decision-making style. It should be noted that each successive question in the quality and acceptance sets of variables asks more specific information concerning the variable—it is similar to programmed history taking when an answer of "history of familial diabetes," for example, results in more specific questions concerning this matter being asked.

The decision model is conceptually saying the following:

1. If acceptance of decision by followers is crucial, then get the group involved in solving the problem.
2. If quality is important, with expertise being a requirement, then find people who have the expertise and solve the problem.
3. When both quality and acceptance are required, then bring the experts and the group together for problem solving.

The purpose of the tree, however, is to integrate these variables and to suggest a decision-making style that will take the shortest amount of time, considering the requirements of the task. Time increases as one moves down from AI to GII. Hence, if style CII is suggested at the end of the tree, quality and acceptance are important so one could not use styles AI, AII, or CI because the group would not be involved to the degree required in these styles. But one could use GII or DI if the leader thought that the group was mature enough to solve the problem using those styles *and* had the time available. The problem would be solved more quickly in style CII than in style GII. Simply, any decision-making style under the one indicated by the decision model is fine to use; more time would be needed to solve the problem. Decision-making styles above the one indicated by the decision model should not be used.

Let us walk through the case example using the decision model to see if Vroom agrees with your choice for the best style to use given the nature of the task. Start at the left and answer question A.

Question A: Quality—Yes
There is quality requirement in this case. A number of possible solutions to the problem exist, and one could be better than another; there are several ways to solve this problem, and one way could result in more effective outcomes than another.

Follow the "yes" line on the tree to the next node; question B must be answered.

Question B: Manager's information—No
The assistant director obviously has neither the information nor the expertise to make a high-quality decision and solve the problem.

Follow the "no" line to the next node and answer a further question on quality.

Question C: Structure—No
This question requires explanation. A structured problem is one in which the decision is based on quantitative (objective) data, and the location of those data is known. An unstructured problem has a subjective element; the decision is a qualitative assessment—a value judgment—and/or the location of the information is unknown. In the case example, information that is required for solving the problem is qualitative and its specific location is unknown.

Follow the "no" line to the next node and answer question D.

Question D: Acceptance—Yes
Another way of asking question D is: Do followers have to do anything in order for the problem to be solved? In this case, acceptance is critical. In fact, one reason the system is failing may be that personnel were not involved in the initial planning.

Follow the "yes" line to question E.

Question E: Prior probability of acceptance—No
An autocratic decision in this case probably would not be tolerated.

Follow the "no" line to question F.

Question F: Goal congruence—Yes
Another way of asking this question is: If the problem is solved, will it benefit the people working in the environment? Obviously, the people will benefit in this case if the unit manager system works.

The resulting style that is suggested by the model is GII. Bring the two supervisors together with the four head nurses and proceed in solving the problem as a group.

Does the style you chose match Vroom's choice? If so, your intuition was on target. Now you can up your batting average continuously by using the theory. If no match existed, it would be advisable to follow Vroom's suggestion over your own. Vroom and Jago (1978) reported on an experimental study suggesting that managers who apply the decision model have significantly more effective outcomes—more technical quality and more follower acceptance—than managers who do not use the model.

DISCUSSION OF THE MODEL

The decision model just discussed is used to diagnose the task; this is just one part of the environmental diagnosis. Diagnosis of the system and self-diagnosis must be considered in determining leader behavior.

Suppose that the system diagnosis in the case example resulted in followers being assessed at the M1 level of maturity, thereby requiring high structure and low consideration leader behavior. The diagnosis of the task in the case suggested that group decision making is indicated—high consideration and low structure (see Figure 6.1). What should the manager do?

The best course for the leader is to bid for more time by presenting evidence to the superior that the nature of the task demands that the group become involved in solving this problem in order to have the best probability for an effective outcome. Further, the group is not mature enough to handle a group problem-solving activity. More time is needed to help the group mature to the level required for solving the problem. The manager's best bet, therefore, is to try to get the task tabled until the group is mature enough to handle it—get more time.

The manager should try, to the degree possible, to match the decision-making style required by the task with the leader behavior suggested by the group maturity level—this is ideal. It is also a way to determine the problems/goals that should be the focus of group work at a given point in time. Tasks should be given to groups according to the group's ability to accomplish them effectively. Decision styles (AI through DI) can be used by the manager to help followers progressively mature in group problem solving. Decision styles are a ladder to maturity in this area.

If the superior of the manager says "the task must be done even though the group is not ready to handle it," even though a case against this has been made repeatedly and with strength, then the manager must act. Given that the situation is far from ideal, every effort must be taken to ensure the highest probability for success. The group must be involved even though the experts must maintain control of the group's process because quality and acceptance are both critical. The manager's best bet in this instance is to move into a leader behavior style that falls between what the system requires and what the task requires—high structure and high consideration—CI or CII.

It must be noted that group decision making in the case example, indicated as best by the decision model, means that the manager presents the problem for the group members to solve. The problem is to determine how to make the unit manager system work effectively, producing the anticipated outcomes. The problem must be presented with clarity. Group members should not be given the opportunity to say that they do not want the system. The system exists, and now it must be made effective. This principle applies in all group decision-making processes.

Foresight in management is always better than hindsight. The manager should always try to prevent the situation just discussed by a complete and accurate diagnosis of essential elements in the environment. However, when prevention has not worked (and prevention does not always work), then the manager must do the best possible in the given situation.

Self-diagnosis must also be matched because a manager who is most easily suited to the requirements of the system and task will have the smoothest journey through solving the problem. Should the leader's personal style not match, two alternatives are possible, given that the task must be accomplished by the system: (1) delegate leadership for solving the problem to an assistant whose personal leadership style matches the requirements or (2) provide the leader behavior style that is required by the system and task by being conscious that one's behavior must follow the style needed. In the second alternative, the manager must be diligent in thinking about the leader behavior that must be provided for the system because one's personal inclination may be different from the desired behavior.

SUMMARY

The task is the third aspect of the environment that must be diagnosed in order to determine leader behavior. Vroom and Yetton's (1973) managerial decision-making model was discussed for this purpose. The variables of quality, acceptance, and time are considered important in specifying the task's requirements. A decision model (tree) can be used to integrate elements of quality and acceptance for a given situation and to suggest a decision style that requires the least amount of time and has the highest probability for effective outcome. One case was followed and discussed applying the decision model. The experiential exercises in this part of the book contain three additional cases for practice using the model. The manager should try to match the decision-making style required by the task with the leader behavior suggested by the system's maturity level. The manager can use the model to decide on task priorities for a given group.

The next chapter contains a case application of the management process and problem-solving method.

REFERENCES

Field, R. H. G. (1982). A test of the Vroom-Yetton normative model of leadership. *Journal of Applied Psychology, 67*(5), 523–532.

La Monica, E., & Finch, F. (1977). Managerial decision-making. *Journal of Nursing Administration, 7,* 20–28.

Vroom, V. (1973). A new look at managerial decision-making. *Organizational Dynamics, 1,* 66–80.

Vroom, V., & Jago, A. (1974). Decision-making as a social process. *Decision Sciences, 5,* 743–769.

Vroom, V., & Jago, A. (1978). On the validity of the Vroom-Yetton model. *Journal of Applied Psychology, 63,* 151–162.

Vroom, V., & Jago, A. (1988). *The new leadership: Managing participation in organizations.* Englewood Cliffs, NJ: Prentice-Hall.

Vroom, V., & Yetton, P. (1973). *Leadership and decision-making.* Pittsburgh: University of Pittsburgh Press.

CHAPTER 7

Applying the Management Process and the Problem-Solving Method

PROBLEM IDENTIFICATION
PROBLEM DEFINITION
PROBLEM ANALYSIS
  Diagnosing Self
  Diagnosing the System
  Diagnosing the Task
  Synthesizing the Diagnosis
ALTERNATIVE ACTIONS
RECOMMENDED ACTION
IMPLEMENTATION AND EVALUATION
THE MANAGEMENT PROCESS
SUMMARY

This chapter provides an application of the theory that has been presented in Chapters 1 through 6. A case example is studied by following the steps of the problem-solving method, each of which has been discussed in separate chapters. As a review, this problem-solving method involves:

1. Problem identification
2. Problem definition and/or goal statement
3. Problem analysis
4. Alternative solutions
5. Recommended action
6. Implementation and evaluation

The management process—which is comprised of planning, organizing, motivating, and controlling—will then be interrelated in response to the manager's activities in the case example.

Box 7.1 contains a description of the case that forms the basis for this chapter. Assume the role of the leader/manager in this environment, reviewing the data presented in Box 7.1 in order to carry out the problem-solving method.

BOX 7.1 Case Example

You are the head nurse of a 54-bed orthopedic unit in a 400-bed general hospital located in a northeastern capital city. You have held the position for five years and work the day shift. During the ski season, which lasts from December to April, the unit maintains a full capacity and often overflows with clients who are set up in the halls and in the solarium.

Clients are generally healthy, robust people who are forced into dependency by various incapacitating fractures, most frequently the broken tibia and/or fibula. Clients fall into two categories: those who require a short hospital stay (one to two days) and those who need a long stay (two to four weeks) due to the severity of the injuries.

The organization is old and traditional, sporting an excellent reputation for the quality of its services. There is a bureaucratic hierarchy of control in nursing, with power and authority belonging to the position rather than to the incumbent—there is a right way of doing things and a wrong way of doing things. The director of nursing generally makes the decisions regarding policy and passes the information down.

Team nursing is the model of nursing care delivery that is practiced. Nurses have made team nursing into a packaged procedure, dividing the labors of the team, using flow charts, setting up informal routines for getting the work done, and compartmentalizing all team responsibilities. Nursing histories and care plans have been made up so that they can be applied to all clients; nurses simply check what applies to the particular client. Giving medications to all clients on the unit is the responsibility of one registered nurse on each shift. Since the task is perceived as boring, it is rotated on a weekly schedule.

The quality of nursing care is considered good at the present time. Each team has 18 clients, and there is usually one registered nurse, one licensed practical nurse or nurse's aide, and one orderly assigned to each team during the day shift. The staff has been fairly stable over the past year.

You meet with the staff every morning and afternoon for report and again for team conference when time permits. If there are problems, the team leaders come to you for assistance and vice versa. Otherwise you generally leave the team leaders alone. You try to make rounds every day but that is not always possible because managerial responsibilities have been increasing since the nursing organization was decentralized.

For the past several weeks, you have noticed increasing tardiness at morning report. Then, staff seemed to be concerned with the functions of their position rather than the gestalt. You believe that nursing care is not as individualized as it could be. Staff members are spending more and more time talking and complaining with each other in the conference room, reporting that their "work is finished." You check on this and they are right—the work they set out to do is done, and the clients seem happy.

Source: Selected aspects of this case were originally prepared by Anita R. Madea, Doctoral Candidate, Teachers College, Columbia University, Department of Nursing Education, 1981.

PROBLEM IDENTIFICATION

A problem is identified by the difference between what is actually happening in a situation (the actual) and what one would like to have occur (the optimal). The manager should first write down the problem areas. These are then narrowed down to one or two areas and defined succinctly, as shown in Table 7.1.

After thinking about these problem areas, it is necessary to focus on a particular problem. Several questions must be answered: (1) Are the problem areas related to one another? (2) Are any of the problem areas an effect of another problem? (3) Which problem is tractable and can be solved directly?

In looking at the three problem areas just delineated, it is possible that as nursing care is systematized, it is becoming repetitive, boring, and monotonous. Staff members may not have the opportu-

TABLE 7.1 Problem Identification

Actual	Problem	Optimal
1. Tardiness is increasing	Tardiness	1. No tardiness
2. Nursing care is becoming increasingly routine	Routine nursing care	2. Nursing care is becoming increasingly individualized
3. Nursing time spent with the client is decreasing	Decreased time spent with clients	3. Nursing time spent with the client is increasing

nity to develop new skills and capacities, and work is getting done quickly. Innovation and creativity are suppressed as nursing care becomes procedure-bound.

The three problem areas are seen as related. Since nursing care is becoming a tight routine, it gets done fast, leaving the staff with excess time. This may contribute to a lack of enthusiasm, accentuated by the paucity of creativity, that is present in nursing care planning. The head nurse must now use the knowledge available and make a decision on the problem.

PROBLEM DEFINITION

The priority problem area of those stated in the previous portion of this chapter is that nursing care was becoming increasingly routine. The goal should be for nursing care to become more individualized. This problem area includes many aspects of nursing care. Since problem statements should be specific, what aspect of nursing care requires the first emphasis? Suppose the head nurse decides that the client should become involved in developing the care plan, using the established core care plans as baseline information and cues to nursing responsibilities in caring for clients with orthopedic problems. The problem and goal might sound like the following:

> *Actual:* The client has no input into the nursing care plan, which is routine for all clients with orthopedic problems.
>
> *Optimal:* The client and the team leader develop an individualized nursing care plan using the routine care plan as minimal expectations.
>
> *Problem:* Routine nursing care plans are not individualized; clients do not plan with the team leaders.
>
> *Goal:* To individualize nursing care plans by having the team leader and the client build on the routine care plan.

PROBLEM ANALYSIS

In problem analysis, the environment must be diagnosed in order to choose a leader behavior style that has the highest probability for success in motivating the system to accomplish the task. It is the pivot upon which all solutions are based. In order to diagnose the environment, the system must first be specified.

In the case example, the head nurse decides to work with the three day shift team leaders since they are mainly responsible for taking nursing histories and personalizing the routine care plan. The two regular staff nurses who cover the team leaders on days off are also considered part of the system. Nothing will be added to the normal material resources in solving the problem. In essence, the system consists of three team leaders and two staff nurses who act as team leaders when necessary. The environment can be diagnosed as follows.

Diagnosing Self

The manager sits back and considers why this problem has been specified—routine nursing care has always been considered boring and dull. As a client several years ago, the manager had found routine care dehumanizing and ritualistic—in other words noncaring, which is the antithesis of nursing practice.

Thinking more, the manager realizes that the staff has generally been left alone concerning their task responsibilities; support was offered often and the presence of a manager was constant. This style of leadership seemed easy and was most enjoyable and rewarding.

Diagnosing the System

The manager decides to use the following two theories to diagnose the system: (1) Maslow's hierarchy of needs to diagnose motivational needs and (2) Hersey and Blanchard's (1988) levels of readiness to diagnose educational needs. Staff members are diagnosed individually regarding their ability and willingness to fulfill the goal and/or to solve the problem. Remember that Hersey and Blanchard's theory requires a "yes" or "no" response—if not totally "yes," then the answer is "no."

> Team leader 1 is a bright, energetic Associate Degree graduate with four years experience on this unit who has learned the position's responsibilities quickly but lacks ability to solve problems scientifically. The person has procedures for everything.
> *Diagnosis:*   M2—Social
>   R2—Unable but willing or confident
>
> Team leader 2 is a baccalaureate graduate who has been on the unit in this position for seven years. Responsibility for establishing a routine history form rested predominantly with this team leader, who always enjoys starting new things once a cue has

been given. Planning nursing care with the client, however, has never been part of nursing practice. This nurse spends the most time sharing information about clients with associates.

Diagnosis: M2—Social
                R2—Unable but willing or confident

Team leader 3 is a graduate of this hospital's School of Nursing and adores team nursing. The nurse is flexible and goes along with all new ideas, giving much of self to accomplishing new projects especially if she is working with friends. This nurse has had little experience since graduation.

Diagnosis: M2—Social
                R2—Unable but willing or confident

Staff nurse 1 is a baccalaureate graduate who has a wide knowledge base but seems bitter. The nurse always carries out and individualizes responsibilities with pride and makes thoughtful comments in reports about clients, yet often resists group efforts toward change.

Diagnosis: M3—Self-Esteem
                R3—Able but unwilling or insecure

Staff nurse 2 is a new graduate of a humanistic program in nursing. This nurse's chief complaint on the unit is insufficient time to sit and talk with clients. This nurse is used to having the time to collaborate with the client in developing the care plan, being a graduate of a school of nursing that used Orem's (1985) theory of nursing as a conceptual framework. However, this nurse always seems frustrated and she rarely feels satisfied with the work completed.

Diagnosis: M1—Safety
                R2—Unable but willing or confident

The manager must identify the modal level of maturity/readiness. The majority of people in the system are at R2 and M2—unable but willing or confident and motivated at the social level. The leader behavior style that is indicated for an M2/R2 level of maturity/readiness is leader behavior style two (LB2), high structure and high consideration. This style becomes the pivot upon which alternative actions and the recommended action are based. The level of maturity of the system suggests that the leader must give direction to the group concerning the task—what is to be done—and also involve them in problem-solving activities. The leader should meet with the group on a regular basis, suggesting solutions to issues as they arise and offering directions after receiving the group's advice. When talking with the two staff nurses individually, the manager can behave according to the leader behavior style that is indicated by their individual levels of maturity. But, when communicating with the group, LB2 is indicated as the best beginning leader behavior style on the journey to goal accomplishment.

Diagnosing the Task

The last diagnosis to be made by the leader is of the nature of the task. Using the Vroom and Yetton managerial decision model (Vroom, 1973; Vroom & Jago, 1974, 1978, 1988; Vroom & Yetton, 1973), the questions shown in Figure 6.2 must be answered, starting with question A.

> *Question A: Quality—Yes.* Clearly, there are a number of possible solutions, and one could be more effective than another.
>
> Follow the "yes" line to the next node and respond to question B.
>
> *Question B: Manager's information—No.* The manager would certainly have ideas on how this can best be accomplished. Given that there are a variety of client problems and that the system has been directly involved in planning care, the staff would obviously have information and expertise that is not possessed by the leader.
>
> Follow the "no" line and answer question C.
>
> *Question C: Structure—No.* The manager has to make a subjective decision on how this problem will be solved. The decision will not be based on objective (quantitative) data. Further, the exact location of the data that will be used to solve the problem is unknown.
>
> Follow the "no" line to question D.
>
> *Question D: Acceptance—Yes.* The team leaders must accept the decision in order for the goal to be accomplished.
>
> Proceed to question E.
>
> *Question E: Prior probability of acceptance—No.* This is a sticky question in this case. There are neither data to suggest that the manager's decision would be followed nor that the managers decision would be rejected. The "no" response is based on the team leaders' deep involvement in developing and implementing the current procedure. Moreover, when in doubt on this question, always favor group discussion; this covers the possibility of group rejection, and the only thing lost is a little time.
>
> Follow the "no" line to question F.
>
> *Question F: Goal congruence—Yes.* The staff will certainly gain from the experience of collaborating with clients and from the feeling of helping another in this personalized way. The resulting style

that is suggested by the model is GII. Bring the system together and solve the problem as a group. As shown in Figure 6.1, GII is LB3, high consideration and low structure.

Synthesizing the Diagnosis

As the manager, you diagnose yourself as committed to solving the problem because of personal and managerial reasons. You enjoy LB3, and that seems to be the one in which you function most often with the team leaders.

Upon diagnosing the system, you find that the modal level of maturity readiness is M2/R2 (socially motivated and unable but willing or confident), requiring LB2, high structure and high consideration. This is moving one quadrant back from your preferred style of LB3. The nature of the task requires LB3, group decision making with high consideration and low structure. The group should be involved in how the problem will be solved.

The manager must first follow the leader behavior style suggested by the system's maturity—LB2. It must be recognized that the problem cannot be totally solved until the system understands the "whys" and "hows" of collaborating with clients in developing nursing care plans. Once this is accomplished, then the group will be both able and willing; the manager can then go into LB3, which is required by the task. Even though an able and willing group requires LB4, remember that once in the leadership model, you move one quadrant forward for a progressing group or one quadrant backward for a regressing group. This provides reinforcement for learning (change). The manager must also be aware that conscious effort must be made to give the initial high task behavior to the group—given the preferences of this manager, such a style may be neither involuntary nor most pleasing for the manager even if necessary. In introducing the problem to the staff, the manager should share the cues that led to the problem definitions, including one's own feelings. This is included in high relationship behavior. Also, a social flavor to the meetings should be staged.

ALTERNATIVE ACTIONS

The alternative actions should be ways of solving the problem that use the indicated leader behavior style—high structure and high consideration. Expected positive and negative results should be delineated for each alternative action (see Table 7.2).

TABLE 7.2 Alternative Actions and Results

Action	*Possible Results*
1. Set up an informal potluck dinner at the leader's house, inviting the system members. Introduce the problem after dinner. Explain everythng that has led up to the problem as you see it—tardiness, lack of creativity, and so forth. Positively reinforce the excellent care plans that are being done and suggest that collaboratively planned individualized care seems like the next step in growth.	Staff nurse 2 offers to develop a protocol and try it with several clients. The nurse will report on the strengths and weaknesses of the protocol and revise it with all of the team leaders before going any further.
	− This result may dampen group involvement in learning about the problem.
	+ It may be a good idea later on.
	− All of the system does not come to the informal dinner.
Explain your perception of the problem solution and stress that this is just one way to solve the problem. What you would like is to spend time discussing concerns and getting and sharing information about the problem; the team leaders would develop a plan for designing the new care plan protocol and implementing it. Prior to leaving, a series of information sessions is planned.	+ The group decides to meet once a week in order to get more information about what they are going to do, prior to designing or implementing anything.
	+ The three regular team leaders express insecurity in their ability to do this; they request help from someone who has done this before.
In this action, the manager is being high task in delineating the problem and its rationale. Knowledge is the first priority, and then the manager states that group problem-solving is expected. The manager provides reinforcement in a group discussion. This all characterizes starting at LB2, high structure and high consideration, with a planned shift to LB3, high consideration and low structure.	− Staff nurse 1 expounds that it will not work because clients expect to be told what to do.
	+ The group openly discusses the problem, asking questions of the manager and of each other.
2. Announce a meeting for team leaders during the conference time slot on the regular shift. Then introduce the goal and	− Those nurses not scheduled on that day will not attend.
	+ All positive possible results stated in the first alternative.

(continued)

TABLE 7.2 (continued)

Action	Possible Results
follow the same agenda as in the first alternative. Provide coffee and snacks.	− The negative result from the first alternative concerning staff nurse 1.
3. Invite the unit supervisor to the first meeting that has been set up during a team conference time slot. The problem and goal is introduced in the same way as alternative actions one and two. In addition the supervisor emphasizes that the goal is favorable with administration.	+ The staff members may be encouraged by support from higher administration. − The staff members may be resentful that an authority figure not in the direct system was aware of the problem/goal before they were.

Note. + Possible positive outcome
      − Possible negative outcome

RECOMMENDED ACTION

The manager decides that alternative action two is the most favorable because the team leaders are not accustomed to meeting together socially. Further, they never meet outside of the work environment, even for work-related issues. The meeting would be scheduled, if possible, on a day that all members of the system were working. If not possible, the greatest number in the system would be on duty. The person(s) not on would be asked whether it would be possible to come in for this meeting. Compensation time would be offered. The manager should attempt to neutralize negative outcomes of this alternative action.

Following delineation of the recommended action, it must be implemented and then evaluated.

IMPLEMENTATION AND EVALUATION

To implement simply means "to do" or "to put into action." It follows that after one has specified a recommended action, it must be implemented. Prior to implementation, evaluation emerges as a responsibility and continues to be important until after the action is completed.

Evaluation is most effective when it includes all three types. These are discussed by Newman (1975) as types of control, a broader concept that includes evaluation.

1. *Steering controls.* In this form of evaluation, results are predicted prior to implementation. If things are not going along as desired, corrective action is taken during implementation.

   Referring back to the example, if at the team conference the nurses were not responding in general accordance with the expected positive results, the manager might change the action strategy immediately.

2. *Yes-no controls.* This is a check point where action does not proceed to another step until quality and effectiveness with the previous step are confirmed.

   Again going to the case example, all members should generally be satisfied with the first meeting's outcomes and be clear and agreed on the agenda for the next meeting prior to adjourning.

3. *Post-action controls.* This form of evaluation is after-the-fact—action has been completed; the problem is solved. Now accomplishments and what is being done regarding care plan development are compared with the leader's original intent.

THE MANAGEMENT PROCESS

Chapter 1 contained a discussion of the four components of the management process—planning, organizing, motivating, and controlling. These relationships are discussed regarding the case example.

In order to plan for all of these areas, the areas requiring attention had to be organized logically. What was to be done first and why? Further, the system was organized to contain only the people who were primary in solving the problem.

The determination of a leader behavior style that responded to the modal level of maturity of the system was a planned intervention that intended to motivate the system to accomplish by giving the nurses what they needed. The manager had to (1) plan for behaviors that filled the indicated leader behavior style requirements and (2) organize alternative actions and a recommended action to respond to the group's needs.

In each of the three components of the management process, the manager is also comparing accomplishments with intent. Are all necessary nurses included in the system? Should anyone be added? Is my diagnosis accurate—do I need more data? Did my recommended action provide a structured taking-off place for the system? Did it kindle interest in the problem? Will high structure be required for the second session? Was the entire group involved?

SUMMARY

This chapter used a case study to apply all of the material in Chapters 1 through 6. Theory was applied in the problem-solving method. The chapter concluded with a discussion of the interrelatedness of the management process given the described case example. The experiential exercises at the conclusion of Part II contain guidelines for applying the problem-solving method to a case from the learner's real world.

REFERENCES

Hersey, P., & Blanchard, K. (1988). *Management of organizational behavior: Utilizing human resources* (5th ed.). Englewood Cliffs, NJ: Prentice-Hall.

Newman, W. (1975). *Constructive control*. Englewood Cliff, NJ: Prentice-Hall.

Orem, D. (1985). *Nursing: Concepts of practice* (3rd ed.). New York: McGraw-Hill.

Vroom, V. (1973). A new look at managerial decision-making. *Organizational Dynamics, 1,* 66–80.

Vroom, V., & Jago, A. (1974). Decision-making as a social process. *Decision Sciences, 5,* 743–769.

Vroom, V., & Jago, (1978). On the validity of the Vroom-Yetton model. *Journal of Applied Psychology, 63,* 151–162.

Vroom, V., & Jago, A. (1988). *The new leadership: Managing participation in organizations*. Englewood Cliffs, NJ: Prentice-Hall.

Vroom, V., & Yetton, P. (1973). *Leadership and decision-making*. Pittsburgh: University of Pittsburgh Press.

Managerial Ethics

Elizabeth M. Maloney, Ed.D. *

In May 1922, 68 years ago, The American Academy of Political and Social Science devoted an entire issue to the ethics of the professions and business. It is clear that concern with ethics is far from new. However, it is the content of that concern that has changed so much

*Elizabeth M. Maloney, Ed.D., R.N., is an Associate Professor of Nursing Education at Teachers College, Columbia University, New York. She is a former member of the New York State Nurses Association Council on Ethical Practice and she currently teaches ethics for health care professionals. Dr. Maloney has written and spoken extensively in the area of ethical nursing practice and in psychiatric nursing.

over the years in both nursing and in related health fields. The individual struggle with justice—right and wrong—remains essentially the same. Meanwhile, in the last two decades particularly, there has been mounting concern with the ethical management of society's organizations. This concern ranges from national government to structures closer at hand, particularly the health care system. Specifically this chapter is concerned with nursing management in the spectrum of organizations devoted to health and illness.

BACKGROUND FOR ETHICAL CONCERNS IN NURSING

It is of interest to note that almost from the beginning of nursing in the United States, a measure of concern for ethical behavior was manifested. Aroskar (1987b) identified that the first objective of the American Nurses Association in the late 1890s was to establish and maintain a code of ethics. There is little doubt also that the old "service to humanity" credo contained most of the elements of the Christian-Judeo belief system that undergirds ethics in the Western world.

The first ethics book by a nurse (Robb, 1901) is often described as more of a book on etiquette or good behavior than what would be accepted as ethics today. Perhaps the term "ethics" at that time encompassed all of professional behavior, including demeanor, dress, hair, and desertion of patients. Robb noted, on the other hand, concern with behavior:

> One occasionally hears a nurse boast that it is her custom to nurse patients through the critical periods of their illness and then leave them to the care of others. Such conduct—the willingness to desert a patient before the work is finished—is not only a breach of nursing ethics but also shows a want of perseverance on the part of the nurse. (p. 83)

As late as 1974, Pellegrino noted that the ethical codes of both the American Medical Association and the American Nurses Association were a mixture of ethics and etiquette.

Almost without exception, early literature in this area was a blend of commenting on professional organizations and their structure, admission standards, and legal aspects of licensing. There were, of course, no discussions of ethical dilemmas in a high technology illness system as one knows of them today.

It is highly probable that early content was emphasized precisely because there existed a natural limit to what health workers could do (or were expected by the public to be able to do). Indeed, the early 1900s was an era when it was freely acknowledged at some identifiable point what was good nursing care. There was, in short, a limit to the possibilities. At the edge of the limit was death, when it could no longer be held at bay. It is important to recognize that this was the generally held opinion or consensus; a matter of public acknowledgment. Today there is a vast array of available technology and there is high expectation of more to come. The increased debates in the public realm are best measured by the flood of literature in the press, both popular and professional. Ethics is in fact one of the persistent themes of our time.

Emmanuel (1987, p. 16) indicated that people now live "in a liberal polity" where a multiplicity of views are entertained as to what constitutes the meaning and value of life. Directly associated with these terms is another: the "quality" of life. Hypothetically, part of the discussions around and about the patient's right to die have to do with this latter concept. However, to simply discuss "quality" of life is to say little. Anyone capable of rational thought has a different definition of the quality of life. Basically, as in all ethical decisions, the final outcome of care is dependent on reconciliation of multiple personal value systems. These systems are in turn based on religious and family experiences and the specific context in which the "quality" must be defined. Briefly it all depends on whose ox is being gored, as the saying goes—whose life; whose family; and under what circumstances? And what are the restrictions legally?

It is important to note here again, that cultural concerns have a great deal more to do with attitudes about right and wrong than any of us realize. Assuming that professional literature reflects the immediate concerns of a profession, it can clearly be seen that these concerns ebb and flow over time. For example, Anderson (1949) reviewed articles on ethics in the *American Journal of Nursing* in 10 year intervals starting with 1900 and ending in 1948. Briefly, a curve peaking in the years 1930 to 1940 showed 30 articles; the number of articles descended to zero from 1941 to 1945, indicating a national concern with other matters, most likely the years at war. Certainly speculation could be pursued also with the unprecedented concern with ethical matters manifested in the 1970s and 1980s. This concern, grounded in the use of ever more sophisticated, expensive technology and its use, has culminated in the employment of philosophers in medical centers and in the rise of ethical committees in well over half of the nation's hospitals. It has also resulted in the development of a group of nurses commonly called nurse-ethicists. It is of interest that many (but not all) came from a psychiatric nursing background. Working with philosophers and studying at centers dealing with ethical concerns, these experts have produced a solid body of literature aimed directly at problems found in nursing practice. It is these same problems that the nurse manager confronts each day. The solution to these ethical dilemmas is almost never clear cut and oftentimes remains open-ended. Still, from the currently available theoretical material, there are strong markers for the resolution of some of these dilemmas. It is reasonable to emphasize that the more pressing ethical dilemmas are, in the end, so urgent that they are concretized into law, thus providing relief from ambiguity for all concerned personnel. For example, there is the New York State law, effective in 1988, which requires that health care facilities have a written policy on "do not resuscitate" (or DNR) orders (Brawer & Miller 1987).

As well as the foregoing legal direction, professional codes are helpful in counteracting institutional pressures. Recognition of the part played by these pressures has increased in the literature of managerial ethics. Utilizing the argument that the "most obvious link between nursing and the great moral ideas is health," Packard and Ferrara (1988, p. 60) objected to the conventionally held idea that nurses' moral freedom is constrained by institutional and other pressures so great as to restrict their ethical freedom. Citing the need for a code of ethics for corporate employees, Rue and Byars (1986) noted that "a code of ethics also reduces the organizational pressures to compromise personal ethics for the sake of organizational goals" (p. 2). It would seem then that there are almost universal pressures— political, organizational, and others—that militate against moving toward the right and just solution to ethical dilemmas. Managers everywhere share common problems.

ETHICS AND MORALITY DEFINED

Rue and Byars (1986) defined ethics as "standards or principles of conduct used to govern the behavior of an individual or group of individuals" (p. 2). Ethics are generally concerned with questions of right and wrong or with moral duties. Hosmer (1987) pointed out that the term ethics is used in the plural since most people have a system of beliefs rather than one single value by which to live.

What then is morality? Hosmer (1987) stated that morality is a

set of standards by which people judge one another. He noted also
that one usually speaks of "moral standards of behavior and systems
of belief" (p. 92). One could say then that morals are the way that
people expect other people to behave, according to established group
norms.

Aroskar (1987a, 1987b) added that ethics, as an area of philosophy, refers to moral conduct; not what is *actually* done, but what
ought to be done. She further cited some of the realities that act as
barriers to doing what should be done. Some of these constraints are
constant in the daily lives of nurse managers: cost-containment factors, limitations and shortages of personnel, internal and external
politics, and others. Germane to the work of the nurse manager is
Aroskar's comment that ethics in nursing is concerned with moral
decision making both in day-to-day affairs and in the larger world of
policy making. Modern day nursing practice and management is rife
with situations where value-laden conflicts arise. As Benjamin (1988)
and others have pointed out, it has not been widely recognized that
nurses are involved in pivotal and complex ethical situations and that
willingly or not, they are involved in and often make ethical decisions. These decisions are made within an intricate system of formal
and informal relationships where conflicting value systems are often
found. These problems are compounded by an organization whose
goals at any given time may be in conflict with those of individuals
or groups within it. It is managerial leadership that often must set
the scene for the ethical decisions that the total group must make.

Peculiar to nurses among professionals is the fact that the majority of nurses are employees of health organizations. As employees,
they are bound to accede to lawful demands of the employing institutions. Compounding this is the presence of the physician, who most
frequently is not hospital-employed but who uses hospital facilities
primarily for nursing care and multiple other technological personnel
and/or resources. The fact is that there are many examples where
nurses have been caught between their own personal values and
legal demands to obey the lawful orders of physicians or superiors.
Even more important are situations where demands may be lawful,
but they conflict with other moral values and emphasize the legal-
moral conflict that will continue to occupy students of moral dilemmas. For example, it may be lawful to have an order to discontinue
aggressive treatment, but in the day-to-day care of the patient, it
might be that the advocate's role would imply a different stance. The
legalities are not always clear as to what constitutes interference in
the patient-physician role, as amply demonstrated in the now famous

Tuma case (Veatch & Fry, 1987). There are a number of writers in the field who have considered the major world views from which primary ethical systems arise (Kant, 1909; Rawls, 1971; Ross, 1939). Their work serves as a starting point for the formulation of a coherent set of principles or guidelines for decision making in the ethical realm.

PRINCIPLES OF ETHICS—GUIDELINES

Principles arise from the ethical system that have developed from a lifelong exposure to fundamental beliefs about how a human being behaves in a given situation. Obviously, these go back to a group of beliefs in one of the two major ethical systems. Add to that a particular cultural system of beliefs and some normative directions for what to do come into being. It would seem that the concept of "normative" comes into consideration immediately in ethical dilemmas. The principles are as follows: autonomy, beneficence, nonmaleficence, veracity, justice, and confidentiality. A brief discussion of each principle follows.

Autonomy

Basically, this is the freedom to decide what persons will or will not do with their lives, their bodies, and their selves, all of course within the limits of what is possible and what does not infringe upon the rights of others. It does mean that one accords others the same freedom and independence of action as accorded self and that one respects the dignity of others. Autonomy means never looking upon another as a means to some end unless that person is in entire agreement with the clearly understood end. For example, in the health field informed consent emerges from this concept. If, as in some past instances, patients have become part of a research study without consenting and without being informed, then this is a clear violation of an ethical principle. Freedom to act upon information given is an integral part of informed consent. If by one means or another the element of coercion enters the situation, then free choice cannot be exercised. Sometimes professionals are not entirely aware that their position intimidates their lay audience, the patient, and that patients will go along because they think they have received what amounts to a definitive statement about their condition.

Beneficence

This is a situation where one is not only minimally responsible for doing no harm; rather, in various service professions, one is bound also to do good. Hospitals, physicians, and nurses exist "to do no harm" but also to institute activity that will be beneficial to all of the clients encountered. Since patients enter the health care system for the solution of a health problem, to do nothing about their problems is acting counter to the principle of beneficence. Of course, in the instances where doing nothing is of therapeutic value, there is an exception to this principle.

Nonmaleficence

This principle requires the professional to prevent harm whenever possible and to never use a particular treatment or medication to harm patients. Lifton (1986) in *The Nazi Doctors* described in detail how a whole group cooperated in the malevolent use of formerly benevolent treatment and research efforts. The process by which this took place is worthy of study, particularly the concepts of climate or milieu or the importance of the context in which malevolent actions take root. The idea of the "slippery slope" is important here and can partially be described as that having accepted the possibility of what once was unthinkable, the rapid descent into unethical activity becomes commonplace. The unacceptable becomes acceptable. If unit staff decides that it is too time consuming to take all of the vital signs of recovering patients, then this nonactivity at some point becomes institutionalized or commonplace; the next step may be to enter fictitious figures.

Veracity

In the health care field, truth-telling has long been debated in the literature. In recent years, opinion has come down hard on the patient's right to know the truth. Certainly the professional's obligation to present the full array of information to patients is unquestioned, with however some notable exceptions. There are instances where bald truth telling may destroy the last vestige of hope available to the patient. There are still people who communicate in every manner possible that they do not wish to hear bad news. One could argue that by failing to make certain professional statements, one is in essence lying. Bok (1978) explored the concept of lying in effective detail, including the giving of placebos as lying. Included in her work also is the consideration of references given by management that might, among other things, fail to include serious behavioral deficits on the part of a departing employee. To say nothing then can be to lie.

This has always been a troubled area. In more paternalistic times, the problem did not arise as frequently. The patient was told what he or she was supposed to know. The content of what the patient was offered was based on values and perceptions of the health worker offering the information. Certainly no one would argue today that in most instances autonomy is involved; patients have a right to information about themselves. There are still people who argue that the individual with a terminal health problem simply does not want to know, on the grounds that such information would do more harm than good. Thus the teleological approach is tempting—to produce good feeling without too much thought about the moral value of the patients' right to know, along with the moral duty to make the information available. (In reality, however, there are many combinations possible.) Here also can be summoned Kant's (1909) concept that everyone has the duty to tell the truth, thus answering the question "are lies ever justified?" in the negative.

The bare bones of a common practice dilemma are that situations will arise wherein nurses must make value judgments about whether lying might be the best thing to do for a patient (beneficence). Thus two principles are involved; to do good and to tell the truth. Sissela Bok (1978) said that liars in such circumstances comfort themselves with the thought of their benevolence but that, in the long run, the liar loses some measure of credibility and damages the system that supports the lie. Characteristic of the dilemma is conflict among principles and the need to formulate some personal guidelines as to how one solves the problem, based on, among other things, some alternatives relevant to a moral solution of the dilemma.

Justice

Germane to the health field is the expectation that people with like problems will be treated equally or alike. It is central to the principle of justice that fairness and rights be considered always. Perhaps in no other area is the question so pressing as in how scarce resources will be distributed in the health care field. Faced with cost-containment and ever-rising expectations about the efficacy of modern health technology, the dilemma persists concerning who is to receive the scarce organ or the expensive or novel treatment. Should people for example be moved to the head of the transplant list for any reason at all?

Justice also demands that differences be handled differently if a patient is so unequal in some respect to all of the others for whom a policy has been applied. When then should exceptions be made? If so, on what grounds? Are professionals willing to deny health care to such exceptions because of the rules?

Confidentiality

The contract often unspoken between professional and client and between nurse and patient exists in part because the patient (in this instance) makes the assumption that whatever is divulged will be held in confidence. So sure of this are most people that they do not even think about the matter. In short, all of us make assumptions about our private matters that may be just that—assumptions. Excluding all of the inroads on privacy that have arisen in late years, largely due to computers, situations in the health field certainly exist where the patient's right to keep information private infringes on the rights of others. Nowhere is this more glaring than in the question of Acquired Immune Deficiency Syndrome (AIDS) and the right-to-know of those closest to the patient.

The control of information about ourselves is, whether people are aware of it or not, subject to gradiation—that is, people quantify who will receive what part of our store of information about ourselves and others. The most common way to do this is by degree of closeness. Spouses may know what the outer world does not; but in order to solve various problems, selected others must also know. Every professional group then becomes privy to information that their patients or clients do not wish to have known widely. Confidentiality becomes a duty and the patient or client has a right not to have specified information released. Nurse managers are privy to information about employees that may be confidential. To whom and under what circumstances is such information released?

MANAGEMENT AND THE DEVELOPMENT OF A MORAL CLIMATE

Turning to Aroskar (1987a, 1987b) for a definition of moral and ethical leadership, the following perception is found: leaders describe moral leadership as taking responsibility for one's commitments—taking responsibility for one's choices. Drawing on prominent ethicists,

Aroskar also noted other characteristics that emerged, such as leadership being a particular kind of social-ethical practice evoked by health issues that require caring. Other adjectives invoked are responsibility, involvement, fairness, concern for others—all of these words describing moral leadership. Ethical dilemmas, it goes without saying, do not arise every day but must be part of a carefully defined situation. Bok (1988) and others have, for example, pointed out the fate of "whistleblowers" in our society. It should be an act of last resort; all other reasonable avenues having been exhausted. Whistle-blowers are, in the long run, not treated well in our society.

Although it is seldom discussed overtly, the work environment on a particular plane of behavior makes implicit assumptions. These assumptions are based on cues taken from those already in place on a nursing unit. These cues can be as concrete as a warning from a fellow worker—"never cut a corner when x is here"—to an aura of openness about mistakes; there may be a generalized assumption that "right" and "justice and regard for others" will prevail in that particular environment. Admittedly the "right" attitude or the "just" response are influenced by different value systems. Often responses to ethical dilemmas have to be developed through interdisciplinary debate based on known principles of ethics.

Managers are at a pivotal place in an organizational structure and are expected to accomplish organizational goals as smoothly as possible. Clearly this brings them into conflict at times with staff and patient goals. Indeed, part of the nurse manager's dilemma arises from serving multiple masters. Specifically, the constituencies to be served are: (1) the patient or client for whom the health organization exists; (2) the nursing staff and related others *for* whom management is responsible; and (3) the agency administration *to* whom the nurse in a managerial position is responsible. By way of illustration, a simple situation is described and found in Part II experiential exercises; it is one that is perhaps destined to become more common as the current nursing shortage persists. A series of questions is posed in Exercise 5, Ethics—A Managerial Dilemma, and the opportunity to utilize the answers based on ethical principles is open to the learner.

Framework for Managerial Activity—General Considerations

It would be useful at this point to identify some of the most commonly experienced or perceived ethical problems by nursing staff. With the end in view of establishing a nursing ethics committee, which would provide assistance to professional nursing staff, a survey was conducted by Edwards and Haddad (1988). The purposes of the study were to assess the educational needs and primary ethical problems that were perceived by the nursing staff. It is the identification of the staff members' ethical concerns that may provide guidance to the nurse manager in dealing with ethical dilemmas. The findings were reduced to two factors:

1. The justification of life-support and resuscitative efforts in futile or gravely burdensome cases; and

2. Professional competency issues, such as truth-telling, withholding information, and questioning the competency of the medical staff and nursing colleagues.

In general, all of the available literature in the field bears out the foregoing findings, albeit expressed in somewhat different language. It says little for either medicine or nursing that the most common reason cited by these subjects for compromising their ethical values was a physician's or a superior's request. It does, however, add verisimilitude to the picture of the nurse as the person "caught in the middle" in terms of not only ethical dilemmas but many other situations as well. On the other hand, it is important to point out that many corporations have developed codes of ethics for their personnel, since hierarchical pressure (those perceived to be in authority) and a work climate where corners are cut are by no means unique to the health field.

Health Care Cost-Containment

The control of health care costs eventually translates itself into allocation of scarce resources. The technology that allows for life, where there once would have been death, is extremely expensive. Who then will be designated to receive it—everyone who establishes need? Or, will it be selected individuals based on stated criteria? Who will set the criteria? How long will these criteria be used and who decides when they will be terminated? These are but a few of the significant questions that nurse managers will be obliged to consider in concert with other professionals from the health disciplines. The second problem that emerges in the managerial realm is the pressure to employ less qualified personnel to deal with an increasingly complex care situation. There are two sources for this pressure, the first being a shortage of qualified personnel and the second, the cost of qualified personnel.

Scarce Research and Personnel

Part of the manager's ethical dilemma is generally related to staffing and to the quality of patient care. The increasing impetus to provide cost-effective care may take the form of pressure to employ and use less qualified personnel in situations where greater knowledge and skill are required. The concept that Fry (1985) used to describe this dilemma is based on the idea that nursing and management in nursing are assumed social roles. Not only does one act as an individual or in one's private capacity, but one also bears the moral responsibility for actions carried out in the name of a particular profession. Fry called this the "morality of role acceptance" (pp. 135–136). Fry illustrated this dilemma graphically in describing a nursing home director faced with quality of care concerns (legislation allowing unlicensed personnel to administer medications) and measures to assure cost-effectiveness. Although there were other issues involved, Fry stated that this was a classic example of a common dilemma in health care: "between what is right according to universal moral norms and what is right according to outcomes or consequences" (pp. 135–136). It is right that medications be dispensed, but the situation becomes problematic if lack of expertise leads to undesirable ends. Related to ethical principles, the following principle might be invoked; clearly nonmaleficence is appropriate, that is, do no harm.

As resources become ever more scarce, what is "due" to whom and what are the criteria to determine this? A classic focal point in ethics is the lifeboat dilemma. Briefly, in order to survive as a group, someone must go overboard. On what basis is this decided? Is it age, evidence of a productive life, or possibilities for future contributions to mankind? Who will receive the organ transplant? What are the criteria and who develops them? Are the answers based on a first-come-first-served basis, or do other factors preempt the waiting list? And how does the nursing staff react to the decision? The amount of national resources allocated to the health dollar is finite and probably will always operate in competition with other well-defined national concerns. Since the situation will undoubtedly become more urgent, then the impact will be felt in nursing units and will often become priority staff-management problems. The tendency to solve economic problems by bringing in less skilled workers is evident countrywide in the health field.

Staff Concern with "Do Not Resuscitate" Orders

This area appears to be a focal point for a great many ethical concerns, primarily because decisions one way or the other have such profound implications for everyone concerned. These implications are both moral and legal. Further, they are of extreme importance to nursing since many experts in ethics point out that it is nurses who are caught in the middle. If there are, as has happened in the past, ambiguous unwritten directives, it is nurses who have called the code or not; nurses have dealt with directions for "no codes" and "slow codes," at least before the era of public debate and subsequent clarification of the situation. This clarification has been achieved by a steadily expanding series of legal decisions such as the Quinlan and Fox cases (Jameton, 1984). These were cases where substitute judgments were invoked because of incapacity; but what of the patient who decides that it is time to terminate treatment—or to refuse a specific operation, such as limb amputation? For nurse managers, Tamborlane's (1987) comment concerning the agency and administrative role when a patient makes a personal decision to terminate treatment is to the point: "Agency personnel's moral or ethical beliefs should not be allowed to infringe upon a competent individual's rights to discontinue treatment when he or she wishes to let the disease take its natural course" (pp. 30–31). These are the kinds of decisions that management-instituted ethics committees regularly discuss.

Competence

Managers spend considerable time wrestling with the problem of personnel who for one reason or another may be providing care that does not come up to standard. Recognition of problem personnel generally "comes up" from the unit in the form of an oral or written report. The nature of the incompetence can range from repeated mistakes to lying, and those reported behaviors may have their origin in several sources. One of the most common is substance abuse. Such impairment is expensive in human and monetary terms and gives rise to ethical dilemmas among those who are most closely associated with the individual concerned. The danger to patients is clearly identified to be greater than, for example, the substitution of medication, which is such a frequent outcome of an employees' addiction. This is only one area for concern.

Formerly, attitudes toward substance abuse in the workplace were moralistic and often resulted in harsh disciplinary measures.

People were reluctant to report colleagues and probably still are. At least two studies demonstrated that there remains an apparent disinclination to cooperate with managers in the identification of substance abuses. For example, as late as 1985, *Nursing Life* reported that 53% of the respondents to their survey stated that they would not help management and appeared to perceive such identification as management's responsibility. There are two strong factors working for management in the solution of dilemmas thus presented to colleagues of the abuser. One is the legal necessity in most states to report incompetence and the other is the much more therapeutic approach to such problems that is demonstrated through organization-wide assistance programs. In asking why ethical dilemmas should arise in situations such as the foregoing, a good question is raised. Between the obligation to report and the now very common practice of directing identified abusers into special programs for assistance, why would anyone consider this a dilemma? First, there is the common or shared humanity—what will happen to this person if they lose their job or license? Second, most people have a perceived loyalty to colleagues. As Winslow (1988) noted, most people are unwilling to publically expose the shortcomings of a colleague. Based on the childhood tradition of not telling on a peer or being tagged as a tattletale, there is an element of felt injustice for the other if one does take steps to expose the abuse.

MANAGERIAL OPTIONS

In attempting to provide leadership in situations where ethical dilemmas are identified, there are several things that managers are able to do. Some of these things are concrete, such as establishment of a nursing bioethics committee. Other steps include assurance that everyone for whom management is responsible is aware of guidelines related to confidentiality of sensitive patient material. All personnel need to have complete information about how one begins dealing with incompetence in colleagues and the like. Nurse managers can address the underlying ethical principles through specifically oriented continuing education programs. Perhaps one of the most effective means of maintaining a reasonably open and moral climate is to hold a genuine belief in staff capacity to identify and solve ethical problems. As Aroskar (1987a, 1987b) pointed out, both nurses and patients are persons who are worthy of respect. More to the point, she noted that there may be coercive forces or elements such as threats and peer pressure if one refuses dubious medical orders. "Such actions or an environment that condones such actions may jeopardize an individual nurse's personal and professional integrity in any practice setting and require change" (Aroskar, 1987a, p. 26).

Although nurse managers are sometimes involved as patient advocates, it is more likely that there will be situations where advocacy of an embattled staff nurse may be the issue. Noting the complexity of the nurse's role vis-a-vis the ever expanding technology of patient care, many ethicists writing about nursing have taken note of the great responsibility that many nurses carry which must be based on an equally great degree of necessary skill and knowledge. The same ethicists have noted the lack of power to make decisions—the frequent and classic case of the man or woman in the middle. What are some of the operative ways that the manager can deal with situations involving the foregoing factors?

Establishment of a Nursing Committee

The hospital ethics committee is now commonplace in institutional life. Over 50 to 60% of U.S. hospitals now have such committees; indeed, some of the larger medical centers employ philosophers who have extensive backgrounds in ethics and the solution of ethical dilemmas. In larger practice settings these committees often deal with matters that do not filter down to daily life on the unit. To provide for nursing staff, Edwards and Haddad (1988) described the establishment of an ethics committee specifically for nursing staff. One activity included the separation of ethical problems from management problems. Essentially, tackling ethical problems involves the elements and steps in problem solving, thus allowing for a reasoned and principled solution.

Another similar effort is described by Jaeger (1988). Although confined to one unit staff, many of the elements were the same. First, staff frustration with ethical concerns in which there seemed to be no clear cut means of dealing with these questions was identified. Essentially, the nurse manager described an identification of a staff problem (ethical concerns and no apparent means of dealing with these problems), the mobilization of the staff through unit meetings, the encouragement of staff members' identification of the problem(s) as they saw it, and provision of an environment where staff felt free to verbalize ethical concerns. This was followed by an educational phase. Literature was provided and discussions ensued, thereby tying the abstract literature to the setting. Although the first problem to be clearly defined was the code status of patients, after several months it became apparent that there were many other dilemmas involved. It was at this point that the need for ethical nursing conferences became evident. Therefore, guidelines were set up and the goal of the conferences was to provide a continuing pattern of open communication and mutual support among patients, family, and the health care team. Finally, a structure for data collection was established. The report of both of these efforts emphasized that the support and commitment of the top-level nurse executive is tantamount to survival of such efforts. Thus, as can be seen from a brief summary of two committee efforts, such activity provides one of the most useful means for management to solve ethical dilemmas. Out of such infrastructure comes identification of educational needs in the ethical area. Essentially the classic steps of problem-solving emerge from the foregoing examples.

WHAT OF THE FUTURE?

Jameton (1984), a philosopher who has studied ethics in nursing, wrote that "nursing is the morally central health care profession. Philosophers of nursing, not medicine, should determine the image of health care and its future direction" (pp. 196–197).

Recently two efforts to provide a moral foundation for nursing and another to ground the "nursing ethic in a convenantal relationship" may offer a glimpse of where a specifically nursing ethic may be going. In one direction Yarling and McElmurry (1986) called for the reform of the hospital and the social structure it embodies as being essential to autonomy for nursing practitioners, and thus to a moral basis for nursing. Bishop and Scudder (1987) objected on the grounds that nursing autonomy is secondary to the nurse's primary concern, that of patient welfare.

Winslow (1988) argued that there is a need to be aware of and to change metaphors about nursing, noting that such metaphors interact with nursing ethics (stated rules or principles), which in turn interact with the more explicit features of nursing ethics. The metaphors touch on roles in that, for example, the traditional loyal, servant-mother roles are being slowly replaced by contractual advocacy roles. Concomitant alterations in expectations will eventually create a focus on different realities in the nurse-patient-institutional context. It is to be noted that these are only a few of the many roles played in an ever-changing health care scene.

SUMMARY

Ethical dilemmas in the health care field, hospital, community, and home can be expected to intensify in the future. As new technology is perfected and as resource allocation becomes a more acute problem, nursing management will predictably draw more and more on ethical committees as devices for support and as development vehicles for at least working consensus among staff when ethical dilemmas present themselves. Some of the dilemmas will be at least partially resolved (after prolonged public debate) by legal means. Certainly euthanasia is much on the public mind and is closely allied to its more concrete form labeled "do not resuscitate." As Edwards and Haddad (1988) noted, a basic knowledge of ethical theories and related principles is a necessity both for the practicing nurse and the nurse manager. It is a necessity to deal with the moral-ethical issues that arise in the work day. Certainly every barometer reads that there will be more, not less, technology; therefore there will be probably more, not less, concern with moral and ethical problems in the future.

REFERENCES

American Academy of Political and Social Sciences. (1922). The ethics of professions and business. *The Annals, C1.*

Anderson, B. (1949, July). Discussion of ethics in the curriculum. Lecture at Teachers College, Columbia University, New York, NY.

Aroskar, M. (1987a). Commentary. *Hastings Center Report, 17*(2), 26.

Aroskar, M. (1987b, September). *Ethics in the leadership equation.* Distinguished Lecture at Columbia University Health Sciences Campus, New York, NY.

Benjamin, M. (1988). Nursing ethics: An emerging integrity. *Hastings Center Report, 18*(2), 38–39.

Bishop, A., & Scudder, J. (1987). Nursing ethics in an age of controversy. *Advances in Nursing Science, 9*(3), 34–37.

Bok, S. (1978). Lying: Moral choice in public and private life. New York: Pantheon.

Bok, S. (1988). Whistleblowing and professional responsibilities. In J. Callahan (Ed.), *Ethical issues in professional life.* New York: Oxford Press.

Brawer, I., & Miller, T. (1987). New York to provide comprehensive guidelines for do not resuscitate orders. *Journal of the New York State Nurses Association, 18*(5), 3.

Edwards, B., & Haddad, A. (1988). Establishing a nursing bioethics committee. *Journal of Nursing Administration, 18*(3), 30–33.

Emmanuel, E. (1987). A communal vision of care for incompetent patients. *Hastings Center Report, 17*(5), 15–20.

Fry, S. (1985). Political activities and the professional role. In S. Talbot & D. Mason (Eds.). *Political action*. Menlo Park, CA: Addison-Wesley.

Hosmer, L. (1987). *The ethics of management*. Homewood, IL: Irwin.

Jaeger, T. (1988). A head nurse's approach to multidisciplinary ethical conferences. *Nursing Management, 10*(1), 61–62.

Jameton, A. (1984). *Nursing Practice: The ethical issues*. Englewood Cliffs, NJ: Prentice-Hall.

Kant, I. (1909). *Critique of practical reason*. London: Longmans.

Lifton, R. (1986). *The Nazi doctors*. New York: Basic Books.

Nursing Life. (1985). What our readers said about entrapping a colleague. *Nursing Life, 3*(5), 54–55.

Packard, J., & Ferrara, M. (1988). In search of the moral foundation of nursing. *Advances in Nursing Science, 10*(4), 60–71.

Pellegrino, E. (1974). Educating the humanist physician: An ancient ideal reconsidered. *Journal of the American Medical Association, 227*, 1288–1294.

Rawls, J. (1971). *Theory of justice*. Cambridge, MA: Belknap.

Robb, I. (1901). *Nursing ethics*. Cleveland: S.B. Savage.

Ross, W. (1939). *The right and the good*. Oxford: Oxford University Press.

Rue, L., & Byars, L. (1986). *Management: Theory and application* (4th ed.). Homewood, IL: Irwin.

Tamborlane, T. (1987). A patient's right to refuse or discontinue treatment. *Caring, 4*, 30–31.

Veatch, T., & Fry, S. (1987). *Case studies in nursing ethics*. Philadelphia: Lippincott.

Winslow, G. (1988). From loyalty to advocacy: A new metaphor for nursing. In J. Callahan (Ed.). *Ethical issues in professional life*. New York: Oxford Press.

Yarling, R., & McElmurry, B. (1986). The moral foundation of nursing. *Advances in Nursing Science, 8*(2), 63–73.

Part II

Manager Responsibilities: Experiential Exercises

EXERCISE 1   **Diagnosing Personal Leader Behavior Style***

Purposes   1. To diagnose one's personal leader behavior style.

2. To identify one's expectations of leader behavior.

3. To explore the implications of one's personal leadership style.

4. To explore the similarity or disparity between one's personal style and one's expectations of leader behavior.

Facility   Classroom.

Materials   Worksheet A: Leader Behavior (Self) Questionnaire.

Worksheet B: Scoring Key for "Initiating Structure."

Worksheet C: Scoring Key for "Consideration."

Worksheet D: Locating Scores on the Ohio State Leadership Studies Model.

Pencil or pen.

Time Required   Forty-five minutes to one hour.

Group Size   Unlimited.

Design   1. Instruct members to respond individually to the items in Worksheet A, following the directions on the instrument.

2. After completing Step 1, go to Worksheets B and C and follow the directions for scoring.

(continued)

---

*Adapted by permission from La Monica, Elaine L., *The Nursing Process: A Humanistic Approach*, pp. 376–384. Copyright © 1979 by Addison-Wesley Publishing Company, Inc., Menlo Park, Calif.

EXERCISE 1 *(continued)*

3. Go to Worksheet D and interpret scores on the model.

4. Discuss findings. Compare self with expectations.

Variations

Worksheet A can be given to an associate, a superior, and/or a follower. Their task is to rate you on how they feel you behave. Instruments can then be scored and compared with perceptions of self. Since behavior is as perceived by others, ratings scales filled out on your behavior lend support to your perceptions of self. A discussion of differences in perceptions among raters can be an excellent consciousness-raising activity. The mean score of different raters (including self) is the best indicator of leader behavior style.

EXERCISE 1
WORKSHEET A: Leader Behavior (Self) Questionnaire

This questionnaire is to determine your leadership style. Following is a list of items that may be used to describe your behavior as you think you act. This is not a test of ability. It simply asks you to describe how you believe you act as a leader of a group.

DIRECTIONS:

a. Read each item carefully.

b. Think about how frequently you engage in the behavior described by the item.

c. Decide whether you *always, often, occasionally, seldom,* or *never* act as described by the item.

d. Draw a circle around one of the five letters following the item to show the answer you have selected: A = always, B = often, C = occasionally, D = seldom, E = never.

When acting as a leader, I:

1. Do personal favors for group members.	A	B	C	D	E
2. Make my attitudes clear to the group.	A	B	C	D	E
3. Do little things to make it pleasant to be a member of the group.	A	B	C	D	E
4. Try out my new ideas with the group.	A	B	C	D	E
5. Act as the real leader of the group.	A	B	C	D	E
6. Am easy to understand.	A	B	C	D	E
7. Rule with an iron hand.	A	B	C	D	E
8. Find time to listen to group members.	A	B	C	D	E
9. Criticize poor work.	A	B	C	D	E
10. Give advance notice of changes.	A	B	C	D	E
11. Speak in a manner not to be questioned.	A	B	C	D	E
12. Keep to myself.	A	B	C	D	E
13. Look out for the personal welfare of individual group members.	A	B	C	D	E
14. Assign group members to particular tasks.	A	B	C	D	E
15. Am the spokesman of the group.	A	B	C	D	E

(continued)

EXERCISE 1
WORKSHEET A *(continued)*

16. Schedule the work to be done.   A B C D E
17. Maintain definite standards of perform-
    ance.   A B C D E
18. Refuse to explain my actions.   A B C D E
19. Keep the group informed.   A B C D E
20. Act without consulting the group.   A B C D E
21. Back up the members in their actions.   A B C D E
22. Emphasize the meeting of deadlines.   A B C D E
23. Treat all group members as my equals.   A B C D E
24. Encourage the use of uniform procedures.   A B C D E
25. Get what I ask for from my superiors.   A B C D E
26. Am willing to make changes.   A B C D E
27. Make sure that my part in the organization
    is understood by group members.   A B C D E
28. Am friendly and approachable.   A B C D E
29. Ask that group members follow standard
    rules and regulations.   A B C D E
30. Fail to take necessary action.   A B C D E
31. Make group members feel at ease when
    talking with them.   A B C D E
32. Let group members know what is
    expected of them.   A B C D E
33. Speak as the representative of the group.   A B C D E
34. Put suggestions made by the group into
    operation.   A B C D E
35. See to it that group members are working
    up to capacity.   A B C D E
36. Let other people take away my leadership
    in the group.   A B C D E
37. Get my superiors to act for the welfare of
    the group members.   A B C D E
38. Get group approval in important matters
    before going ahead.   A B C D E
39. See to it that the work of group members
    is coordinated.   A B C D E
40. Keep the group working together as a
    team.   A B C D E

Source: Worksheets A, B, and C copyright Ohio State University. Developed by staff
members of the Ohio State Leadership Studies, Center for Business and Economic
Research, Division of Research, College of Administrative Science, Ohio State University, Columbus. Reproduced by permission.

EXERCISE 1
WORKSHEET B: Scoring Key for "Initiating Structure"

SCORING INSTRUCTIONS: On the Leader Behavior (Self) Questionnaire, draw a circle around the questionnaire item numbers noted below (2, 4, 7, 9, etc.). On the left side of the questionnaire, beside each such item, write the score you get for each item. The appropriate score is determined by noting, as indicated below, the points for the response you made on the questionnaire. For example, if your response to question 2 was "seldom" you would put a "1" by question number 2 on your questionnaire. Do this for each of the 15 questions below. Add these 15 scores together. The total is your score for initiating structure. Transcribe the score in the space provided on Worksheet D.

Item No.	A Always	B Often	C Occasionally	D Seldom	E Never
2	4	3	2	1	0
4	4	3	2	1	0
7	4	3	2	1	0
9	4	3	2	1	0
11	4	3	2	1	0
14	4	3	2	1	0
16	4	3	2	1	0
17	4	3	2	1	0
22	4	3	2	1	0
24	4	3	2	1	0
27	4	3	2	1	0
29	4	3	2	1	0
32	4	3	2	1	0
35	4	3	2	1	0
39	4	3	2	1	0

(continued)

EXERCISE 1 *(continued)*
WORKSHEET C: Scoring Key for "Consideration"

SCORING INSTRUCTIONS: On the Leader Behavior (Self) Questionnaire, circle the questionnaire item numbers noted below (1, 3, 6, 8, etc.). On the left side of the questionnaire, beside each circled item, write the score you get for each item. The appropriate score is determined by noting, as indicated below, the points for the response you made on the questionnaire. For example, if your response to question 1 was "often" you would put a "3" by question number 1 on your questionnaire. Do this for each of the 15 questions below. Add the 15 scores. The total is your score for consideration. Transcribe this score in the space provided on Worksheet D. (Note that there are 10 questions "left over," which are not scored. These are in the questionnaire in order to maintain conditions comparable to when the questionnaire was standardized.)

Item No.	A Always	B Often	C Occasionally	D Seldom	E Never
1	4	3	2	1	0
3	4	3	2	1	0
6	4	3	2	1	0
8	4	3	2	1	0
12	0	1	2	3	4
13	4	3	2	1	0
18	0	1	2	3	4
20	0	1	2	3	4
21	4	3	2	1	0
23	4	3	2	1	0
26	4	3	2	1	0
28	4	3	2	1	0
31	4	3	2	1	0
34	4	3	2	1	0
38	4	3	2	1	0

EXERCISE 1
WORKSHEET D: Locating Scores on the Ohio State Leadership Studies Model

Self

Initiating Structure Score   _____
Consideration Score   _____

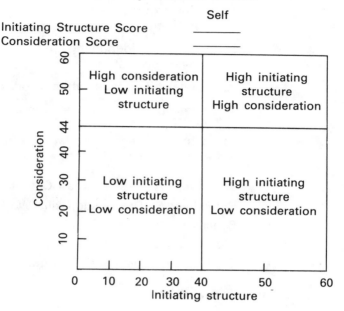

DIRECTIONS: After scoring the instrument, Worksheets B and C, indicate where your initiating structure scores place on that continuum, followed by your consideration scores. Draw the horizontal and vertical line from each axis until both meet. The box in which lines meet indicates your leadership style. Scores above 40 on the initiating structure dimension indicate you are above the mean. If you scored above 44 on the consideration dimension, you would also be above the mean.

The purpose of using this instrument is to begin the process of gaining awareness of your leader behavior. The Leader Behavior (Self) Questionnaire is a rough indicator. If your scores conform to your experience in dealing with others and their perception of you, then the instrument provides an excellent basis for further self-study.

Source: Copyright Ohio State University. Developed by staff members of the Ohio State Leadership Studies, Center for Business and Economic Research, Division of Research, College of Administrative Science, Ohio State University, Columbus. Reproduced by permission.

EXERCISE 2   Diagnosing the System

Purposes

1. To gain experience in specifying the priority problem in a case.

2. To practice identifying particular leader behavior styles.

3. To determine leader effectiveness.

4. To develop a problem solution.

Facility

Large room to accommodate learners working around tables of six to eight.

Materials

Worksheet A: Case—Urban City Hospital.

Worksheet B: Diagnostic Skills Worksheet.

Pencils or pens.

Blackboard and chalk.

Experts' Diagnosis and Rationale

Time Required

Two and one-half hours.

Group Size

Unlimited groups of six to eight.

Design

1. Each individual working independently and viewing self as an outside consultant is to:
   A. specify the priority problem goal in Urban City Hospital;
   B. identify the dominant leader behavior styles used by George Jones and May Conte;
   C. determine the organizational effectiveness of Urban City Hospital under the management of George Jones and May Conte;
   D. develop a problem solution; and

Source: Adapted by permission from La Monica, Elaine L., *The Nursing Process: A Humanistic Approach*, pp. 385–394. Copyright © 1979 by Addison-Wesley Publishing Company, Inc., Menlo Park, Calif.

E. write down detailed rationale for A–D. The rationale will serve as a basis for discussion in reaching group consensus (Step 2). Record individual determinations on the Diagnostic Skills Worksheet (30 minutes).

2. Following the individual diagnosis, each work group of six to eight should then reach consensus as to the problem goal, solution, leader behavior styles of the characters, and their organizational effectiveness. The group should attempt to reach unanimous consensus. A group recorder must be chosen to record the group decisions (45 minutes to one hour).

3. Form into a total group and have each recorder share the work group's decisions and discuss rationale. Record decisions on a blackboard using the following suggested format:

PROBLEM/GOAL	LEADERSHIP STYLE		EFFECTIVENESS		SOLUTION
	Jones	Conte	Jones	Conte	
Group 1					
Group 2					
Group 2					

4. Refer to the discussion section and share the interpretations from the experts' diagnosis and rationale.

5. Discuss the experience.

(continued)

EXERCISE 2 *(continued)*

Variations

1. The individual diagnosis can be given as a homework assignment.
2. The exercise can be used only to identify leader behavior styles and leader effectiveness, deleting the aspects of specifying a problem and developing a solution. This is recommended if the exercise is used after studying Chapters 4 and 5 and prior to completing Chapters 6 and 7.

*Discussion Based on Experts' Diagnosis and Rationale:**

Problem/Goal

The problem is that the time clock policy is being applied inconsistently. There may be other potential problems in the case, but managers should identify the simplest, most tractable present problem and attack it. The time clock problem has the potential for erupting in such a way that people may be labeled dishonest or commanded to attend to a policy under threat; such would undoubtedly decrease productivity.

Leadership Styles

Leader behavior is as perceived by others. George Jones exhibited low structure and low consideration behavior—he was not constantly telling followers what needed to be done, how to do it, when to do it, and so forth. Neither was he observed involving staff members in two-way communication or in establishing interpersonal rapport.

Given the data provided, May Conte was considered to be high consideration and low structure because she was observed relating with the group, giving support and reinforce-

*The experts are K. Blanchard and P. Hersey. Oral presentation, School of Education, University of Massachusetts, 1974.

ment, and establishing a team. One did not observe Conte defining facets of task accomplishment. Even though the case did not portray Conte as high task, it could be assumed safely that such a manager also directed the task. It can be said, therefore, that Conte's basic style was high consideration and low structure, while her supporting style was high structure and high consideration.

Effectiveness

Organizational effectiveness under the management of May Conte and George Jones should be evaluated on the four variables discussed in Chapter 5. It is easy to create a halo or horn effect and judge a manager's overall effectiveness on the basis of one or two traits that are important to the evaluator. If the manager has the trait, then the manager is good in everything, and vice versa. This effect is tempered significantly by rating a manager on each variable, summing the ratings and dividing by the number of variables to get an average effectiveness rating.

Since the scale of −4 to +4 is arbitrary, it is simplest to say that Jones and Conte were +4 unless a negative point in the area is noted. Remember that manager effectiveness should be judged on the basis of the majority of who or what is being evaluated. There will always be the unreachable or the spurious.

Both managers were considered excellent. Jones, however, was slightly more effective than Conte. The case is designed to bring out the halo-horn effect because most groups see Conte as the more effective manager. Conte is certainly more likeable because one gets a feel for her personality and one knows more about her. Also, it is easy

(continued)

EXERCISE 2 *(continued)*

to say that Jones should not be credited with success because he does not do anything. Such a conclusion relates only to the evaluator's past experience with a low structure and low consideration manager who behaved that way because she or he did not care. LB4, however, is a legitimate strategy, and one must believe that Jones is behaving this way because that is what his followers require. To think otherwise would be aiming to perpetuate a previous negative experience. What would have happened to Conte's group if Jones had started to tell Conte what to do and sought invitation to the group's social events? This author sees beginning disaster.

Solution

The solution is to get rid of the time clock or to appoint a committee to make recommendations on this problem. Policies are placed because of a need by the majority of the group. Once passed, policies tend to live forever, even though this should not occur. Policies need to be reevaluated to see if they best serve the majority of people in the organization. Is the policy what is needed given their level of maturity? A time clock is a high task intervention and obviously is not required given the majority at Urban City Hospital. The hospital is running beautifully, and the work is getting done. There will always be a couple of freedom abusers as will there be obsessive workers. *Policies, however, must reflect the needs of the majority.*

Experts' Diagnosis of Organizational Effectiveness

Variable	Jones	Conte	Discussion
1. Causal Variables • Leadership strategies • Management's decisions • Organizational philosophy, policies, and objectives.	+2		Two points were deducted because Jones had a policy in the hospital that was abused. His management style was appropriate given the level of maturity of his immediate followers.
		+2	Two points were deducted because Conte did not attend to the time clock policy. While a policy is in effect, it should be supported. If the policy seems inappropriate, do something to change it—it should not be ignored. Conte's management style was appropriate given the follower's level of maturity.
2. Intervening Variables • Employees' personal commitment to objectives and growth • Motivation and morale	+4	+4	The majority of people being led by Jones and Conte were happy, committed, and growing within the organization.
3. Output variables • Production • Costs • Earnings • Turnover	+4	+4	From the perspective of both managers, output was excellent. The hospital was not in the red, clients were satisfied, quality of care was very good, and people would rather work there than any place else. Conte's group also always got their work done.
4. Long-term and short-term goals	+4		Immediate output of the hospital was excellent, and there is no reason not to believe that this

(*continued*)

EXERCISE 2 *(continued)*

Experts' Diagnosis of Organizational Effectiveness

Variable	Jones	Conte	Discussion
			would continue. Jones's followers functioned effectively when he was in LB4—low structure and low consideration.
		+3	Output of Conte's group was excellent, and this would most likely continue. Conte's group was not able to function effectively without steady input from her, however, which is evident since Conte was appropriately in LB2 or LB3—high structure and consideration or high consideration and low structure.
Totals:	14 +4 = 3.50	13 +4 = 3.25	

Generally speaking, Urban City Hospital was an effectively running organization and both Conte and Jones were excellent leaders. There is every reason to believe that this time clock issue would be handled effectively and that both managers would continue to improve.

EXERCISE 2
WORKSHEET A: CASE—Urban City Hospital*

Janis Monroe, Executive Director of Urban City Hospital, was concerned by reports of absenteeism among some of the staff. From reliable sources, she had learned that some of the staff were punching the time cards of fellow workers who were arriving late or leaving early. Monroe had only recently been appointed to head Urban City Hospital. She judged from conversations with the previous director and other administrators that people were, in general, pleased with the overall performance of the hospital.

Urban City Hospital has a reputation for quality medical care with a particularly good reputation in the areas of coronary care, intensive care, and emergency care. Located in the center of Urban

---

*Source: The author of this case is unknown. This author received it at the School of Education, University of Massachusetts, 1974.

City, the hospital draws many lower socioeconomic families from that area but also services many clients from the suburban areas. The staff, with various educational backgrounds and training, were generally from the small state in which Urban City is located. In fact, a number of nurses are graduates of the hospital's nursing program.

It is thought that clients usually enter Urban Hospital for one of the following reasons:

■ High quality of care

■ Somewhat lower costs than other nearby facilities

■ Variety of medical care available.

George Jones, a long-time employee in the hospital, was administrator of Urban City Hospital. He generally left the staff alone, spending most of his time scheduling personnel, procuring funds and supplies, overseeing budget matters, and tending to related issues. Jones had an assistant, Rudy Lucas. When he needed to communicate with people in a particular area, George would just call them together or talk to an individual in the area and ask him to "pass the word." The latter was his usual approach.

Work situations at the hospital were quite varied. Some laboratories were cramped and less than adequate by some standards for the job required, whereas others more than met minimum criteria. Work efficiency did not seem to be related to these circumstances.

It should be noted that as far as hospitals are concerned, Urban City Hospital was one of the finest in the area. Clients generally liked their care and spoke highly of the facility.

The pay scale for the staff was low compared with other similar facilities. The average starting salary for a nurse was about $600 per week, and the age of the building made working conditions generally more difficult than might be desirable.

Judy Mulry, a first-year administrative assistant to the director, provided the data for this case. After she had been working at the hospital for a month or so, Mulry noted that certain members of the staff tended to seek each other out during free time and after hours. She then observed that these informal associations were enduring, built upon common activities and shared ideas about what was and what was not legitimate behavior in the hospital.

(continued)

EXERCISE 2
WORKSHEET A (continued)

Her estimate of these associations is diagrammed in Exhibit 1. The hospital responsibility for each person is given.

The Conte group, so named because May Conte was its most respected member and the one who seemed to take responsibility for maintaining good relations within the group, was the largest. The group invariably tried to eat lunch together and operated as a team, regardless of the differences in individual assignments. Off the job, Conte's group members often joined parties or got together for weekend trips. Conte's summer camp was a frequent rendezvous.

Conte's group was also the most cohesive one in the hospital in terms of its organized punch-in punch-out systems. The time clock system for the staff had been started three years before by the Board of Trustees, which had been taken over by a conservative element. There might be times, however, when an individual staff member would have completed any specific responsibilities from one-half to three-quarters of an hour prior to the scheduled time to leave. If there were errands or other things to do that extra free time would help, another member of the group would punch out for the one who left early. The "right" to leave early was informally balanced among the members of the group. In addition, the group members would punch a staff member "in" if he or she were unavoidably late.

Conte explained the logic behind the system to Mulry.

"You know we don't get paid as well here as in other hospitals," she said. "What makes this the best hospital to work in is that we are not continually bothered by administrators. When things are under control, as they are now, and the clients are satisfied, the top brass seems to be happy. It seems silly to have to stay to punch out on those few occasions when a little extra free time would be of help to you. Of course, some people abuse this sort of thing. . . like Marsha. . . but the members of our group get the job done and it all averages out."

"When there is extra work, naturally I stay as late as necessary. So do a lot of others. I believe that if I stay until the work is done and everything is in order, that's all the administration expects of us. They leave us alone and expect the job to get done. . . and we do."

McBride
  Executive
  housekeeper

Harris
  Assistant
  housekeeper

Mulry
  Administrative
  assistant

Smith
  Accountant

Blanche
  Food service
  manager

Kane
  Dietician

Lucas
  Assistant
  administrator

G. Jones
  Administrator

Roberto
  Assistant
  laboratory
  manager

Conte
  Laboratory
  manager

Pellegrini
  Pharmacist

Luciano
  In-service
  education

Venko
  Pharmacist

Impolitto
  Physical
  therapist

Nappa
  X-ray
  technologist

Roberts
  Controller
          Leighton
          Credit
          manager
Parant
  Business office
  manager

Manfred
  Director, plant
  operations

Proctor
  Operating room
  supervisor

Pope
  Assistant
  supervisor,
  registered nurse

Patti
  Supervisor,
  admitting

Roman
  Supervisor, records

Johnson
  Supervisor,
  registered nurse

Jones
  Supervisor,
  registered nurse

Spaulding
  Discharge planner
  registered nurse

EXHIBIT 1:   Urban City Hospital Staff, Informal Groupings

(*continued*)

EXERCISE 2
WORKSHEET A (continued)

When Mulry asked Conte if she would not rather work at a newer hospital at a higher salary, she just laughed and said, "Never."

The members of Conte's group were explicit about what constituted a good job. Customarily, they cited Marsha Jones, who happened to be the administrator's sister, as a woman who continually let others down. Mulry received an informal orientation from Marsha during her first few days at the hospital. As Marsha put it: "I've worked at this hospital for years, and I expect to stay here a good many more. You're just starting out, and you don't know the lay of the land yet. Working in a hospital is tough enough without breaking your neck. You can wear yourself out fast if you're not smart. Look at Manfred, the director of plant operations. There's a guy who's just going to burn himself out, and for what? He makes it tough on everybody and on himself, too."

Mulry reported further on her observations of the group activities: "May and her group couldn't understand Marsha. While Marsha arrived late a good deal of the time, May was usually early. If a series of emergency situations had created a backlog of work, almost everyone but Marsha would spend extra time to help catch up. May and members of her group would always stay later. While most of the staff seemed to find a rather full life in their work, Marsha never got really involved. No wonder they couldn't understand each other."

"There was quite a different feeling about Bob Manfred, the director of plant operations. Not only did he work his full shift, but he often scheduled meetings with maintenance and other plant personnel on other shifts to consider better ways of getting their jobs done. He was also taking courses in the evening to complete the requirements for a degree. He often worked many Saturdays and Sundays. . . and all for 'peanuts.' He hardly got paid a cent extra. Because of the tremendous variance in responsibilities, it was hard to make comparisons, but I'm sure I wouldn't be far wrong in saying that Bob worked twice as hard as Marsha and 50% more than almost anyone else in the hospital. No one but Marsha and a few old-timers criticized him for his efforts. May and her group seemed to feel a distant affection for Bob, but the only contact they or anyone else had with him consisted of brief greetings."

"To the members of May's group, the most severe penalty that could be inflicted was exclusion. This they did to both Manfred and Marsha. Manfred, however, was tolerated; Marsha was not. Evidently, Marsha felt her exclusion keenly, though she answered it with derision and aggression. Marsha kept up a steady stream of stories concerning her attempt to gain acceptance outside working hours. She wrote popular music, which was always rejected by publishers. She attempted to join several social and literary clubs, mostly without success. Her favorite pastime was attending concerts. She told me that 'music lovers' were friendly, and she enjoyed meeting new people whenever she went to a concert. But she was particularly quick to explain that she preferred to keep her distance from the other people on the staff at the hospital."

"May's group emphasized more than just effort in judging a person's work. Among them had grown a confidence that they could develop and improve on the efficiency of any responsibility. May herself symbolized this. Before her, May's father had been an effective laboratory manager and helped May a great deal. When problems arose, the director and other staff would frequently consult with May, and she would give counsel willingly. She had a special feeling for her job. For example, when a young lab technician couldn't seem to get off the ground, May was the only one who successfully stepped in and probably saved a promising young technician. To a lesser degree, the other members of the group were also imaginative about solving problems that arose in their own areas."

"Marsha, for her part, talked incessantly about her accomplishments. As far as I could tell during the year I worked in the hospital, there was little evidence to support these stories. In fact, many of the other staff members laughed at her. What's more, I never saw anyone seek Marsha's help."

"Willingness to be of help was a trait the staff associated with Conte and was prized. The most valued help of all was a personal kind, though the jobs were also important."

"The members of Conte's group were constantly lending and borrowing money, cars, and equipment among themselves and, less frequently, with other members of the hospital staff."

"Marsha refused to help others in any way. She never tried to aid those around her who were in the midst of a rush of work,

(*continued*)

EXERCISE 2
WORKSHEET A (continued)

though this was customary throughout most of the hospital. I can distinctly recall the picture of the day supervisor trying to handle an emergency situation at about 3 PM one day while Marsha continued a casual telephone conversation. She acted as if she didn't even notice the supervisor. She, of course, expected me to act this same way, and it was this attitude in her I found virtually intolerable."

"More than this, Marsha took little responsibility for breaking in new nurses, leaving this entirely to the assistant supervisor. There had been four new nurses on her shift in the space of a year. Each had asked for a transfer to another shift, publicly citing personal reasons associated with the 7—3 shift but privately blaming Marsha. May was the one who taught me the ropes when I first joined the staff."

"The staff who congregated around Pat Johnson were primarily nursing supervisors, but as a group tended to behave similarly to the Conte group, though they did not quite approach the creativity or the amount of helping activities that May's group did. They were, however, all considered 'good' in their jobs. Sometimes the Johnson group sought outside social contact with the Conte group. Even though they worked in different areas, both groups seemed to respect each other; and several times a year, the two groups went out on the town together."

"The remainder of the people in the hospital stayed pretty much to themselves or associated in pairs or triplets. None of these people were as inventive, as helpful, or as productive as Conte's or Johnson's groups, but most of them gave verbal support to the same values as those groups held."

"The distinction between the two organized groups and the rest of the hospital was clearest in the punching-out routine. McBride and Harris, Blanche and Kane, and Roberts, Parant, and Leighton arranged within their small groups for any early punchouts. George Jones was frequently out of the building during any punch-outs, and he didn't seem to pay attention to such things like the time clock anyway. His assistant, Lucas, although always in the hospital, wasn't seen by many people. He seemed to 'hide' in his office. Jones and Patti had no early punch-out organization to rely upon. Marsha was reported to have established an arrangement with Patti whereby the latter would punch Marsha out for a fee.

Such a practice was unthinkable from the point of view of Conte's group. Marsha constantly complained about the dishonesty of other members of the staff in the hospital."

"Just before I left Urban City to take another position, I casually met Ms. Monroe on the street. She asked me how I had enjoyed my experience at Urban City Hospital. During the conversation, I learned that she knew of the punch-out system. What's more, she told me she was wondering if she ought to 'blow the lid off the whole mess'."

(continued)

EXERCISE 2
WORKSHEET B: Diagnostic Skills Worksheet (*continued*)

Problem (Individual Diagnosis) _____

_____

_____

Problem (Group Diagnosis) _____

_____

_____

LEADER BEHAVIOR STYLE—Indicate dominant style with a checkmark for each character.

LEADERSHIP STYLE	INDIVIDUAL DIAGNOSIS		GROUP DIAGNOSIS	
	George Jones	May Conte	George Jones	May Conte
High structure and low consideration				
High structure and high consideration				
High consideration and low structure				
Low structure and low consideration				

EFFECTIVENESS DIMENSION—Indicate by a checkmark your determination of the degree of effectiveness or ineffectiveness for each character in the case.

	Ineffective							Effective
	−4	−3	−2	−1	+1	+2	+3	+4
INDIVIDUAL DIAGNOSIS: George Jones								
May Conte								
GROUP DIAGNOSIS: George Jones								
May Conte								

Solution (Individual) _____

_____

_____

Solution (Group) _____

_____

_____

EXERCISE 3   Diagnosing the Task

Purpose

To practice applying the Vroom and Yetton managerial decision-making model.

Facility

Large room to accommodate learners working in groups of six to eight.

Materials

Table 6.1: Management Decision Styles.
Worksheet A: Cases 1, 2, and 3.
Figure 6.2: Decision Model.
Blackboard and chalk.

Time Required

One and one-half hours.

Group Size

Unlimited groups of six to eight.

Design

1. Individuals working alone are to read each case on Worksheet A and choose the decision style they (as individuals) would use if they were the manager in each situation. Record responses and rationale for decisions in the spaces provided after each case (15 minutes).

2. After completing Step 1, individuals in each work group of six to eight should then discuss their choices for decision styles with each other, citing reasons for each selection. A recorder for each group should write down the group consensus by majority vote (30 to 45 minutes).

3. Following discussion in small groups, form into a total group and have the recorders share the group's decisions and rationale. Record decisions on a blackboard using the following suggested format:

(continued)

EXERCISE 3 *(continued)*

	Case 1	Case 2	Case 3
Group 1			
Group 2			
Group 3			

4. In the total group, use the decision model to determine the diagnosis of each task. Refer to the discussion section and hold an open discussion case by case for each of the three examples. Compare decision styles arrived at by consensus (displayed on the blackboard) with those determined by application of the decision model.

Discussion

Case # 1:

A. Quality	Yes
B. Manager's information	Yes
C. Acceptance	No
Minimum-time decision style	AI

There is a quality requirement, and since the head nurse has been in that position for ten years, it is reasonably certain that he or she would possess the information to make a high-quality decision. The nurses are only concerned that supplies be available; therefore they have to accept nothing. Once supplies are ordered and stocked, the problem is alleviated; people must live with the results. Since AI can be used given the task, all styles could be used depending on how much time is available. A head nurse who wanted to develop problem-solving skills in followers could use this task to accomplish it.

Case #2:

A. Quality   No

B. Acceptance   Yes

C. Prior probability of acceptance   No

Minimum-time decision style   GII

There is no quality requirement since who attends the conference does not affect staffing. The decision must be accepted by the staff, and it is doubtful whether a supervisor's judgment would be accepted. The wise supervisor, therefore, would not use any style above GII and might even delegate the task (DI) by letting the nurses make a decision among themselves.

Case #3:

A. Quality   Yes

B. Manager's information   No

C. Structure   No

D. Acceptance   Yes

E. Prior probability of acceptance   Yes

Minimum-time decision style   CII

There is definitely a quality requirement; one location may be better than another. The manager needs to have the staff assess the district in order to make a wise choice. The problem is not structured because there is a subjective element in making the decision—"what feels right"—and the executive director does not know exactly what information is needed to make the decision. The case says that the staff are willing to accede to the director's judgment. CII is the decision style that would require the least amount of time but GII might be used, especially if the manager wishes the group to

(*continued*)

EXERCISE 3 *(continued)*

mature so that there is less of a need for manager reliance.

Variations

1. Teaching designs for in-service education
   and for ongoing units can be found in the
   original article: La Monica, E., & Finch, F.
   (1977). Managerial decision-making. *Journal
   of Nursing Administration, 7,* 20–28.

2. Further cases that have been adapted from
   business examples are in the following: Tay-
   lor, A. (1978). Decision making in nursing: An
   analytical approach. *Journal of Nursing Administration, 8,* 22–30.

3. Cases can be developed by individuals as a
   homework assignment and then discussed in
   small groups.

EXERCISE 3
WORKSHEET A: Case 1

You are the head nurse of a 50-bed orthopedic unit that is the first group to move to a new wing in one week. You must estimate the supplies and medications necessary to stock on the new floor so that nursing care can be maintained smoothly and without interruption.

Since you have been head nurse for ten years on this unit, you have the knowledge and experience necessary to evaluate approximately what you will need. It is important that nothing be forgotten since surgery will be uninterrupted, and fresh postoperative patients will be arriving from surgery as well as preoperative patients needing preparation. Absent supplies may result in delayed surgery, confusion, frustrated personnel, and poor nursing care. It is your practice to meet regularly with your managerial subordinates to discuss the problems of running the floor. These meetings have resulted in the creation and development of a very effective team.

Decision style you would use: _____
Rationale: _____
_____
_____

Case 2

You are the nursing coordinator of 12 registered nurses in an intensive care unit. Their formal education, responsibilities, and experience are very similar, providing for an extremely close-knit group who share responsibilities. Yesterday, your director of nurses informed you that she would supply funds for four of your nurses to attend the National Critical Care Nursing Association Convention for five days in San Francisco.

It is your perception that all of your nurses would very much like to attend, and from the standpoint of staffing there is no particular reason why any one should attend over any other. The

(*continued*)

EXERCISE 3
WORKSHEET A (continued)

problem is somewhat complicated by the fact that all of the nurses are active officers and members of the local organization.

Decision style you would use: _____

Rationale: _____

_____

_____

Case 3

You are the executive director of a small but growing midwestern Visiting Nurse's Association. The rural location and consumer needs are factors that contribute to the emphasis on expanded roles in nursing practice at all levels.

When you took the position five years ago, the nursing care was poor, and finances were slim. Under your leadership, much progress has been made. You obtained state and federal monies and personally educated your nursing resources. This progress has been achieved while the economy has moved into a mild recession, and, as a result, your prestige among your colleagues and staff is very high. Your success, which you are inclined to attribute principally to good luck and to a few timely decisions on your part, has, in your judgment, one unfortunate by-product. It has caused your staff to look to you for leadership and guidance in decision making beyond what you consider necessary. You have no doubts about their capabilities, but wish they were not quite so willing to accede to your judgment.

You have recently acquired a grant to permit opening a satellite branch. Your problem is to decide on the best location. You believe that there is no formula in this selection process; it will be made by assessment of community needs, lack of available resources, and "what feels right." You have asked your staff to assess their districts since their knowledge about the community in which they practice should be extremely useful in making a wise choice.

Their support is essential because the success of the satellite will be highly dependent on their willingness to initially staff and then educate and assist new nurses during its early days. Currently, your staff is small enough for everyone to feel and function as a team; you want this to continue.

The success of the satellite will benefit everybody. Directly they will benefit from the expansion, and indirectly they will reap the personal and professional advantages of being involved in the building and expansion of nursing services.

Decision style you would use: _____

Rationale: _____

_____

Source: La Monica, E., & Finch, F. (1977). Managerial decision-making. *Journal of Nursing Administration, 7*, 21–22. Reproduced by permission.

The first two nursing situations were adapted from business examples. The original material is presented in Vroom, V. H. (1973). A new look at managerial decision making. *Organization Dynamics, 1*, 72–73. The third adaptation is originally found in Vroom, V. H., & Jago, A. G. (1974). Decision making as a social process. *Decision Sciences, 5*, 750.

EXERCISE 4   **Term Project—Independent Case Analysis**

Purposes

1. To carry out the steps of the problem-solving method.

2. To apply theory and research findings in analyzing a nursing situation.

3. To report the results formally.

Facility

A clinical setting where learners work with a group of people (professional and nonprofessional) in the delivery of health care.

Materials

Worksheet A: Evaluation of Written Assignment.

Paper and a typewriter.

Time Required

Variable, but generally a term project.

Group Size

Not applicable.

Design

1. Each learner is to develop a personal case experience as a leader, a follower, or a consultant, and analyze what is happening (or has happened) in the situation.

2. The problem-solving method should be applied using individually selected theories to diagnose the system and choose the appropriate leader behavior style.

3. The paper is a formal project. It must be typed doublespace, using an approved style and format. References must be included and the paper's maximum length should be 30 pages.

4. Worksheet A: Evaluation of Written Assignment will be the basis on which the paper will be graded. This worksheet can be used as an outline for the paper.

Variation

Grade determinations can be adjusted according to teacher preference.

EXERCISE 4
WORKSHEET A: Evaluation of Written Assignment

I. Synthesis of Theoretic Framework Used in Analysis (10 points)

II. Problem Identification and Definition (20 points)

III. Problem Analysis (30 points)

IV. Alternative Actions with Anticipated Results for Each (20 points)

V. Recommended Action and Rationale (10 points)

VI. Style and Format (10 points)

(*continued*)

EXERCISE 4
Worksheet A (*continued*)
GRADING SCALE:

A+	100	B+	90–92	C+	80–82
A	97–99	B	87–89	C	77–79
A–	93–96	B–	83–86	C–	73–76
				F	72 and below

EXERCISE 5   Ethics—Managerial Dilemma

Purpose

To gain experience in discussing and problem-solving managerial dilemmas that have ethical implications.

Facility

Large room to accommodate participants seated in groups of six.

Materials

Worksheet A: A Managerial Dilemma
Paper and Pencil or Pen

Time Required   One hour

Group Size   Unlimited groups of six

Design

1. Participants should consider themselves as nurse managers. Using the managerial dilemma described in Worksheet A, ask participants to individually respond to the following questions:
   A. What is the problem? Is there an ethical problem?
   B. Who is involved?
   C. What is the context?
   D. Is anything interfering or possibly interfering with an individual's rights to freedom while away from the employing organization? Is privacy invaded or potentially invaded?
   E. Are patient's rights involved? Are staff member's rights involved?
   F. What alternatives exist?

2. In groups of six, participants should share and discuss their responses. Different per-

(continued)

Source: The content for this exercise was prepared by Elizabeth M. Maloney, author of Chapter 8 on Managerial Ethics. The exercise was put into the format used in this book by Elaine L. La Monica.

EXERCISE 5 (*continued*)

ceptions between/among learners should receive particular attention.

3. Small groups should report on their thoughts to the large group of the whole.

Variations

1. Step 1 may be done as a homework assignment.

2. Individuals or small groups can develop other managerial dilemmas and use the same process for discussion and problem-solving. The dilemmas may be done as part of a homework assignment.

3. The entire exercise can be a written homework assignment that is carried out by individual learners or dyads.

EXERCISE 5
WORKSHEET A: A Managerial Dilemma

Due to the shortage of registered nurses, your agency employs nurses three days a week, in twelve hour shifts. Susan Jones, one of these employed nurses, begins to make small but important errors at work. She oversleeps and is often late enough that co-workers have begun to complain. Susan also seems irritable and tired.

It comes to your attention indirectly that this individual, Susan Jones, is working the same 3-day pattern at another hospital. You feel strongly that it is only a matter of time before serious mistakes in patient care will occur. There are no regulations prohibiting such employment practices.

Part III

MANAGEMENT SKILLS

The purpose of Part III of this book is to discuss the skills managers need to carry out the steps of the management process—planning, organizing, motivating, and controlling—described in Part I.

Chapter topics are related specifically to management and leadership and are not meant to be all-inclusive. A conceptual framework is provided for each area, and discussion focuses on basic skills that can be augmented and amplified by the manager through experience and continued education. The basic management skills are discussed in separate chapters even though all of the topics are interrelated. Areas that are covered in this part of the book are: communication, change, power, teaching, interviewing, assertiveness, group dynamics, conflict resolution, time management, and performance evaluation. Experiential exercises for topics conclude Part III.

Communication

Communication is the most important skill in nursing management and leadership. As a matter of fact, it is probably the most important concept in life. Communication occurs in every step of the management process; **everything** that a manager does involves communication—with followers, with superiors, and with associates. Kepler (1980) accepted communication as the most critical task that leaders must master; this position has been widely supported in research investigations (Anderson, 1984; Pincus, 1986; Tjosvold, 1984).

Chapter 9 begins with a definition of communication followed by a theoretic perspective on the communication process and the purposes of communication. Types of communications are then presented; how leaders communicate concludes the chapter.

DEFINITION OF COMMUNICATION

Communication would not be necessary if human beings existed in a vacuum, autonomously going through life in an impermeable cell; if they were born, lived, and died in isolation from others; or if individuals reached only within the self to fulfill needs. Humans are social beings who are dependent, independent, and interdependent on others in the environment. The only vehicle for reaching out to closely related others in the environment is communication through languages—both verbal (French, Italian, German, and so forth) and nonverbal (body language and gestures understood by particular cultures) (La Monica, 1985).

Shannon and Weaver (1949) defined communication as all that occurs between two or more minds. Since behavior is what other people perceive, all behavior is communication, and all communication produces behavior. Davis and Newstrom (1985) defined communication as "the transfer of information and understanding from one person to another person" (p. 424). It is the bridge between people. Johnson (1986) saw the concept as a means for one person to relay a message to another, expecting a response.

Communication, therefore, always involves a sender and a receiver. Even though Gibran (1951) said that one can verbally speak with self, communication in organizations always includes at least two people and both roles of sender and receiver. Davis and Newstrom (1985) aptly pointed out that a manager sending a written message to a follower has communicated the message only when the follower receives, reads, and understands the message.

THE COMMUNICATION PROCESS

The communication process involves five basic steps, portrayed in Figure 9.1 (Berlo, 1960; Chartier, 1981; Davis & Newstrom, 1985; Hein, 1980; Hewitt, 1981; Johnson, 1986; Long & Prophit, 1981; Miller, 1966; Pluckhan, 1978).

The sender has an idea and a wish to communicate that idea to another person. Davis and Newstrom (1985) cogently asserted that senders must think before sending a message; this step is critical. Once a sender has the idea clearly in mind, then the appropriate language(s) for communicating the idea must be selected. It is necessary to consider nonverbal body language as well as verbal language. Remember that management and leadership involve conscious, identifiable strategies for all behaviors. Choose language that has the highest probability for sending the message accurately and for being received accurately.

After a message has been encoded, it is transmitted by the sender over selected nonverbal and/or verbal channels. The receiver, who must be tuned into the sender's channels, receives the message and decodes it back from language to an idea. The receiver acts in

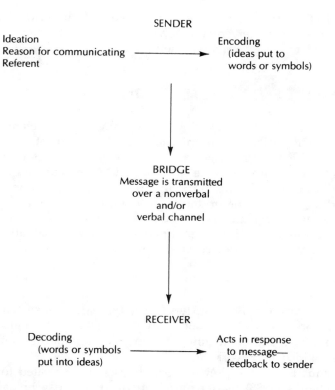

Figure 9.1 The communication process.

response to the decoded message. The message may be stored or ignored; the receiver may communicate another idea back to the sender, or the receiver may simply perform a task in response to the message.

Whatever the receiver does in response to the sender's message is called feedback, which is a message sent back to the sender. The receiver then becomes the sender and the communication process begins again. Such circularity continues until communication ceases.

Evaluating feedback is a way for the sender to validate that the message has been perceived according to intent. The goal of any communication, of course, is congruence between the sender's intended message and the receiver's perceived message. Validation is essential because people communicate and perceive in response to individual attitudes, knowledge, and experience (Berlo, 1960). Perception is selective. Hence, what is transmitted on "the bridge" (Figure 9.1) may not be perceived as such. If necessary, further messages may be used to clarify original intent.

PURPOSES OF COMMUNICATION

The overall purpose for managing and leading is to motivate systems to accomplish goals. Communication to and with others is "the bridge" by which the manager and the human resources in a system relate. A manager must be able to communicate effectively in order to truly fulfill the role. Furthermore, it is the manager's responsibility to build and to maintain the bridge even though other human resources participate in its design and structure; the manager is the leader. Davis and Newstrom (1985) identified the following equation when discussing the purposes of communication:

The skill to work + the will to work = teamwork

It is evident from von Bertalanffy's (1968, 1975) general system theory that teamwork has a high probability for resulting in high quality, decreased costs, and high employee morale. Communication is the bridge on which teamwork rests.

The equation in the previous paragraph can be related to Hersey and Blanchard's (1988) theory on job maturity and psychological maturity. In the theory, the manager wishes to have human resources in a goal-directed system both willing and able. Then the system will accomplish the task because the people are intrinsically motivated and have the required knowledge and experience. Hersey and Blanchard's label *ability* seems parallel with Davis's (1985) term *skill*. Human resources who are not able must be provided with the information necessary to make them skillful. The attitude of willingness, which fosters teamwork, motivation, and job satisfaction, is communicated also.

Hewitt (1981) delineated more specific purposes for which communication processes are used. It is pointed out that the following purposes are rarely, if ever, used in isolation of one another.

1. To learn or to teach something;
2. To influence someone's behavior;
3. To express feelings;

4. To explain one's own behavior or to clarify another's behavior;
5. To relate with others;
6. To untangle a problem;
7. To accomplish a goal;
8. To reduce tension or to resolve conflict; and
9. To stimulate interest in self or in others.

TYPES OF COMMUNICATION

There are two basic types of communication: verbal and nonverbal. Each type can be further broken into one-way or two-way communication. Figure 9.2 illustrates these points.

Everything that is written or spoken is included in verbal communication. Verbal interactions between/among superiors and followers, associates and associates, nurses and patients, nurses and other members of the health-care team, and so forth, form the bases for verbal communication. Written memoranda, bulletin board notices and meeting announcements, newspaper items, written requests, written assignments, and other similar items are also verbal communications.

Nonverbal communication is body language—it is unspoken and unwritten but nevertheless powerfully communicated through the body's behavior. People nonverbally communicate through gestures,

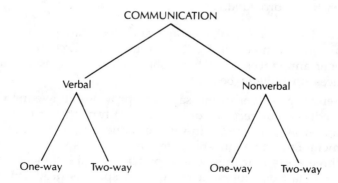

Figure 9.2 Types of communication.

posture, eye contact, facial expressions, space variations, voice volume and tone, and so forth. Both the content and the intensity of interactions between or among individuals is greatly influenced by nonverbal communication. Differences between what a speaker is feeling and saying are often nonverbally communicated to the listener. Even though nonverbal communication amplifies, contradicts, and/or augments what is being communicated verbally, nonverbal communication, like silence, can stand alone.

James (1932) attempted to organize available information into a method for analyzing behavior. It was suggested that leaning the body forward communicated a positive attitude toward the addressee whereas leaning the body backward communicated a negative attitude. There are many early research findings in this area: Fast (1970), Hall (1966), Mehrabian (1968, 1969), and Scheflin (1964), to name a few. Walters (1977) concisely specified research findings in various nonverbal attending skills with effective and ineffective uses of each—Table 9.1.

One-way communication means that the message is sent from the sender to the receiver; it involves no feedback from the receiver back to the sender. Two-way communication uses feedback. Johnson (1986) continued this basic definition by saying that one-way communication occurs when the sender cannot perceive how the receiver is decoding the message. Two-way communication takes place when the sender receives feedback or validation. Referring back to the components of leader behavior discussed in Chapter 5, structure involves one-way communication, and consideration involves two-way communication. Both types of communication are used for verbal and nonverbal interactions in leadership and management. Some examples of each are provided.

1. Sender gives verbal message and does not provide an avenue or time for feedback (one-way). *Example:* Manager announces a luncheon staff meeting by posting notices on bulletin boards.

2. Sender gives verbal message and provides an avenue for feedback but receiver does not comply with the request (one-way). *Example:* In-service educator sends out a memorandum requesting staff nurses to specify one of three areas that they would prefer to be the topic of the next staff development meeting. A space is provided on the memorandum to respond. No responses, however, are received.

TABLE 9.1 Attending Skills

Ineffective Use	Nonverbal Modes of Communication	Effective Use
Doing any of these things will probably close off or slow down the conversation.		These behaviors encourage talk because they show acceptance and respect for the other person.
Distant; very close	Space	Approximate arms-length
Spread among activities	Attention	Given fully to talker
Away	Movement	Toward
Slouching; rigid; seated leaning away	Posture	Relaxed but attentive; seated leaning slightly toward
Absent; defiant; jittery	Eye contact	Regular
You continue with what you are doing before responding; in a hurry	Time	Respond at first opportunity; share time with them
Used to keep distance between the persons	Feet and legs (in sitting)	Unobtrusive
Used as a barrier	Furniture	Used to draw persons together
Sloppy; garish; provocative	Dress; grooming	Tasteful
Does not match feelings; scowl; blank look	Facial expression	Matches your own or other's feelings; smile
Compete for attention with your words	Gestures	Highlight your words; unobtrusive; smooth
Obvious, distracting	Mannerisms	None, or unobtrusive
Very loud or very soft	Voice: volume	Clearly audible
Impatient or staccato; very slow or hesitant	Voice: rate	Average, or a bit slower
Apathetic; sleepy; jumpy; pushy	Energy level	Alert; stays alert throughout a long conversation

Source: From "The Amity Book: Exercises in Friendship and Helping Skills," by R. Walters. In G. Gazda, F. Asbury, F. Balzer, W. Childers, & R. Walters (Eds.) (1977), *Human Relations Development: A Manual for Educators.* Copyright © 1977 by R. Walters. Boston: Allyn & Bacon. Reprinted by permission of the author.

3. Sender gives verbal messages and waits for a response; receiver replies (two-way). *Example:*

Director to supervisor: "You have been using primary nursing on your unit for six months. Have you had any reactions from the clients?"

Supervisor to director: "Not specifically to primary nursing, but our recent survey of patient satisfaction shows that our clients are generally more satisfied now than they were when surveyed last year at this time."

The literature is replete with discussions of types of communications. Basics have been discussed in this chapter. The next section looks at how managers communicate.

HOW MANAGERS COMMUNICATE

Managers communicate in the following ways: telling, selling, participating, delegating, listening, and giving and receiving feedback. Figure 9.3 portrays the relationship between how managers communicate and the Ohio State leadership model that was discussed in Chapter 5. The leadership model represents how leaders behave toward followers; leaders behave by communicating to (one-way communication) and with (two-way communication) followers.

Telling, Selling, Participating, and Delegating

Hersey and Blanchard (1988) used situational leadership theory to specify and explain the active verbs for each leader behavior style:

High Structure and Low Consideration (LB1) is referred to as "telling" because this style is characterized by one-way communication in which the manager defines the roles of followers by telling them what, how, when, and where to do the identified tasks. The manager guides and structures.

High Structure and High Consideration (LB2) is referred to as "selling" because most of the direction is provided by the manager, even though dialogue and clarification is encouraged. Through two-way communication and socio-emotional support, the manager tries to get the follower(s)

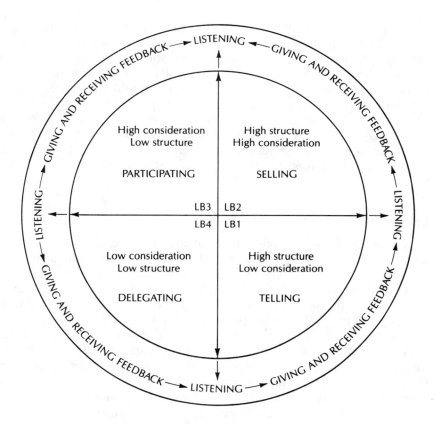

Figure 9.3 How leaders communicate in the Ohio State leader behavior model.

psychologically to buy into decisions that have to be made. This is often called persuasion (Kipnis & Schmidt, 1985).

High Consideration and Low Structure (LB3) is called "participating" because the manager and follower(s) jointly share in decision making through two-way communication, discussion, group process, and problem-solving. The manager reinforces, encourages, and calms.

Low Consideration and Low Structure (LB4) is labeled "delegating" because the style involves letting follower(s) develop and implement their own goal-accomplishing strategies. General supervision is minimal since the follower(s) are high in ability, willingness, and security.

Listening and giving/receiving feedback are represented in Figure 9.3 as a circle that runs around all of the leader behavior styles. A manager behaves by communicating to and with followers in the leader behavior style that has the highest probability for motivating them to accomplish the task. The manager should then listen to the feedback that is verbally and nonverbally provided by followers in response to the message given by the leader through one of the leader behavior styles. Then the manager decodes the feedback and sends another message to the followers. This process occurs until communication ceases; hence, no further message is required at that time.

Listening

Listening involves the ability to tune into people, the environment, and the meanings of messages that are spoken and unspoken (La Monica, 1985). Davis and Newstrom (1985) asserted that one hears with one's ears but listening occurs in the mind. Listening is the ability to perceive the exact message that the sender intended, to the degree that is humanly possible. When messages are perceived accurately, better decisions result because the information inputs are sounder. Time is also saved when people listen because more— qualitatively and quantitatively—is learned in a given period of time. Davis and Newstrom further pointed out that good listening skills represent good manners and are forms of behavior modeling that may enable others to listen more effectively in return. Table 9.2 provides guides for effective listening.

Giving and Receiving Feedback

Wang and Hawkins (1980) suggested that effective communication requires feedback. The purposes of feedback are to increase shared understanding about behavior, feelings, and motivations; to facilitate development of a trusting and open relationship among people; and to give information concerning the effects of individual behavior on others (La Monica, 1985). Feedback is also "the process of adjusting future actions based upon information about past performance" (Haynes, Massie, & Wallace, 1975, p. 260). It refers to the return of generated behavior (Luft, 1984). Feedback can be verbal and/or nonverbal.

Feedback can be given and received in a variety of formal and informal ways. Time can be set aside at the conclusion of meetings for the group to discuss how it functioned. The exercises at the

TABLE 9.2 Ten Guides for Effective Listening

1. *Stop talking!*
   You cannot listen if you are talking.
   Polonius *(Hamlet):* "Give every man thine ear, but few thy voice."
2. *Put the talker at ease.*
   Help the person feel free to talk.
   This is often called a permissive environment.
3. *Show the talker that you want to listen.*
   Look and act interested. Do not read your mail while someone talks.
   Listen to understand rather than to oppose.
4. *Remove distractions.*
   Don't doodle, tap, or shuffle papers.
   Will it be quieter if you shut the door?
5. *Empathize with the talker.*
   Try to help yourself see the other person's point of view.
6. *Be patient.*
   Allow plenty of time. Do not interrupt the talker.
   Don't start for the door or walk away.
7. *Hold your temper.*
   An angry person takes the wrong meaning from words.
8. *Go easy on argument and criticism.*
   This puts people on the defensive, and they may "clam up" or become angry.
   Do not argue: Even if you win, you lose.
9. *Ask questions.*
   This encourages the talker and shows that you are listening.
   It helps to develop points further.
10. *Stop talking!*
    This is first and last, because all other guides depend on it.
    You cannot do an effective listening job while you are talking.
    - Nature gave people two ears but only one tongue, which is a gentle hint that they should listen more than they talk.
    - Listening requires two ears, one for meaning and one for feeling.
    - Decision makers who do not listen have less information for making sound decisions.

Source: Davis, K., & Newstrom, J. (1985). *Human Behavior at Work: Organizational Behavior.* New York: McGraw-Hill, p. 438. Reproduced by permission.

conclusion of this section of the book provide some paper and pencil instruments for encouraging this form of feedback. People can ask for feedback in formal or informal interactions. Performance appraisals at six-month intervals involve feedback; a simple comment like "you have really worked hard today" is also feedback. A casual, understanding nod (nonverbally) is feedback, too. Feedback, therefore, occurs whenever the receiver of a message sends a message back to the sender regarding the message received. In a casual sense, feedback is given constantly. In a more designed sense, however, feedback should be elicited and given by managers so that information on which decisions are based is as accurate as possible.

Napier and Gershenfeld (1985) believed that feedback involves upward communication, thereby making it a high-risk activity for followers. Giving and receiving feedback can do more damage than good by increasing risk and defensiveness if certain criteria are not followed. Managers can dampen this risk factor, minimizing defenses and maximizing acceptance. This is accomplished if feedback is useful; giving and receiving feedback is a skill. The National Training Laboratory (NTL) Institute for Applied Behavioral Science suggested characteristics of useful feedback *(Laboratories in Human Relations Training,* 1971, pp. 27–28):*

1. *It is descriptive rather than evaluative.* By describing one's own reaction, it leaves the individual free to use it or not to use it as he sees fit. By avoiding evaluative language, it reduces the need for the individual to react defensively.

2. *It is specific rather than general.* To be told that one is "dominating" will probably not be as useful as to be told that "just now when we were deciding the issue you did not listen to what others said, and I felt forced to accept your arguments or face attack from you."

3. *It takes into account the needs of both the receiver and giver of the feedback.* Feedback can be destructive when it serves only our own needs and fails to consider the needs of the person on the receiving end.

4. *It is directed toward behavior which the receiver can do something about.* Frustration is only increased when a person is reminded of some shortcoming over which he has no control.

5. *It is solicited, rather than imposed.* Feedback is most useful when the receiver . . . has formulated the kind of question which those observing can . . . answer.

---

*Source: Adapted with permission from NTL Institute, "Feedback: The Art of Giving and Receiving Help," by Cyril R. Mill, pp. 18–19, *Reading Book for Laboratories in Human Relations Training*, edited by Cyril R. Mill and Lawrence C. Porter, copyright 1972.

6. *It is well-timed.* In general, feedback is most useful at the earliest opportunity after the given behavior (depending of course on the person's readiness to hear it, support available from others, etc.).

7. *It is checked to ensure clear communication.* One way of doing this is to have the receiver try to rephrase the feedback he has received to see if it corresponds to what the sender had in mind.

SUMMARY

Communication is the most important skill in management and leadership; everything that a manager does involves relating with others. It is defined as a process of passing information (messages) between or among people. Therefore, it involves a sender, a message, and a receiver who may give feedback to the sender on the message that was received. Since the purpose of managing is to motivate systems to accomplish goals, communication is necessary to give the system the skill to work and to facilitate the system's will to work as a team in goal accomplishment.

Two types of communication exist: verbal and nonverbal. In each type, communication can be one-way or two-way. Verbal communication involves the written or spoken word. Nonverbal communication involves body language. One-way communication means that a message is sent from a sender to a receiver, and it involves no feedback. Two-way communication also involves a sent message, but it includes feedback. Managers communicate by telling, selling, participating, delegating, listening, and giving and receiving feedback.

REFERENCES

Anderson, E. (1984). Communication patterns: A tool for memorable leadership training. *Training, 21*(1), 55–57.

Berlo, D. (1960). *The process of communication.* New York: Holt, Rinehart, & Winston.

Chartier, M. (1981). Clarity of expression in interpersonal communication. *Journal of Nursing Administration, 11*, 42–46.

Davis, K., & Newstrom, J. (1985). *Human behavior at work: Organizational behavior* (7th ed.). New York: McGraw-Hill.

Fast, J. (1970). *Body language.* New York: M. Evans.

Gibran, K. (1951). *The prophet.* New York: Knopf.

Hall, E. (1966). *Hidden dimension.* Garden City, NY: Doubleday.

Haynes, W., Massie, J., & Wallace, M. (1975). *Management: Analysis, concepts, and cases.* Englewood Cliffs, NJ: Prentice-Hall.

Hein, E. (1980). *Communication in nursing practice.* Boston: Little, Brown.

Hersey, P., & Blanchard, K. (1988). *Management of organizational behavior: Utilizing human resources* (5th ed.). Englewood Cliffs, NJ: Prentice-Hall.

Hewitt, F. (1981). Introduction to communication. *Nursing Times, 77,* center pages.

James, W. (1932). Study of the expression of bodily posture. *Journal of General Psychology, 7,* 405–437.

Johnson, D. (1986). *Reaching out: Interpersonal effectiveness and self-actualization* (3rd ed.). Englewood Cliffs, NJ: Prentice-Hall.

Kepler, T. (1980). Mastering the people skills. *Journal of Nursing Administration, 10,* 15–20.

Kipnis, D., & Schmidt, S. (1985). The language of persuasion. *Psychology Today, 19*(4), 40–44 +.

Laboratories in human relationship training: Book of readings. (1971). Washington, DC: National Training Laboratory Institute for Applied Behavioral Science.

La Monica, E. (1985). *The humanistic nursing process.* Boston: Jones and Bartlett.

Long, L., & Prophit, P. (1981). *Understanding—responding: A communication manual for nurses.* Belmont, CA: Wadsworth.

Luft, J. (1984) *Group processes: An introduction to group dynamics* (3rd ed.). Mountain View, CA: Mayfield Publishers.

Mehrabian, A. (1968). Influence of attitude from the posture, orientation, and distance of a communication. *Journal of Consulting and Clinical Psychology, 32,* 296–308.

Mehrabian, A. (1969). Significance of posture and positions in the communication of attitude and status relationships. *Psychological Bulletin, 71,* 359–372.

Miller, G. (1966). *Speech communication: A behavioral approach.* Indianapolis: Bobbs-Merrill.

Napier, R., & Gershenfeld, M. (1985). *Groups: Theory and experience* (3rd ed.). Boston, Houghton-Mifflin.

Pincus, J.D. (1986). Communication: Key contributor to effectiveness—The research. *Journal of Nursing Administration, 16*(9), 19–28.

Pluckhan, M. (1978). *Human communication: The matrix of nursing.* New York: McGraw-Hill.

Scheflin, A. (1964). The significance of posture in communication systems. *Psychiatry, 27,* 316–331.

Shannon, C., & Weaver, W. (1949). *The mathematical theory of communication.* Urbana: University of Illinois Press.

Tjosvold, D. (1984). Effects of leader warmth and directiveness on subordinate performance on a subsequent task. *Journal of Applied Psychology, 69*(3), 422–427.

von Bertalanffy, L. (1968). General system theory. New York: Braziller.

von Bertalanffy, L. (1975). *Perspectives on general system theory: Scientific-philosophical studies.* New York: Braziller.

Walters, R. (1977). The amity book: Exercises in friendship and helping skills.

In G. Gazda, F. Asbury, F. Balzer, W. Childers, & R. Walters. *Human relations development: A manual for educators* (2nd ed.). Boston: Allyn & Bacon.

Wang, R., & Hawkins, J. (1980). Interpersonal feedback for nursing supervisors. *Supervisor Nurse, II,* 26–28.

Everyone exerts influence on another—changes another—implicitly and explicitly, covertly and overtly. This fact is especially important in management and leadership. At an informal level, each time a person interacts with another by sending a message, the receiver's response to the sender is shaped by the message received. In a sense, the receiver has formed a response to fit a message sent by another. The sender, therefore, has influenced the receiver. To influence another means that a person elicits something from another or engenders something in another. This is change, and recalling from previous chapters, change is learning, and learning is change. Humans do not interact in a vacuum; people are part of a system that exerts constant influence over individual behavior. This is a sociological perspective, of course, and contemporary management practice embraces this approach.

At a more formal level, managers are constantly attempting to change a system—to move the system from where it is in a given area (the actual) to where the manager wishes it to be in a particular area (the optimal). The processes for accomplishing this change were discussed in Parts I and II of this book. At this point, a major assumption (a given) of this book is that managers change people and people change managers. Changing a system is not simply one aspect of a managers responsibilities—if one is managing and leading, one **is** changing people.

In the pursuit of knowledge and in order to more thoroughly understand leader behavior and, therefore, be able to exert greater productive control over oneself and others, the following theories and concepts on change are presented and discussed in this chapter: force field analysis (field theory), levels of change, the change process, strategies of change, resistance to change, and combatting this resistance.

FORCE FIELD ANALYSIS

Lewin's (1951) force field analysis is a useful theory for understanding what is happening when a manager wishes to move a system from actual to optimal in a particular area. A problem was defined in Chapter 1 as the difference between actual and optimal (see Figure 1.3). This "difference" can be further explained using force field analysis. An example might help in explaining this concept. The problem definition is:

Actual: Staff nurses on Unit 5 are continuously tardy to the day shift.

Optimal: Staff nurses arrive on time for the day shift so that report can be given and the night staff released.

Problem: Tardiness on the morning shift.

Goal: To have day staff nurses arrive on time.

A manager wants to move actual to optimal, thereby eradicating the problem and accomplishing the goal. Figure 10.1 portrays this

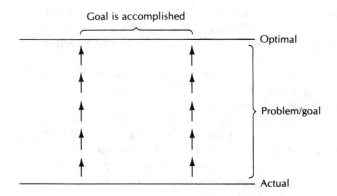

Figure 10.1 Movement for goal accomplishment.

movement. Imagine the line symbolizing actual as a state that is suspended between forces that are working toward moving actual to optimal (driving forces) and forces that are working against the move from actual to optimal (restraining forces). Weights can be added to these forces to portray the relative importance of each force. Figure 10.2 contains such a force field.

If an equal amount of restraining and driving forces were operative in the field, there could be no movement in the actual line, which would be in a state of equilibrium. If driving forces outweigh

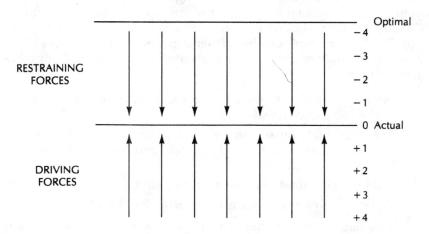

Figure 10.2 Force field.

Change

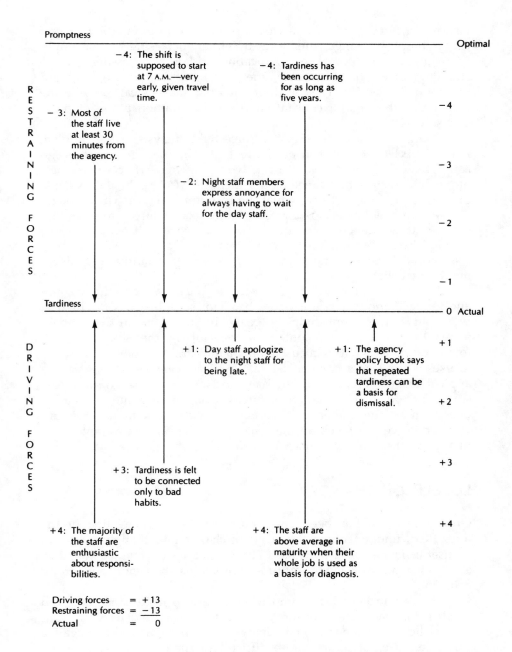

Figure 10.3 Driving and restraining forces in a case example

restraining forces, then actual would shift toward optimal. A manager can accomplish change, therefore, by either increasing and/or amplifying the driving forces or eradicating and/or suppressing the restraining forces. In either case, the actual line would move toward the optimal line. This type of discriminating analysis can provide the manager with items of concentration for the solution phase of problem solving.

Going back to the example, a force field analysis of the problem might look like that shown in Figure 10.3. The manager must assign a weight to each force—it is a relative figure that reflects one's best judgment on the importance of the identified forces. In the example provided, the driving forces equal the restraining forces. The manager can focus on either set of forces or both sets of forces to engender change. It is the belief of this author, however, that the positive should always be amplified. When this is done, the negative looks less formidable. Force field analysis is a way to quantitatively document this belief.

A problem must still be analyzed to diagnose self, the system, and the task and arrive at a leader behavior style that has the highest probability for accomplishing the goal. The manager can then choose forces that become the content in developing the solutions. The forces relate to what is focused on in the strategy; how a manager focuses is the leader behavior style. Any leader behavior style can be applied to any force; *what* and *how* coexist as separate entities. Any single force or a combination of forces, even driving and restraining ones, can be the content of a problem solution. A manager is advised, however, to focus on the forces with the highest weights since they have the greatest impact on producing change.

LEVELS OF CHANGE

Once a problem has been analyzed including a delineation of the force field, understanding the levels of change and change cycles can be useful. Hersey and Blanchard (1988) cited and discussed four levels of change: knowledge, attitudes, individual behavior, and group behavior.

Changes in knowledge tend to be easiest to make since they can result from reading a book or listening to a respected lecturer. Attitude structures are emotionally charged in a positive and/or negative way. They are, therefore, more difficult to change than knowledge. Moving to greater difficulty, individual behavior comes next. A man-

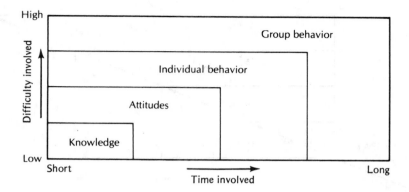

Figure 10.4 Change levels.
Source: This figure was adapted from one used by Paul Hersey and Kenneth H. Blanchard, *Management of Organizational Behavior: Utilizing Human Resources*, 5th ed., p. 4, © 1988. Reprinted by permission of Prentice-Hall, Inc., Englewood Cliffs, NJ.

ager may know about and understand primary nursing, for example, like it, and still not behaviorally apply it for a variety of reasons, like feeling uncomfortable with the behaviors. Group behavior is the hardest to change because of the numbers of people. Trying to change customs, mores, and traditions is also difficult (Hersey & Blanchard, 1988). Figure 10.4 shows the four change levels.

Two change cycles are identified from the four levels of change; participative change and directive or coercive change (Hersey & Blanchard, 1988).

Participative Change

A participative change cycle occurs when change proceeds from knowledge to group behavior, as shown in Figure 10.5. Followers are first provided with knowledge, with the intent that they will develop positive attitudes on a subject. Since research suggests that people behave on the basis of their attitudes, a manager's desire is that this hold true. Once individuals behave in a certain way, these people become teachers and therefore influence others to behave accordingly—group behavior then tends to change also. Participative change cycles can be used by managers with personal and/or positive power. Change is somewhat slow and evolutionary, but it tends to last because followers generally believe in what they are doing—the

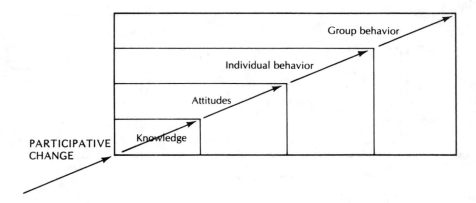

Figure 10.5 Participative change cycle.
Source: This figure was adapted from one used by Paul Hersey and Kenneth H. Blanchard, *Management of Organizational Behavior: Utilizing Human Resources,* 5th ed., p. 340, © 1988. Reprinted by permission of Prentice-Hall, Inc., Englewood Cliffs, NJ.

change is intrinsically imposed rather than extrinsically demanded (Hersey & Blanchard, 1988).

Directive (Coercive) Change

Figure 10.6 shows that directive change occurs in the opposite direction from participative change. Using position power, higher management gives directions about the mode of behavior for the system of concern; actually an entire organization may be the focus. The dicta are set into place and followers are expected to attend to and abide by them. The hope of managers is that once followers see the plan in operation, they will develop positive attitudes about it and then gain further knowledge. This type of change is volatile; it tends to disappear when managers are not present to enforce it (Hersey & Blanchard, 1988). Position power is essential in this cycle.

Implications for Change Cycles

There is informal agreement among managers that participative change is the best. There are, however, specific instances when a leader must use a directive style. These instances relate to the implications for different leader behavior styles (Haffer, 1986).

    A directive style is necessary when an organization is in crisis and when people must behave in a certain way immediately in order

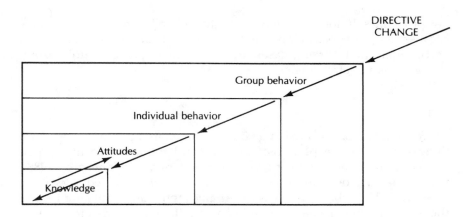

Figure 10.6 Directive (coercive) change cycle.
Source: This figure was adapted from one used by Paul Hersey and Kenneth H. Blanchard, *Management of Organizational Behavior: Utilizing Human Resources,* 5th ed., p. 341, © 1988. Reprinted by permission of Prentice-Hall, Inc., Englewood Cliffs, NJ.

for the organization to continue viably. The participative cycle is usually appropriate for followers who are average to above average in maturity, whereas those followers who are below average to average in maturity may need and prefer a directive cycle.

These two change cycles can be used by a manager regardless of the maturity of the system. A participative cycle, for example, can be used with followers who require high structure and low consideration leader behavior. The solution or strategy for accomplishing a goal simply starts with knowledge—the manager can require followers to attend lectures, to read, and so forth. A directive cycle can be used with mature followers even though such an intervention is risky. The benefits of this intervention must outweigh the probable consequences. If a manager used a participative change cycle with followers who required high consideration and low structure leader behavior, the group might sit together and plan how they would like to gain the knowledge—maybe they could suggest guest speakers and so forth.

THE CHANGE PROCESS

The change process, as defined and discussed by Lewin (1947), Schein (1968), and Kelman (1958), lended further understanding to the experience of changing. It also can guide the manager in developing problem solutions that have a high probability for being effective because they are based on what is known about human behavior. Lewin identified three phases in the change process: unfreezing, changing, and refreezing.

Unfreezing

Unfreezing involves breaking down the normal way people do things—interrupting patterns, customs, and routines—so that a person is ready to accept new alternatives (Hersey & Blanchard, 1988). Forces that act on and within an individual are "melted down" or "thawed." This phase involves externally motivating someone to take the journey toward goal accomplishment. (If necessary, refer back to Chapter 2 for a discussion on motivation.)

Changing

Once people are motivated to change, they are primed to accept new patterns of behavior. Taking on these new behaviors involves changing attitudes. Kelman (1958) suggested three ways this happens: compliance, identification, and internalization.

Compliance occurs when change is forced by someone with position power who manipulates rewards and punishments. Identification means that role models for the new behavior are available and individuals learn by identifying with them and trying to be like them. Internalization occurs when individuals are left to change on their own power. The need and desire to change is present, and people must learn the new patterns of behavior by employing intrinsic resources. Self-learning and self-discovery fall into this last category.

Refreezing

Refreezing occurs when new behaviors become part of one's personality. The behavior occurs because one has knowledge, positive attitudes, and experience with these new behaviors. Refreezing has occurred in followers when a leader has accomplished long-term goals whereby followers function effectively in a task when the leader is in LB4—low structure and low consideration. New behaviors should be positively reinforced by leaders to ensure that refreezing occurs within followers (Ferster & Skinner, 1957).

STRATEGIES OF CHANGE

Problems of change can be approached by individuals and groups in a variety of ways, and each strategy by each manager is unique—one's strategy did not, cannot, and will not exist again in an exact form. Strategies are usually a melding of a variety of methods, modes, and substrategies that are employed by the leader. Themes in change strategies, however, are evident. Olmosk (1972) identified and discussed the following seven pure strategies of change: fellowship, political, economic, academic, engineering, military, and confrontation. Some of these may sound familiar. In reality, a manager's strategy combines two or more of these pure strategies; however, one may stand out over the others.

Fellowship Strategy

Everyone is treated equally and emphasis is placed on team building in a group, getting to know group members, and building social bonds among members. This strategy is ideal for followers who have high social and esteem needs. Hence, it is ideal when LB3 is required by a system—high consideration and low structure. Getting people together at an informal dinner party to discuss new directions for a unit is an example of this strategy.

Political Strategy

A political strategy means identifying the formal and informal power structures. Once these structures are identified, efforts are made to influence those in power. The assumption of this strategy is that something will get accomplished if the influential people in a system wish it to be carried out. Directors who want to change from having nurses write separate notes to having them record on the progress notes might identify the key people in hospital policy-making and discuss with them individually prior to bringing the recommendation to a formal gathering.

Economic Strategy

Money talks! Emphasis is on acquiring or controlling material goods. With material resources, anything and anybody can be influenced—that is, bought and sold. Inclusion in a group is often based on possession or control of marketable resources. Fundraisers often employ this strategy.

Academic Strategy

In academics, knowledge or the pursuit of knowledge is the primary influencer. The belief is that people are logical, rational, and objective; that decisions will be based on what research suggests is the best path to follow. Emotions are not usually acknowledged in an academic strategy, even though it is known that people can never be entirely objective on anything. A bias that can range from narrow to wide always exists. In suggesting ways that result in more effective outcomes of nursing care, a manager might cite research studies that support the identified goal for a unit.

Engineering Strategy

This method for facilitating change in people tends to ignore the subjects by attending to the surrounding environment. It is, therefore, a sociological approach with the belief that if the surroundings change, the people in those surroundings will also change. Health-care planners use this strategy when designing patient units so that beds are in close proximity to the nurse's station. The logic is that if nurses are close to patients, they will spend more time "at the bedside," and the quality of care will increase.

Military Strategy

Physical force and real threats are the names of this game. "Ruling with an iron hand" and "running a tight ship" describe the climate in this environment. Position power is used in the form of threats and punishment if the leader's wishes are not obeyed. This is a high-structure strategy. The iron hand may be disguised in a warm, sweet velvet glove; all concerned, however, are fully aware that the iron fist exists and will be used if necessary. An example in this area is hardly needed. Be cognizant, however, that physical force may be used in hospitals by health-care personnel on patients. Posey restraints are one such example. A nurse must assess the need for such a strategy—it should be the last possible approach.

Confrontation Strategy

This approach induces nonviolent and nonphysical conflict within people. By doing this, a manager forces people to hear and see what is happening in a situation. The intent is that once people are aware of what is occurring, change will follow. People are often polarized into groups or cults as a result of this strategy. When groups feel that they will not or cannot be heard in any other way, this strategy is often employed. A union strike is one example.

RESISTANCE TO CHANGE

Nursing literature is and has been riddled with articles on the nurse's responsibility for changing the health-care system and on the nurse as the "change agent" (Beyers, 1984; Claus & Bailey, 1979; Lancaster, 1980; Levenstein, 1979; New & Couillard, 1981; Smith, 1970; Spradley, 1980; Stevens, 1977, 1985). Just the term *change agent* can arouse defensiveness in the subjects of change and can threaten the agent. No one really wants to change, because people like the comfort of behaviors that have worked in the past. Who wants to trade in their security blankets, and who wants to be "the one" to say that old security blankets must be burned in favor of new ones?

To say that people will change or that someone is a change agent engenders resistance. Davis and Newstrom (1985) explained this resistance as one of two types: resistance based on rational opposition to change and resistance based on emotional and selfish desires. In the former type of resistance, followers may believe and provide evidence substantiating their belief that the costs of the change exceed the benefits. The term *costs* is used literally and figuratively. In the latter type of resistance, followers ignore the benefits of the outcomes of change because of their own personal needs and fears.

COMBATTING RESISTANCE TO CHANGE

One of the best ways to combat resistance to change is by believing that change is a natural process that occurs continuously in everyone's life at every minute. The label of change is the insidious wart; the process of changing is simply cell regeneration—it happens without cognitive awareness, and no one really feels it. Managers should do their job, lead people, and forget labels. Change will happen.

Moving away from a philosophical but most important approach that should underlie the more concrete ways to combat resistance, various authors offer suggestions. Stevens (1975) suggested providing answers to the following questions that are commonly felt by those being changed: Will the change cause my position to be different? Will my status, power, job content, freedom, and so forth be affected? Will my financial status be improved? Schweiger (1980) stated that the manager should make the tangible benefits of change clear. Furthermore, the change should reflect the followers' existing values and ideas. Davis and Newstrom (1985) and Stogdill (1974) both believed that follower participation is the best way to gain support for change. This principle is also evident in the theory for diagnosing the task that was discussed in Chapter 6 (Vroom, 1973; Vroom & Jago, 1974, 1988; Vroom & Yetton, 1973). If followers must accept a decision, that is, if followers must do something in order to solve the problem, then they must be involved in problem solving.

SUMMARY

Change occurs constantly. Change is learning, and learning is change. Managers are constantly trying to move a system from one point to another—to solve a problem. Managers, therefore, are constantly developing strategies to change people and to solve problems. This is leadership.

The force field analysis theory is used to explain the forces that operate within the discrepancy between where a system is on an issue (the actual) and where a manager wishes it to be on that same issue (the optimal). Driving and restraining forces are identified, and change can occur by amplifying the driving forces, and/or suppressing the restraining forces.

The four levels of change are knowledge, attitudes, individual behavior, and group behavior. A participative change cycle moves from knowledge to group behavior, and a directive cycle moves in the opposite direction. The change process involves unfreezing old patterns of behavior, introducing a change, and refreezing the new mode of behavior.

Strategies for change in a given situation are all unique and usually involve several approaches, with one or two dominant approaches. Seven pure strategies were identified and discussed: fellowship, political, economic, academic, engineering, military, and confrontation. Resistance to change can be expected. Philosophical and concrete approaches to combatting this resistance were offered in conclusion of this chapter.

REFERENCES

Beyers, M. (1984). Getting on top of organizational change: Part 1. Process and development. *Journal of Nursing Administration, 14,* 32–39.

Claus, K., & Bailey, J. (1979). Facilitating change: A problem-solving decision-making tool. *Nursing Leadership, 2,* 30–39.

Davis, K., & Newstrom, J. (1985). *Human behavior at work: Organizational behavior* (7th ed.). New York: McGraw-Hill.

Ferster, C., & Skinner, B. (1957). *Schedules of reinforcement.* New York: Appleton-Century-Crofts.

Haffer, A. (1986). Facilitating change: Choosing the appropriate strategy. *Journal of Nursing Administration, 16*(4), 18–22.

Hersey, P., & Blanchard, K. (1988). *Management of organizational behavior: Utilizing human resources* (5th ed.). Englewood Cliffs, NJ: Prentice-Hall.

Kelman, H. (1958). Compliance, identification and internalization: Three processes of attitude change. *Conflict Resolution, 2,* 51–60.

Lancaster, J. (1980). An ecological orientation toward change: Considerations for leadership in nursing. *Nursing Leadership, 3,* 12–15.

Levenstein, A. (1979). Effective change requires a change agent. *Journal of Nursing Administration, 9,* 12–15.

Lewin, K. (1947). Frontiers in group dynamics: Concept, method, and reality in social science; social equilibria and social change. *Human Relations, 1,* 5–41.

Lewin, K. (1951). In D. Cartwright (Ed). *Field theory in social science.* New York: Harper and Row.

New, J., & Couillard, N. (1981). Guidelines for introducing change. *Journal of Nursing Administration, 11,* 17–21.

Olmosk, K. (1972). Seven pure strategies of change. In J. Pfeiffer, & J. Jones (Eds.). *The 1972 annual handbook for group facilitators.* La Jolla, CA: University Associates.

Schein, E. (1968). Management development as a process of influence. In D. Hampton (Ed.). *Behavioral concepts in management.* Belmont, CA: Dickinson Publishing.

Schweiger, J. (1980). *The nurse as manager.* New York: Wiley.

Smith, D. (1970). Change: How shall we respond to it? *Nursing Forum, 9,* 391–399.

Spradley, B. (1980). Managing change creatively. *Journal of Nursing Administration, 10,* 32–37.

Stevens, B. (1975). *The nurse as executive.* Wakefield, MA: Contemporary Publishing.

Stevens, B. (1977). Management of continuity and change in nursing. *Journal of Nursing Administration, 7,* 26–31.

Stevens, B. (1985). *The nurse as executive* (3rd ed.). Rockville, MD: Aspen.

Stogdill, R. (1974). *Handbook of leadership.* New York: Free Press.

Vroom, V. (1973). A new look at managerial decision-making. *Organizational Dynamics, 1,* 66–80.

Vroom, V., & Jago, A. (1974). Decision-making as a social process. *Decision Sciences, 5,* 743–769.

Vroom, V., & Jago, A. (1988). *The new leadership: Managing participation in organizations.* Englewood Cliffs, NJ: Prentice-Hall.

Vroom, V., & Yetton, P. (1973). *Leadership and decision-making,* Pittsburgh: University of Pittsburgh Press.

CHAPTER 11

Power

POWER DEFINED
TYPES OF POWER
  Position Power
  Personal Power
SOURCES OF POWER
USES OF POWER
POWER IN THE NURSING PROFESSION
SUMMARY

Nurse managers and leaders must have knowledge about the phenomenon of power and be astutely able and willing to put its forces to work effectively in accomplishing specified goals. A manager without such ability and willingness is relatively impotent. The purpose of this chapter is to discuss power by first looking at various definitions of the concept. The types and sources of power followed by uses of power are then presented. The chapter is concluded with a look at power in the nursing profession.

POWER DEFINED

Power is simply the exercise of control or influence over another person or over a group. Given the spirit of inquiry, however, researchers have been diligent in specifying more discriminating theories of social power.

Early theorists define power as intentional force or control (Adler, 1938, 1964; Ansbacher & Ansbacher, 1956, 1964; Bierstedt, 1950; Russell, 1938; Wrong, 1968). Others believe that power is inferred from observing the effects of interactions on those engaged. Simon (1957) called this an asymmetrical influence relation. Still another school of thought describes power as a social exchange (Adams & Romney, 1959; Blau, 1964; Gouldner, 1960; Harsanyi, 1962a, 1962b;

Homans, 1958; Thibaut & Kelley, 1959). Contemporary theorists conceptualized power as one's potential for influencing another person (Hersey & Blanchard, 1988; Rogers, 1973; Nyberg, 1983).

TYPES OF POWER

Etzioni (1961) delineated two types of power: *position power* and *personal power*. He viewed power as one's ability to induce or influence behavior of another person.

Position Power

Position power is derived from within an organization. A manager who can influence a group to accomplish a goal because of one's position in an organization is said to use position power (Etzioni, 1961). Hersey and Blanchard (1988) asserted that position power flows down in an organization—superiors delegate authority and responsibility to followers, who repeat the process again. In a sense, one's position power may be related to the amount of authority and responsibility that is given to and/or taken from one's superior. Simply having a position of management, therefore, does not always mean that one has position power.

An essential aspect of position power is the concept of authority. Bennis (1959) saw authority as "the process by which an agent induces a subordinate to behave in a desired manner" (p. 295). In a sense, authority is thereby granted to a leader—it is a legitimate right (Moloney, 1979) that may or may not be given by superiors in an organization. Authority is also granted by right of office—parent, manager, bishop—and by right of knowledge—lawyer, physician, nurse (Francis, 1982). Power is the intrinsic ability to influence or control others; authority is a possession of granted or delegated power; leader behavior or any behavior is required in order to use or operationalize power. Power can only be communicated through behavior.

Personal Power

According to Etzioni (1961), personal power is derived from followers. It flows upward to a manager and is the extent to which followers respect and are committed to their leader (Hersey & Blanchard, 1988). Personal power is informal power and position power is formal power. Informal power is seen as a day-to-day phenomenon since it can be earned from followers and also can be taken away (Hersey & Blanchard, 1988). Informal leaders in groups are examples of people who have been given and/or have taken personal power.

Reference has been made in the preceding paragraphs to power being given and/or taken. Each person has control over his or her own power—not complete control because of the social interacting system, but control nevertheless. Superiors give position power by delegating authority and responsibility to a manager; a manager earns the trust of superiors by behaving in a confident, able, willing, and trustful manner. Followers give personal power to a manager— they allow themselves to be led. A manager earns personal power by treating people with respect, by being fair, and by having and using the knowledge and experience necessary to lead others in accomplishing goals.

Power is a tension between or among people. To say that one is given power puts power in the control of the giver, not the receiver. To say that power is taken implies that the giver has none. Power can and usually does exist implicitly in all parts of a system. Behavioral evidence of its existence, however, is observable in different people at different times in various contexts. All people cannot exert control at the same time—not without a massive, dysfunctional power struggle.

Etzioni (1961) and Machiavelli (1950) believed that it is best to have both position power and personal power—to be both feared and loved at the same time. What happens if such a combination is not feasible? Hersey and Blanchard (1988) said that if one cannot have both position and personal power, then personal power alone is better than position power alone. This author tends to agree with this assertion—a manager soon becomes impotent if followers collectively choose not to follow. Machiavelli (1950) believed that a relationship based on fear of retaliation (position power) tends to endure longer than one based on love because the latter relationship can be terminated quickly with no sanction or price. Terminating the former relationship may carry a price. Even though contemporary managers do not follow Machiavellian guidelines as principles for their behavior, Machiavelli made statements that all managers should understand.

SOURCES OF POWER

Power is derived from a variety of sources. These sources are also called power bases (Hersey & Blanchard, 1988; Stogdill, 1974). Each source is discussed separately, even though a manager may possess and use several sources at any given time.

Coercive Power—This power source is based on fear. Compliance is induced because failure to comply will result in punishment or penalties (French & Raven, 1959).

Connection Power—A manager with connection power has bonds with influential and important people within and outside of an organization. By complying with the manager, followers believe that favor will be gained with the important people connected with their leader (Hersey, Blanchard, & Natemeyer, 1979).

Reward Power—This is grounded on the belief of followers that the manager can provide rewards for them. Compliance with the manager's strategies results in gains such as increased pay, recognition, and so forth (French & Raven, 1959).

Legitimate Power—Based on a manager's position, followers believe that the manager has the right to influence them; their compliance follows. The higher one's position, the more legitimate power one possesses (French & Raven, 1959).

Referent Power—This source is based on the manager's personality trait; it is a part of one's personal power. A manager who is admired, liked, and identified with can induce compliance from followers (French & Raven, 1959).

Information Power—Information power is based on possession of or access to information. This can influence people because of the belief that compliance will result in sharing of information—followers often have the need to be "in on things" (Raven & Kruglanski, 1975).

Expert Power—Competence—knowledge, expertise, and skill—comprise expert power. Followers are influenced because their manager is seen as possessing the ability to facilitate accomplishment of their work assignments (French & Raven, 1959).

Even though these power sources are discussed distinctly, they are related to one another. Coercive power and reward power are two ends of the same continuum; a manager can give rewards to those who comply and can punish those who fail to comply. Such authority may be granted by the nature of a position, that is, legitimate power. Referent power and expert power are contained within a person and

TABLE 11.1 Sources and Types of Power

Sources of Power	Types of Power
Coercive	Position
Connection	Position and/or personal
Reward	Position
Legitimate	Position
Referent	Personal
Information	Position and/or personal
Expert	Personal

therefore can be labeled as personal power. Connection power can involve position or can refer to those connected to the manager regardless of the position held. Connection power, therefore, can be both position power and personal power. Information power also can be both personal and position power because a manager can have access to information given the nature of one's position or because of personal reasons. Table 11.1 provides a list of the sources and types of power.

USES OF POWER

Nursing literature is replete with suggestions that power should be an essential aspect of managers' personalities (Courtade, 1978; Heineken, 1985; Janik, 1984; Masson, 1979; Peterson, 1979; Shiflett & McFarland, 1978). Nurse managers must know about and exercise power.

In addition to the sources from which power is gained, the nurse manager can employ power strategies to accomplish goals.

1. *Rules and regulations* can be used to thwart attempted change by followers that is not in line with specified goals (Claus & Bailey, 1977; Scheff, 1961).

2. *Direct confrontation* in facts and figures is a maneuver that can be used to push toward a desired end (Peterson, 1979).

3. *Attractive personal attributes* can be amplified when selling a position since research has suggested that the more personable and attractive an individual is, the more influence that person has over others (Claus & Bailey, 1977).

4. *Coalitions* or group alliances, formed so that varied resources are pooled and a united front exists, can be used to overcome opposition (Claus & Bailey, 1977; Peterson, 1979).

5. *Social space* is a phenomenon Korda (1975) studied. The position and arrangement of desks and chairs can be a strategy to gain power. Sitting spaciously behind a desk while positioning a visitor or follower in a cramped area decreases the visitor's psychological comfort. Being situated in the "middle of things" also results in power because of access to information.

6. *Assertiveness* is a method of communication that powerful people know about and use in daily interactions. It is vitally important in management and is discussed in a subsequent following chapter.

7. *Reciprocal open consultation*, in which managers and followers are open to be influenced by another. Equality and reciprocity are essential features of this strategy (Mulder, Koppelaar, de Jong & Verhage, 1986).

POWER IN THE NURSING PROFESSION

Leininger (1977) asserted that "there is probably no discipline so deeply involved in power, politics, and territoriality as nursing" (p 6). She understood the need for powerful, dynamic leaders in educational systems, service systems, and policy-making groups. These three systems are really subsystems in nursing's power structure. Figure 11.1 portrays this point.

The three major components of the nursing profession are education, service, and policy-making groups. All three groups, however, move from and to one another. The three subsystems are interdependent on one another, even though they have independent functions. Position power increases as one moves from the bottom of any subgroup toward the top of that same subgroup.

SUMMARY

Power is the ability to exercise control or influence over another person or a group. Two types of power exist: (1) position power, which is formally derived, and (2) personal power, which is informally derived. Authority is part of position power.

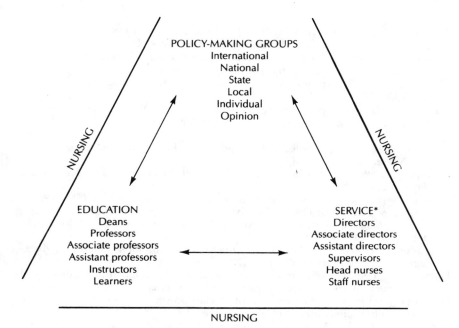

Figure 11.1 Nursing's power structure.
*Titles in institutions vary; the author simply wishes to portray the organizational structure of nursing service by using commonly understood labels for nurse managers and leaders in education and service.

Seven sources of power are noted in the literature: coercive power, connection power, reward power, legitimate power, referent power, information power, and expert power. Various strategies for using power were discussed. These include confronting directly, falling back on existing rules and regulations, amplifying attractive personal attributes, forming coalitions, and using space powerfully. The nursing profession's power structure consists of three subsystems that have independent functions, yet are interdependent. These subsystems are education, service, and policy-making groups.

REFERENCES

Adams, J., & Romney, A. (1959). A functional analysis of authority. *Psychological Review, 66,* 234–251.

Adler, A. (1938). *Social interest.* London: Faber & Faber.

Alder, A. (1964). *Social interest: A challenge to mankind* (J. Linton & R. Vaughn, Trans.). New York: Capricorn Books.

Ansbacher, H., & Ansbacher, R. (Eds.). (1956). *The individual psychology of Alfred Adler.* New York: Basic Books.

Ansbacher, H., & Ansbacher, R. (Eds.). (1964). *Superiority and social interest: A collection of later writings.* Evanston, IL: Northwest University Press.

Bennis, W. (1959). Leadership theory and administrative behavior: The problem of authority. *Administrative Science Quarterly, 4,* 259–301.

Bierstedt, R. (1950). An analysis of social power. *American Sociological Review, 15,* 730–736.

Blau, P. (1964). *Exchange and power in social life.* New York: Wiley.

Claus, K., & Bailey, J. (1977). *Power and influence in health care.* St. Louis: Mosby.

Courtade, S. (1978). The role of the head nurse: Power and practice. *Supervisor Nurse, 9,* 16–23.

Etzioni, A. (1961). *A comparative analysis of complex organizations.* New York: Free Press.

Francis, E. (1982). Using your power. *Health Services Manager, 15*(5), 7–9.

French, J., & Raven, B. (1959). The bases of social power. In D. Cartwright (Ed.), *Studies in social power.* Ann Arbor: Institute for Social Research, University of Michigan.

Gouldner, A. (1960). The norm of reciprocity: A preliminary statement. *American Sociological Review, 25,* 161–178.

Harsanyi, J. (1962a). Measurement of social power, opportunity costs, and the theory of two-person bargaining games. *Behavioral Science, 7,* 67–80.

Harsanyi J. (1962b). Measurement of social power in *n*-person reciprocal power situations. *Behavioral Science, 7,* 81–91.

Heineken, J. (1985). Power: Conflicting views. *Journal of Nursing Administration, 15*(11), 36–39.

Hersey, P., & Blanchard, K. (1988). *Management of organizational behavior: Utilizing human resources* (5th ed.). Englewood Cliffs, NJ: Prentice-Hall.

Hersey, P., & Blanchard, K., & Natemeyer, W. (1979). *Situational leadership, perception, and the impact of power.* La Jolla, CA: Learning Resources Corporation.

Homans, G. (1958). Social behavior as exchange. *American Journal of Sociology, 63,* 597–606.

Janik, A. (1984). Power base of nursing in bargaining relationships. *Image: The Journal of Nursing Scholarship, 16*(3), 93–96.

Korda, M. (1975). *Power: How to get it, how to use it.* New York: Random House.

Leininger, M. (1977). Territoriality, power, and creative leadership in administrative nursing contexts. In *Power: Use it or lose it.* New York: National League for Nursing.

Machiavelli, N. (1950). *The prince and the discourses.* New York: Modern Library.

Masson, V. (1979). On power and vision in nursing. *Nursing Outlook, 27,* 782–784.

Moloney, M. (1979). *Leadership in nursing: Theory, strategies, action.* St. Louis: Mosby.

Mulder, M., Koppelaar, L., de Jong, R., & Verhage, J. (1986). Power, situation, and leaders' effectiveness: An organizational field study. *Journal of Applied Psychology, 71*(4), 566–570.

Nyberg, D. 1983). Power over power. *Teachers College Record, 84*(3), 768–773.

Peterson, G. (1979). Power: A perspective for the nurse administrator. *Journal of Nursing Administration, 9*, 7–10.

Raven, B., & Kruglanski, W. (1975). Conflict and power. In P. Swingle (Ed.), *The structure of conflict.* New York: Academic Press.

Rogers, M. (1973). Instrumental and infra-resources: The bases of power. *American Journal of Sociology, 79*(6), 1418–1433.

Russell, B. (1938). *Power.* New York: W.W. Norton.

Scheff, J. (1961). Control over policy by attendants in a mental hospital. *Journal of Health and Human Behavior, 2*, 93–105.

Shiflett, N., & McFarland, D. (1978). Power and the nursing administrator. *Journal of Nursing Administration, 8*, 19–23.

Simon, H. (1957). *Models of man.* New York: Wiley.

Stogdill, R. (1974). *Handbook of leadership.* New York: Free Press.

Thibaut, J., & Kelley, H. (1959). *The social psychology of groups.* New York: Wiley.

Wrong, D. (1968). Some problems in defining social power. *American Journal of Sociology, 73*, 673–681.

Teaching

All nurse managers and leaders are teachers. The purpose of teaching is behaviorally to facilitate learning in another person. Learning is an intrinsic experience for the receiver. It denotes an integration of knowledge, attitudes, and experience in a person's past and present (La Monica, 1985). When someone learns, change occurs in that individual. The manager's primary goal is motivating others to accomplish goals. Managers should constantly be developing strategies to change what people would normally do if uninfluenced to what they need to do to accomplish the goals of an organization. To effect this change, followers must *learn* what the task requires; managers must facilitate this learning by *teaching*. Being a teacher is a subrole of being a manager. The intent of a teacher is to facilitate learning. The focus of this chapter is to discuss the teaching methods and processes that are available to nurse managers.

Teaching can be formal or informal. Formal processes occur when teaching programs are explicit—planned, organized, and evaluated. Staff development, continuing education, or in-service education are all common labels for teaching units in health-care agencies. Such departments predominantly run formal programs in the following areas: orientation, ongoing education, executive development, and patient education (Donovan, 1975; Littlejohn, 1980). Teaching formal

TABLE 12.1 The Problem-Solving Method in Management and in Teaching

Teaching	Management
Identifying learning needs ———————— Problem identification	
Stating the teaching priorities ————⟍ ⟍ Problem definition	
Developing program objectives ——————⟍➤ Problem analysis	
Exploring teaching strategies ———————— Alternative solutions	
Recommending a program ————————— Recommended action	

programs becomes the responsibility of nurse managers when teaching units and their staff are not separate components in an agency.

Incidental teaching (informal) is also done through teaching units but on a much smaller scale. This type of teaching is often called coaching (Darling & McGrath, 1983; Fournies, 1978; Hersey & Blanchard, 1988; Myers, 1966; Phillips-Jones, 1982). Coaching involves the daily or almost daily reinforcement and development carried out by a manager as an employee is guided through the learning (change) process.

Nurse managers often participate in formal educational programs, which may draw learners from an array of agency units or which may be targeted to one specific group. Usually, however, managers have greater responsibility for on-the-spot teaching of their immediate system. In this sense, more informal teaching is involved. This type of teaching can be impromptu or can be planned, organized, and evaluated. The target system is usually those people who are led by the manager, or it may be only a portion of them.

Teachers can use the problem-solving method to increase their probability for effectiveness in their teaching outcome goals. This process can be thought about quickly, as in impromptu teaching situations, or it can be applied over a period of months. Teachers involved in formal and/or informal teaching would use the same process—the detail to which each would become involved as well as the amount of time devoted to the teaching project would differ. The problem-solving method in teaching is analogous to the problem-solving method that was presented in Chapter 1. Table 12.1 compares these two methods. The five teaching areas shown in Table 12.1 are discussed separately in this chapter.

IDENTIFYING LEARNING NEEDS

Identifying learning needs is the first step in the problem-solving method. Sovie (1981) called this "investigate before you educate."

The process of diagnosis is appropriate for diagnosing learning needs of others and of self—O'Connor (1978) discussed the latter in detail. A learning need is identified by the difference between what a system actually knows (actual) and what one should know in order to accomplish a goal (optimal). Figure 12.1 illustrates this point.

Suppose that a head nurse observed that during the past six months an increasing number of patients on chemotherapy protocols were received on the unit. The head nurse would first need to identify the system responsible for care of these patients. Then information would have to be gathered, examined, and interpreted from primary and secondary sources on whether the system had the knowledge and experience to provide quality individualized nursing care to patients on chemotherapy protocols. A comparison of the outside standard for quality care—what should be known and experienced according to experts—with what is known by the system would result in the specification of a difference that is the learning need. If no difference exists, then a learning need does not exist either. For example:

> *Actual:* A new chemotherapeutic agent is being used in treatment protocols. Nurses are used to working with clients who receive chemotherapy but the nurses are unfamiliar with the new drug and the different protocol and record-keeping system required for research purposes.
>
> *Optimal:* All nurses caring for patients on chemotherapy protocols must have knowledge and understanding of drug actions and side effects, administration regimen, special orders, nursing implications, and record-keeping systems.
>
> *Learning Need:* Knowledge and understanding in all areas of the new chemotherapeutic agent.

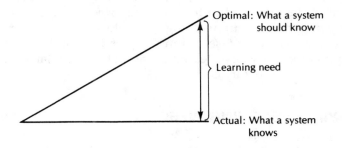

Figure 12.1 Identifying a learning need.

STATING THE TEACHING PRIORITIES

Systems of human resources most often have many learning needs. How does a manager decide what to teach first? Obviously, all learning needs cannot be priorities. Maslow's (1970) hierarchy of needs (refer to Figure 2.3) can be used to answer this question.

A nurse manager should attempt to identify all of the learning needs for all followers given a specific context and period of time. The number of people who have the learning need in focus should be specified; this is the size of the system. Learning needs can then be placed into one of Maslow's five levels: physiological, safety/security, social/affiliative, esteem/recognition, and self-actualization. Table 12.2 provides a format for accomplishing this process; the procedure for stating teaching priorities is discussed more fully in the following paragraphs.

Learning needs involve two areas: (1) those needs essential to quality, individualized nursing care (areas of nursing's clinical responsibility) and (2) those which must be met for the development of the staff (teamwork). Recalling the descriptions in Chapter 4 of the needs in Maslow's (1970) hierarchy, Table 12.3 presents guidelines for classifying areas of nursing responsibility and teamwork needs with Maslow's five levels.

Once the format for stating teaching priorities has been completed, then those learning needs which are first priority—

TABLE 12.2 Format for Stating Teaching Priorities

Learning Needs	Number of Learners (Size of the System)	Maslow's Need Level*
1. _____	_____	_____
2. _____	_____	_____
3. _____	_____	_____
4. _____	_____	_____
5. _____	_____	_____
↓		
n		

*In order of priority: (1) physiological, (2) safety/security, (3) social/affiliative, (4) esteem/recognition, (5) self-actualization.

TABLE 12.3 Maslow's Hierarchy of Needs Paralleled with Areas of Nursing Responsibility and Teamwork Needs

Maslow	Areas of Nursing's Clinical Responsibility*	Teamwork Needs
Physiological	Nutrition Sleep, rest patterns Elimination Prevention of complications Assurance of physiologic status—health maintence	Ongoing clinical education regarding physiological client needs Salary
Safety/Security	Comfort Exercise Personal hygiene Safety Environmental considerations Spiritual comfort and assistance Emotional support, counseling Teaching	Orientation Ongoing clinical education regarding safety/social needs of clients Working conditions Job security Company and administrative policy
Social/Affiliative	Diversional activities Socializing and privacy	Ongoing clinical education regarding social/affiliative client needs Interpersonal relations—superiors, associates, and followers
Esteem/ Recognition	An amplification of what has emerged before, but considering the client's need for achievement	Ongoing clinical education regarding esteem/recognition client needs Executive development Advancement Status Job enrichment
Self-Actualization	The client can take care of self—allow it!	The system can take care of itself—let it!

*Source: La Monica, E. (1985). *The humanistic nursing process*. Boston: Jones and Bartlett.

physiological needs—are immediate concerns. Second, third, and fourth priorities—safety/security, social/affiliative, and esteem/recognition—should be handled in that order. This is not to say that all physiological needs must be filled before a manager thinks of or plans for safety needs, for example. The size of the system becomes important. Small systems containing only a few people or maybe only one person with a specific learning need can be taught much more quickly and more informally than larger systems. When a large number of people require teaching in a certain area, then a more formal program should be developed and priorities for the large program should follow Maslow's theory. Managers, however, can meet a smaller system's needs concurrently. Also, do not forget to use other teaching resources: national, state, and local continuing education programs; in-house programs for people with similar needs; an associate "buddy" system (whereby two managers with the same staff needs split teaching responsibilities, and so forth). Creative use of resources is limitless.

DEVELOPING PROGRAM OBJECTIVES

After a manager decides what is to be taught, several activities are necessary. The more formal the teaching program, the more explicit should be these activities. Mager (1984), in his classic book, said that the goal of a program must first be stated, followed by instructional objectives. The method to evaluate the program's effectiveness should be directly related to the instructional objectives.

The example statement of a learning need that was presented earlier in this chapter is the goal. A description of the course content and procedures may also be given (Mager, 1984). An objective describes the desired outcome of the course, and an evaluation must elicit information on whether the desired outcome has been achieved. An objective should be observable and measurable.

The experiential exercises at the end of Parts I, II, and III of this book contain purposes of the exercises. These purposes are more general than are terminal objectives discussed by Mager (1984). Purposes and a discussion of terminal objectives are presented so that the reader can make an informed decision on the exact type of objective that should be used in a program. The degree of program formality must be considered in making this choice. Applications for continuing education units (CEUs) require explicit terminal objectives and a means for evaluation; implicit objectives and evaluation criteria may only be required, for example, when reviewing colostomy care for a new graduate on the unit.

Mager's (1984)* steps for developing an instructional objective are as follows:

1. Identify the terminal behavior by content name and specify the acceptable behavior indicating that learning has occurred;
2. Define the behavior by stating the conditions under which the behavior should occur; and
3. Specify acceptable performance.

For example:

Orientation Goal: To review pharmacology, dosages, and solutions.

Terminal Objectives:
1. To be able to pass a written 30-item objective pharmacology test at the conclusion of the orientation program with 90% accuracy.
2. To be able to pass a written 25-item objective test on dosages and solutions at the conclusion of the orientation program with 100% accuracy.

Explanation: The content names of the terminal behaviors are pharmacology in the first objective and dosages and solutions in the second objective. The condition under which the behavior should occur is a written test at the conclusion of the orientation program in both objectives. Acceptable performance is the accuracy level required. The evaluative test is the evaluative mechanism.

Evaluating a program is a control process. Newman (1975) specified three types of controls—steering, yes-no, and post-action—as discussed in Chapter 7. The most frequently used method of evaluation is the post-action type, in which the evaluation occurs at the end of a program. Leaders who run programs over a long span of time, however, should employ a yes-no control such as a midpoint evalua-

---

*Mager's programmed instruction on this topic is an easy-to-follow, quick-to-read, fun-to-do, and qualitative classic source for further learning.

tion. An experienced teacher uses steering controls when evaluating a teaching approach by eliciting discussion when people question and by responding to learners' needs during a presentation.

There are many ready-made program evaluation forms that can be applied, adapted, or used as a reference by teachers. The experiential exercises at the conclusion of Part III contain one such form.

EXPLORING TEACHING STRATEGIES

With objectives specified, the content and method(s) for achieving the objectives must be delineated—what will be taught and how it will be taught, our ever-familiar content and process.

Content

It is essential to delineate a detailed outline (at least) of the content that must be taught in order to fulfill program objectives. This is the knowledge base. In the pharmacology example discussed in an earlier section of this chapter, the content would generally include common drug classifications and actions with details on the most commonly used drugs in each category. Specific actions, dosages, administration principles, and side effects would be discussed for the specific drugs. General principles of dosages and solutions would also be taught along with intravenous therapy procedures. The agency's medication procedure would also be content. Given these content areas, what is the best way to teach?

Learning Principles

Learning principles must be considered when deciding how to teach. The literature is replete with discussions of learning theory; a basic overview is provided in this section.

1. A learner must perceive (Bruner, 1960; Conley, 1973; Dewey, 1963, 1982; Ganong & Ganong, 1980).

2. Individual differences such as past experience, intellectual variations, and developmental maturation affect what is learned (Conley, 1973; Ginsburg & Opper, 1969; Wadsworth, 1984; Wertheimer, 1945).

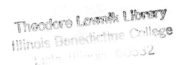

3. The environment influences learning (Conley, 1973; von Bertalanffy, 1968; Watson, 1928).

4. The learner's degree of motivation affects what is learned (Conley, 1973; Hull, 1942; Maslow, 1970).

5. Behavioral reinforcement increases the probability that the desired behavior will recur in another context (Bruner, 1960; Conley, 1973).

6. Repetition facilitates learning (Thorndike [cited in Bower & Hilgard, 1981]).

7. People learn by imitating others (Pohl, 1978).

Rogers (1969) believed that learning has a quality of personal involvement— it is self-initiated and self-reliant. He, therefore, offered the following learning principles that reflect these beliefs:

1. Human beings have a natural potential to learn.

2. Learning is greatly enhanced when learners perceive relevance in the content being taught.

3. Learning that threatens one's self-image tends to be resisted; reduction of external threats eases this effect and facilitates experience.

4. Learning is facilitated when the learner is involved in the process.

5. Self-initiated learning is most powerful—it is lasting and pervasive.

6. Learning the process of learning is most important because it allows one to be continually open to experience.

Within the framework of learning principles, a variety of instructional modes and media—teaching strategies—can be used to fulfill learning objectives.

Instructional Modes and Media

Conley (1973) distinguished modes from media by defining *modes* as types of conversations between the teacher and learner(s); *media* are devices or vehicles to amplify and/or augment various modes of teaching. Various modes and media are presented and explained (Conley, 1973).

Modes

Lecture—This mode is widely used in formal education systems and involves one-way communication from teacher to learners. It is useful when a large group has a particular learning need and is best when followed by small-group discussion to reinforce learning. Content that is in the cognitive domain is often taught by the lecture mode.

Group Discussion—This mode involves two-way communication between teacher and learners and between learner and learners. It is one of the best ways to teach content in the affective domain. Moreover, problems can be shared and support groups or teams can be facilitated. Keenan (1982) referred to this method as a "cooperative goal structure" (p. 487).

Panel Discussion—Expert panel members discuss a topic or an issue among themselves, and/or an interchange among learners and panel members may occur.

Seminar—One or two members present an issue or a problem, and the entire group participates in the discussion. A patient conference is one example of this method. The seminar is useful in self-learning peer groups.

Demonstration—Role modeling in an actual or hypothetical case is one example of demonstration. Any media can be used by the teacher to personify intended learning. Demonstration and laboratory instruction are especially useful when learning involves the psychomotor domain.

Laboratory Instruction—This mode involves learner self-discovery in a safe, low-risk environment. Simulations such as the experiential exercises in this book may be involved. The learner actually "tries on" what is being taught.

Team Teaching—Two or more professionals have responsibility for teaching a particular program; this mode requires coordination and integration of efforts. Learners have the opportunity to hear different points of view on the same issue.

Media

Television—Closed-circuit and public television are becoming increasingly popular. Television specials on topics such as rape and life after death are also media that can be used by a teacher.

Programmed Instruction and Computer-Assisted Instruction— The learner is carried step-by-step through content, using teaching machines or books. The learner receives immediate feedback. Even though this feedback can be thought of as two-way communication, learning occurs better when group or individual discussion follows use of these media.

Motion Pictures—Films on specific content areas can amplify and demonstrate content.

Simulations—Laboratory learning and role modeling are involved in simulations. The preface of this book provides discussion of a rationale for this medium of instruction.

Pictorial Presentations and Printed Language—Pictures, figures, graphs, slides, and overhead transparencies are examples of this category.

Tape and Disk Recordings—These are most useful in seminars and group discussions. They also often augment slides, films, and other similar media.

Models—These are representations of objects needed in demonstrations, such as those used in teaching life support systems.

Different media can be used in the teaching modes. Selection should be guided by what would be most suitable given the objectives, what would be the most well received, and what is most enjoyable for the teacher. Do not overlook the latter statement— people are best at what they like to do, and there is no substitute for a teacher who enjoys what is being done. Learners catch the excitement.

RECOMMENDING A PROGRAM

This step in the problem-solving teaching method is writing out the following in formal teaching situations and rehearsing the following to oneself in informal situations:

- Title of the program (stems from the learning need)
- Description of the program

- Objectives
- Outline of content
- Teaching methods: modes and media
- Faculty/teachers
- Evaluation methods
- Required textbooks and/or reading
- Bibliography
- Handouts (optional)

SUMMARY

Teaching is ubiquitous in management, and all managers and leaders are teachers. Because teachers facilitate learning in people, they change people.

The process of teaching can be informal or formal. Both types should follow the problem-solving method for teaching: identify learning needs, state the teaching priorities, develop program objectives, explore teaching strategies, and recommend a program. Details in each of these areas formed the basis of this chapter. All teaching must reflect knowledge and application of learning principles—what research has suggested has a high probability for facilitating learning as a product of teaching.

REFERENCES

Bower, G., & Hilgard, E. (1981). *Theories of learning* (5th ed.). Englewood Cliffs, NJ: Prentice-Hall.

Bruner, J. (1960). *The process of education.* Cambridge, MA: Harvard University Press.

Conley, V. (1973). *Curriculum and instruction in nursing.* Boston: Little, Brown.

Darling, L., & McGrath, L. (1983). Minimizing promotion trauma. *Journal of Nursing Administration, 13*(9), 14–19.

Dewey, J. (1963). *Experience and education,* New York: Macmillan.

Dewey, J. (1982). *Democracy and education: An introduction to the philosophy of education* (reprint of 1932 ed.). Darby, PA: Darby Books.

Donovan, H. (1975). *Nursing servicing administration: Managing the enterprise.* St. Louis: Mosby.

Fournies, F. (1978). *Coaching for improved work performance.* New York: Van Nostrand Reinhold.

Ganong, J., & Ganong, W. (1980). *Nursing management.* Rockville, MD: Aspen.

Ginsburg, H., & Opper, S. (1969). *Piaget's theory of intellectual development.* Englewood Cliffs, NJ: Prentice-Hall.

Hersey, P., & Blanchard, K. (1988). *Management of organizational behavior: Utilizing human resources* (5th ed.). Englewood Cliffs, NJ: Prentice-Hall.

Hull, C. (1942). Conditioning: Outline of a systematic theory of learning. In *The Psychology of Learning* (Part 2). Forty-first Yearbook of the National Society for the Study of Education. Chicago: University of Chicago Press.

Keenan, M. (1982). Collaboration in students: How can we improve it? *Nursing & Health Care, 3,* 486–488.

La Monica, E. (1985). *The humanistic nursing process.* Boston: Jones and Bartlett.

Littlejohn, C. (1980). What new staff learned and didn't learn. *Nursing Outlook, 28,* 32–35.

Mager, R. (1984). *Preparing instructional objectives* (2nd rev. ed.). Belmont, CA: D.S. Lake Pub.

Maslow, A. (1970). *Motivation and personality,* (2nd ed.). New York: Harper & Row.

Myers, S. (1966). Conditions for manager motivation. *Harvard Business Review, 44*(1), 142–155.

Newman, W. (1975). *Constructive control.* Englewood Cliffs, NJ: Prentice-Hall.

O'Connor, A. (1978). Diagnosing your needs for continuing education. *American Journal of Nursing, 78,* 405–406.

Phillips-Jones, L. (1982). *Mentors and proteges.* New York: Arbor House.

Pohl, M. (1978). *Teaching function of the nursing practitioner.* Dubuque: W.C. Brown.

Rogers, C. (1969). *Freedom to learn.* Columbus: Merrill.

Sovie, M. (1981). Investigate before you educate. *Journal of Nursing Administration, 11,* 15–21.

von Bertalanffy, L. (1968). *General system theory.* New York: Braziller.

Wadsworth, B. (1984). *Piaget's theory of cognitive and affective development* (3rd ed.). New York: David McKay.

Watson, J. (1928). *Psychological care of infant and child.* New York: Norton.

Wertheimer, M. (1945). *Productive thinking.* New York: Harper & Row.

Interviewing*

The interview is the primary procedure used in data collection—this can be for varied purposes such as gathering information on a client for the nursing care plan or gathering information from potential and hired employees. On a smaller scale, a nurse manager can interview an employee informally regarding a situational event.

The process of interviewing is a human interaction during which information is needed and/or is shared. The interactors determine the exact process; the interview has a high interpersonal component and is also seen as a developmental procedure. Gathering data through an interview is a skill that is built on other skills. Observation, listening, and communication are particularly essential.

---

*Much of this chapter is an adaption, replication, and expansion of the chapter on interviewing written by this author in the following source: La Monica, E. (1985). *The humanistic nursing process*. Boston: Jones and Bartlett.

WHAT IS AN INTERVIEW

In many areas of the literature, the interview is recognized as a strategy. Kahn and Cannell (1964) conceived the interview as purposeful conversation. Schatzman and Strauss (1973) agreed with this description even though their perspectives were as field researchers in the areas of sociology and anthropology. Hein (1980) stated simply that interviewing was a human interaction during which information is requested and/or shared.

In discussion of nursing care planning, Bermosk (1966) defined the interview as a special time when the nurse focuses particular attention on the client and/or the client's system or family. Interpreting this definition in nursing management, the manager's client essentially is the employee or follower. The principles of interviewing apply in whatever situation is in focus. The eventual purpose of the interviewing process, according to Keltner (1970), is determined by the people involved in the unique process. Bermosk and Mordan (1973) believed that the interview involved sequenced, directed, and progressive changes in all participants of the interview process.

PURPOSES OF AN INTERVIEW

Perhaps the primary purpose for an interview has been explicated by Hein (1980) in discussion of nursing care planning. This author interprets Hein's original description for nursing management. In the practice of nursing management verbal communication is used to interrelate with a potential or an actual employee with the intent of facilitating, educating, and/or restoring the person to his or her fullest potential. It is therefore a strategy for data collection to help the manager discern another's world, recognize areas requiring assistance or education, and plan an individualized program that is aimed toward accomplishing the stated goals. Marriner-Tomey (1988) termed the interview as goal-directed communication. The following specific purposes for an interview are described. Hiring, promotion, and retention refers to employee interviewing; planning individualized nursing care refers to client interviewing; and describing an event or collecting data refers to both.

Hiring

The interview that occurs prior to employment generally is aimed at collecting and sharing information: (1) to discern whether the person being interviewed has the behaviors necessary for success in the position; (2) to describe the position to the applicant; (3) to sell the job to the applicant; (4) to answer questions from the applicant; and (5) to ascertain the applicant's career committment (Brydon & Myli, 1984).

The interviewer should be keenly aware of the laws governing discriminatory questions since legal action against health care institutions for unlawful preemployment interviews is great (Poteet, 1984). Nurse managers who must conduct interviews should check with the personnel departments in their agencies. Such offices have the guidelines and procedures readily available.

Promotion

Employees are often interviewed prior to the selection of a single person who will be promoted. In this instance, the pre-promotion interview is similar to the interview for hiring. Basically, one wishes to collect information from a candidate that could lead to the best decision regarding success in a designated position.

On the other hand, employees are interviewed upon promotion to collect information on their feelings, goals, and so forth. This type of interview can occur immediately following promotion, and/or can occur as a delayed interview one to two months following promotion in order to discover how the person feels in the new position and what, if any, particular assistance is required as a result of being in the position for a short time.

Retention

The interview that is conducted for the purposes of retention is most often called the performance evaluation. This topic will be discussed in Chapter 18.

Planning Individualized Nursing Care

This interview is often called the therapeutic interview (Bermosk, 1966). Bermosk (p. 205) described this as "a specific kind of communication which is in operation when the professional person (the nurse) focuses . . . attention on the patient (client, subject, group, family) and attends to the business of helping this person to better understand what is happening or what has happened to him at a particular moment in a particular situation . . . [The nurse] encourages him to describe his actions and to express his thoughts and feelings so as to identify needs and to establish goals which will help him to regain, maintain, or improve his health status."

Categories of information that may be obtained during the interview process refer to those areas of the PELLEM Pentagram (La Monica, 1985) (see Figure 3.1, Chapter 3, this volume):

1. Description of the happening;
2. Perceptions of the client regarding the event;
3. Behaviors of the client;
4. Attitudes and beliefs of the client;
5. Client feelings; and
6. Client values.

Questions and statements by the nurse or interviewers should have the purpose of generating information on the categorical guidelines as stated above. They should describe and elaborate, clarify, validate, substantiate, interpret, and compare. In a sense, the interviewer's comments should be levers by which the interviewee can find further self-expression.

Since the nurse manager is often the primary nurse, it is important to see the gathering of client information and the subsequent nursing care plan as an essential function in one's position. As the shortage of nursing personnel continues, as all sources predict, the nurse manager may be found to be the only professional nurse who is guiding nursing care; actual nursing care may be provided by technical nurses and other personnel. Though the above situation is definitely not the wish of this author, increasingly it has been observed as reality. As any good manager knows, contingency planning is the best way to meet demands in any situation.

Describing an Event or Collecting Data

Occasionally, situations occur in which a description is required for records, or just discussion. The purpose of this type of interview is to gather data on the attitudes, feelings, values, and perceptions of interviewees—or those involved in the situation. In a sense, the manager is collecting information so that decisions and actions can be based on a complete record of data that are considered to be valid. This type of interview is usually open-ended with the interviewer stating the situation and asking the interviewee to share what was thought to have occurred. An exit interview is another example of this type of interview.

TYPES OF INTERVIEWS

The interview can be structured, semistructured (Ivancevich, Donnelly, & Gibson, 1989), or unstructured. *Structure* implies that specific questions related to topic areas are posed by the interviewer and are asked of all people being interviewed for a specific purpose. *Semistructure* is less rigid than the structured interview, allowing the interviewer more flexibility; only some questions are prepared in advance (Ivancevich, Donnelly, & Gibson, 1989). An *unstructured* interview relates to the fact that the interviewer's wording of questions is not specified prior to the interview. General content is identified; however, questions flow spontaneously from the interview context. Different interviewees may be asked different questions, depending on the flow of conversation and responses. The purposes of a specified interview may remain constant in all types of interviews. Also, the rule of thumb is that the more experienced the interviewer, the less structure is required in order to obtain the needed information.

   Formal and *informal* are words used to further classify interviewing. Formality broadly represents the fact that time, place, and content are arranged prior to the interaction. It generally involves a longer period for interviewing than does the informal interview. Informal interviewing can be anything from a lengthy, unplanned talk over lunch to a five-minute, spontaneous interaction in a hallway.

CONTINGENCIES OF THE INTERVIEW

Schatzman and Strauss (1973) stated various contingencies that shape the interview's form and content:

1. *Expected duration:* How long is it expected to last? Will it be interrupted? Can it be extended or shortened as guided by the interaction?
2. *Single interview versus a series:* Is this the only one? Is there a series? Where in the series does this one fall?
3. *Setting:* Is this a public or a private place? What does the environment feel like? Is this feeling conducive to the interview's purpose? Is a specific conversational style more appropriate than others in this setting?
4. *Identities:* Is the interviewer an outsider or insider to the system? Can the interviewer and the interviewee be seen as part of the same group?

5. *Style of the respondent:* Is the interviewee comfortable enough to provide responses that are not bathed in a skewer of anxiety?

In addition to these noted above, the author includes the following:

6. *Style of the interviewer*
7. *Harmony between the respondent's style and that of the interviewer.*

Steps in the Interview Process

The following guidelines are provided as a framework for conducting an interview:

1. The interviewer should do the necessary homework prior to the interview. Background information should be available for discussion. Notes on the content of the interview should be delineated. If the interview is formal, time and place should be stated. The interviewee should be instructed on what to study, bring, think about, or prepare.

2. The applicant/interviewee should be greeted. The aim is to quickly establish rapport and put the interviewee at ease. If introductions are necessary, they occur during this step.

3. The purpose(s) of the interview should be stated briefly.

4. Ground rules should be established—boundaries regarding the purpose, time limits, people involved, and so forth.

5. The next step is the exploration phase where data are collected and/or shared. Structured interview questions may be asked during this portion of the interview.

6. The interviewer should review notes to be sure that all information has been covered.

7. The interviewee should be asked if they have any questions. These should be answered as is feasible and within the responsibility and authority of the interviewer.

8. The interview should be closed. Follow-up, if indicated, should be specified regarding time and place—or procedure.

9. The interview should be evaluated to determine if it was successful in accomplishing its purpose(s) or unsuccessful in that the stated goals were not met.

PRINCIPLES OF INTERVIEWING

Kahn and Cannell (1964) viewed the interview as a lengthy conversation in which there are three conditions for success: accessibility, cognition, and motivation. The first requires that the information received by the interviewer be in a conscious, clear, and relevant form. It must relate to the purposes of the interview for each unique interviewee. Cognition requires that the person interviewed understand his/her role, and the reasons for data collection. Finally, motivation, or willingness to interact, is the major requirement for a successful interview.

Since client motivation has been observed as a paramount and necessary condition, much research by social scientists has been devoted to the area. In one example, Kahn and Cannell (1964) postulated both instrumental and intrinsic factors in their motivational framework (Figure 13.1).

It is easy to observe that the interview can and should be regarded as a complex social phenomenon. *Instrumental factors* of motivation focus heavily on the interviewee's belief that the results of the interview will have some positive effect on what happens to him. The second type of motivational factors, *intrinsic* (Kahn & Cannell, 1964), reflect the qualities of the interviewer. Receptiveness, warmth, understanding, and interest are all important. It is also pertinent to note that the principles of communication which were presented in Chapter 9 are also valid for a productive interview.

Certain principles for an effective interview must be integrated into interview techniques. Hein (1980, p. 26) explicated the following essentials; they are adapted for the nurse manager by this author:

1. An interview is effective to the degree that the manager creates an atmosphere that encourages and supports the employee's or potential employee's freedom of expression.

2. An interview is effective to the degree that the manager clearly establishes and understands the goals of the interview.

3. An interview is effective to the degree that the man-

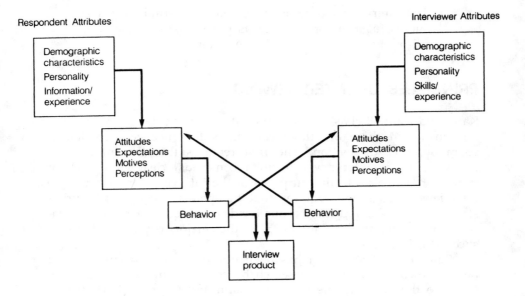

Figure 13.1 Motivational Model of the Interview as a Social Process
Source: *The Dynamics of Interviewing,* by R. Kahn and C. Cannell. Copyright ©
1964 by John Wiley & Sons, Inc. Reprinted by permission.

ager can relate to the follower without using value
judgments.

4. An interview is effective to the degree that the manager examines, encourages, and clarifies mutual
   thoughts and feelings that may affect the issue and
   outcome.

5. An interview is effective to the degree that the manager consistently evaluates needs, goals, and the behavioral responses of the interviewee.

6. An interview is effective to the degree that the manager is able to evaluate her communication behavior
   objectively in relation to the needs and behavioral responses evidenced by the interviewee.

7. An interview is effective to the degree that the man-

ager employs and encourages the use of feedback in conveying, implementing, and evaluating goals.*

In addition, Bermosk (1966, p. 207–210) stated other requisites:

8. The climate the manager creates within the interaction influences the substance of the interview.
9. Professional attitudes of warmth, acceptance, objectivity, and compassion are essential for effective interviewing.
10. The identification and clarification of conflicting thoughts and feelings of the participants lead toward a harmony of goals in the interview.**

The social process involved in the interview can again be noticed by studying the principles; the interpersonal facet involves the nurse interviewer, the client, and the interaction of both.

SUMMARY

It becomes clear that interviewing is a complex social process involving the principal interactors, purposes guided by principles of interviewing, and many extraneous variables that also must be considered. This chapter contained discussion of the primary purposes of an interview along with the types of interviews that can occur, depending on the preference and experience of the interviewer and the reasons for the interview. The section on interview contingencies included the generic steps of the interview process. The chapter concluded with principles of interviewing.

REFERENCES

Bermosk, L. (1966). Interviewing: A key to therapeutic communication in nursing practice. *Nursing Clinics of North America, 1,* 205–214.
Bermosk, L., & Mordan, M. (1973). *Interviewing in nursing.* New York: Macmillan.

---

*From *Communication in Nursing Practice,* by E. Hein. Copyright © 1980 by Little, Brown and Co., Inc. Reprinted with permission.
**Reprinted with permission from *Nursing Clinics of North America,* by Bermosk, L. 1966, Vol. 1, No. 2.

Brydon, P., & Myli, A. (1984). After the interview: Who gets the job? *American Journal of Nursing, 84*(6), 736–738.

Hein, E. (1980). *Communication in nursing practice* (2nd ed.). Boston: Little, Brown.

Ivancevich, J., Donnelly, J. Jr., & Gibson, J. (1989). *Management: Principles and functions* (4th ed.). Homewood, IL: Irwin.

Kahn, R., & Cannell, C. (1964). *The dynamics of interviewing.* New York: Wiley.

Keltner, J. (1970). *Interpersonal speech-communication: Elements and structures.* Belmont, CA: Wadsworth.

La Monica, E. (1985). *The humanistic nursing process.* Boston: Jones and Bartlett.

Marriner-Tomey, A. (1988). *Guide to nursing management* (3rd ed.). St. Louis: Mosby.

Poteet, G. (1984). The employment interview: Avoiding discriminatory questioning. *Journal of Nursing Administration, 14*(4), 38–42.

Schatzman, L., & Strauss, A. (1973). *Field research: Strategies for a natural society.* Englewood Cliffs, NJ: Prentice-Hall.

CHAPTER 14

Assertiveness
by Patricia M. Raskin*

Although the concepts underlying assertiveness training have been gaining increasing popularity, the usefulness of the training model to the helping professions was first noted in 1949. Originally conceived as a limited form of behavior therapy (Salter, 1961; Wolpe, 1958), assertiveness training has been found to have so many applications

---

*Patricia M. Raskin, Ph.D., is an Associate Professor of Counseling Psychology at Teachers College, Columbia University, New York. She is currently Chair of the Department of Social, Organizational and Counseling Psychology. As a psychologist, she consults nationally with industry, health-care systems, and educational institutions. Dr. Raskin is a former coordinator of the Women's Task Force of the American College Personnel Association. She has been teaching assertiveness to various lay and professional groups since 1974.

that it can no longer be considered as a single technique, but rather as an array of techniques designed to be effective with a large and varied number of target populations (Shoemaker & Satterfield, 1977). Most of the strategies and techniques, however, rest on three basic assumptions about human nature (Percell, 1977):

1. That feelings and attitudes relate closely to behavior;
2. That behavior is learned; and
3. That behavior can be changed.

The purpose of this chapter is to define and discuss the concept of assertiveness and its application to nursing. Following a discussion of the definition and the theoretical aspects of the assertiveness paradigm, the goals and components of training are presented. The final section of the chapter is devoted to an application of assertiveness techniques.

WHAT IS ASSERTIVENESS?

It is not unusual for people to make the assumption that the words *assertive* and *aggressive* have the same meaning. According to most dictionary definitions, they are synonyms. Professionals who teach people how to be more assertive, however, make a distinction between those words. A continuum along which assertive behavior can be rated is presented in Figure 14.1.

A *passive* communication is one in which an individual's needs, wishes, desires, or concerns are not expressed explicitly, usually because the sender believes the receiver of the message wants something different, or the sender consciously or unconsciously feels that the receiver is responsible for caretaking or mind-reading. An *aggressive* communication involves pushing one's needs, wishes, desires, or concerns onto another. In *assertive* communication, it is clear that in any given dyad there are two actors; two people may express their needs, wishes, desires, or concerns, and the opportunity exists for

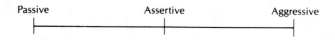

Figure 14.1 Assertiveness continuum

both to listen and respond to one another nondefensively. An assertive message is an open one that facilitates or enhances effective communication, understanding, and/or closure.

People are rarely completely passive, assertive, or aggressive; rather, messages are usually contextually bound. It is entirely possible, for instance, that a staff nurse who is tongue-tied with a supervisor at work can be clear, direct, and confident with family members, children's teachers, and the mechanic at the local garage. The same supervisor, who is an effective, assertive administrator, may have difficulty returning clothing to a store, changing her mind about an order in a restaurant, or asking a family member for a favor.

WHY IS ASSERTIVE BEHAVIOR DESIRABLE?

Both passive and aggressive messages are costly, sometimes only to the conversation in which they occur, but often to relationships as well. A passive communication leaves the sender or responder with thoughts or feelings that still need expression; this often leads to resentment or a belief that one is misunderstood or that what is said is of no consequence to the other. Even with resentment evident, its source may be unclear. A passive message is deficient in information, so it does not help another to understand the needs, wishes, desires, concerns, or limits of the sender as fully as may be possible. The hidden agenda in a passive message is often an unwillingness to take responsibility for the matter at hand, a wish to be taken care of, a set of unrealistic expectations ("If she really cared about me, she'd figure out what I need"), or an unwillingness to accept the consequences for one's own actions.

Aggressive communcations have more directly observable costs to their recipients and therefore are not brought to the attention of the aggressor for some time. Aggressive behaviors tend to elicit "fight or flight" reactions; people either respond with equal or greater aggression or else they withdraw. In both cases, the aggressor ought to be sensitive to the fact that she or he is at least partly responsible for the reaction that occurs; that sensitivity, however, is exactly the trait that is in shortest supply at the moment of aggression.

Extended periods of passivity often lead to an explosion of aggression given the "right" stimulus—the straw that breaks the camel's back. In this instance, the time is long past for discussion and mediation. The statements, "I've had it up to here, and I quit," may reflect a buildup of resentment that resulted from passivity. It is clear that there is not much left to be negotiated when the person making those statements ends the discussion abruptly.

Assertive behavior is desirable from at least two points of view: (1) It represents an open, mature, direct way of communicating that allows the other to learn about one's feelings and identify, while enhancing self-esteem (Percell, 1977), and (2) it is more likely to preserve effective interpersonalrelationships than are either passive or aggressive behaviors.

ASSERTIVE BEHAVIOR IN NURSES

The need for assertiveness training for nurses has been widely documented both in the field and in the literature (Clark, 1978, 1979; Kilkus, 1986; Marriner, 1979; Pardue, 1980). Initially, most of this documentation was limited to nurse leaders and managers. There is increasing evidence that staff nurses, particularly those in the beginning of their careers, can benefit from assertiveness training, especially since most nurses are female and are subject to all of the effects of sex-role socialization that operate to inhibit assertive behaviors (Angel & Petronko, 1983; Jakubowski-Spector, 1973). Further, when assertive behaviors are learned early in a nurse's career, the chances increase that they will develop over time. These mature behaviors enable one to be a better candidate for administrative positions and to be more effective in such positions (MacDonald, 1986).

The occupational characteristics of nursing are changing (Kinney, 1985; Milauskas, 1985), thereby creating demands for greater responsibility and authority at all levels of the profession. Such demands alter both the role concept and professional self-concept of nursing's practitioners.

Super (1957) suggested that choosing a career is a means of implementing one's self-concept. Engaging in work that permits self-expression and is congruent with personal values may therefore be a function of personality and style as well as of exposure and opportunity. Although there are many reasons for choosing nursing as a career, one primary motive is the opportunity to help others. Until recently, nurses have accepted the demands of unquestioning obedience, the maintenance of one's place in the hierarchy, and the dependence of subordinates on supervisors (Valiga, 1982). The historical roots of nursing have led to the widespread view of nurses as submissive handmaidens to physicians, doers rather than thinkers, and reactors rather than initiators (Keller, 1973).

It is reasonable to suggest that people attracted to the old view of nursing might have difficulty adapting to the new demands and altering their behavior to include greater initiative, more persistence, and more autonomy in decision-making. In fact, McIntyre, Jeffrey, and McIntyre (1984) found nurses to be sufficiently subassertive as a group and to be the ideal test population for their comprehensive assertion training package. Speigel, Smolen, and Jones (1985) reported that many medical students had less difficulty being aggressive with nurses than with authority figures or peers. They suggested that this finding might be interpreted in light of Hayes and Patterson's (1975) observation that medical students become domineering, while nurses become submissive early in multidisciplinary groups. There is some evidence, however, that this pattern is changing. Klein and Klein (1984) found that nursing graduates from 1980 felt more independent, felt that they had achieved more, and were more assertive than their 1974 counterparts.

It follows from the preceding paragraphs that there are several reasons assertiveness training is appealing to nurses: (1) Those nurses who are more comfortable in a reactive stance might need to become more at ease with and fluent in the skills and language of more active participation in their work; (2) those who support a professional and primary role for nurses might find the assertiveness training paradigm useful for facilitating the development of attitudes about responsible nursing behavior as well as effective communication skills; and (3) those nursing professionals who are concerned with the public view of nursing might find a way of communicating their attitudes and expectations more clearly.

GOALS OF ASSERTIVENESS TRAINING

Alberti and Emmons (1986) pointed out that the goals of assertiveness training are to teach people how to exercise their rights, to assist them in developing an expanded repertoire of behaviors, and to help them to act in their own best interest. Because assertiveness training is a behavioral (rather than insight-oriented) method, the goals are inductive rather than deductive. There are three levels at which assertiveness occurs: techniques, response style, and lifestyle. Reinforcement occurs as one learns and practices the techniques of assertion. Making requests, saying no, accepting compliments, and expressing concern become easier, rewarding the individual with increased self-respect and improved interactions. In turn, this may lead to an assertive response style, in which being assertive becomes more natural and is characterized by open verbal and nonverbal expression. At the most complex cognitive level, one may develop an assertive lifestyle, one that includes both intra- and interpersonal awareness. If assertiveness training "takes" at this level, the end result is quite similar to the goals of many forms of humanistic psychotherapy: ease in interpersonal relationships; congruence among thoughts, feelings, and behaviors; and a willingness to accept responsibility for one's actions as well as to accept the consequences of those actions.

COMPONENTS OF ASSERTIVENESS

Assertive behaviors can be broadly separated into two components: verbal and nonverbal. In order for a communication to be categorized as assertive, both components must be present. It is entirely possible that an individual says all the right words, for example, "I'd like the sweater back that you borrowed," but does so in either such an aggressive way (hands on hips, eyes glaring, edge to the voice) or in such a passive way (small voice, downcast eyes, pleading tone) that the receiver of the message is either offended or uncomfortable. In order for a message to be truly assertive, the words and the music behind the words have to go together. People have learned, for instance, that tenderness is not expressed in a loud tone of voice, that intimate conversations do not take place between two people who are 15 feet apart, and that anger is not expressed with a smile. As a matter of fact, when the words and the music do not go together, it is difficult to know what to believe. Confusion results, and the natural response of the listener to this mixed message is avoidance, withdrawal, anger, or some other form of interpersonal distance.

Nonverbal Components

Serber (1977) suggested that the nonverbal components of behavior are:

> Loudness of voice,
> Fluency of spoken words,
> Eye contact,

Facial expression,

Body expression, and

Distance from person with whom one is interacting (p. 69).

Loudness of Voice. Neither screaming nor whispering is assertive. Tone of voice does not depend on the content of the message sent. An assertive tone should be loud and firm so that it is heard clearly; it should not, however, be so loud that it is assaultive to the ear of the receiver.

Fluency. Fluency of spoken words also does not depend on the content of the message. People who use too many pauses or "filler" words such as *uh, er, huh, you know, like,* and so forth, are likely to be perceived as hesitant, whereas people who speak too quickly are often experienced as overwhelming. A moderate, unbroken rate of speech is assertive.

Eye Contact. It is imposssible to be assertive when not looking at the intended receiver of one's message. Without eye contact, there is no way of gauging a response, and the receiver of a message is forced to intrude on the sender in order to give feedback about the communication. Staring or glowering, of course, are intrusive by their very nature. Assertive eye contact means that one is able to look at the receiver's face more or less continuously without such intensity that the receiver's gaze is challenged.

Facial Expression. People who giggle when angry or frown when saying loving, affectionate words sabotage the content of their messages. When people are angry, they do not smile; when expressing appreciation, they do. Although facial expression is hard to measure or describe, most people have been socialized to be capable of choosing congruent facial expressions for the meaning of their words. It is often a signal of discomfort or anxiety when one is unable to get the words and music together; since congruence and anxiety are mutually exclusive reactions, being congruent may help to reduce the anxiety.

Body Expression. Like facial expression, how one stands, sits, or moves conveys a complex series of attitudes. A person who is slouching can be perceived as hostile, uninterested, or frightened. Crossed arms may give the impression that one is guarded, armed, or unreceptive. Hands on hips may indicate a combative, patronizing attitude, while a rigid, wooden posture can indicate fear. People who are assertive in their body expression seem relaxed but do not slouch, stand straight without being rigid, and use their hands and shoulders to embellish their conversation without being too forceful or abrupt.

Distance. How far away one stands from the person while interacting varies from culture to culture and individual to individual. The term *bubble* has been applied to the invisible boundary that people use to protect themselves from intrusion (Sommer, 1969). In southern Europe, for example, one may become uncomfortably aware of how close people stand when engaging in a conversation. It is natural for Americans to back away in order to feel more comfortable—to protect their bubble. Although the example just given is of a cultural difference rather than interpersonal style, it is possible to experience new European friends as aggressive or intrusive. The other extreme involves too much distance. A meaningful interpersonal dialogue usually does not occur at a distance of five feet. People who are assertive in their distance from others stand close enough so that not much can pass between them and their receiver (like another person, for instance) but not so close they break the receiver's bubble.

Verbal Components

What is said is just as important as how one says it. It is unlikely, for instance, that someone who makes an unclear statement or request will get an appropriate response. It may not be that the listener is unresponsive, but rather that the message is too ambiguous for a lucid answer. Cooley and Hollandsworth (1977) suggested three verbal components of assertive statements:

1. Saying "no" or taking a stand;
2. Asking favors or asserting rights; and
3. Expressing feelings.

Saying no. Assertive statements can be either initiations or reactions. There are ways to say no assertively in response to another's request or demand. Many people feel backed into a corner when asked to do something that they do not want to do. "I just couldn't say no" is a common complaint. The reasons people cannot or will not say no vary; some are afraid of the other's anger or disapproval;

some are afraid of hurting others' feelings; some are afraid of rejection; and some feel that to say no would violate their self-concept as "nice." Nevertheless, everyone wants to or needs to refuse a favor or a request from time to time; if saying no is uncomfortable, one may unintentionally become aggressive or overjustify a refusal. A crucial aspect of saying no assertively is that the refusal be understood and believed. Saying too much makes one less convincing while saying too little may seem rejecting. The object is to say no firmly and uncompromisingly while acknowledging the other's right to ask. Saying no assertively means that one can refuse a request and give a reason for refusing the request while indicating that the other person has been heard: "I appreciate your need to change shifts with me, but I can't on Thursday because I already have plans."

Taking a Stand. This component of assertion may be either an initiation or a response to a situation. The key elements in this area are the clarity of one's position, the self-respect with which such a position is stated, and an understanding of the other's position: "I know that you believe that Mrs. Lloyd is recovering; I'm not convinced, however, that she's ready for discharge, and I will not support her release."

Asking Favors. Many people believe that they do not have the right to ask for a favor. This is not true. People do not have the right to get everything they request, but permission to ask is unnecessary. If one has trouble asking for favors, it sometimes means that more meaning may be attached to a refusal than is appropriate in the circumstance: "If he says no to this, it means he doesn't love me." Or it may mean that one will feel guilty and obligated for asking: "If she lends me her car, I'll have to do whatever she wants whenever she wants it done." When asking for favors, being assertive means stating the problem clearly and making a specific request. How long to persist with the request is a matter of judgment; the request should end with either its being granted or with the understanding of why it cannot or would not be granted. One should not end a request before this point has been reached.

Asserting Rights. In our society, no human being has the right to take advantage of another; every human being has the right to speak. Differences in power between two individuals do not alter those fundamental rights, although sometimes the less powerful member of the dyad may feel the need to remind the more powerful member that this is the case, and, of course, the consequences of power inequities need to be considered. The key components of asserting one's rights are similar to those in asking favors: stating the problem, making a specific request for resolution or change, and persisting until one has effectively communicated a point. "I understand that you sometimes need me to work later than usual. I don't like it when you simply expect that and don't check with me. If you give me some advance notice, I'm sure I'll be able to accommodate you most of the time."

Expressing Feelings. Although feelings often appear to be obvious from nonverbal behavior, people may have no idea of another's feelings unless they are expressed in words. A colleague may not be aware of making a peer angry, and a friend may be blind to the pain that laughing at a neighbor's handwriting caused that person. Part of being assertive is expressing emotions such as anger and affection. "I appreciate your saying that" is a more assertive way of responding to an expression of gratitude than "it's nothing" or "it's just my job," which belittles both the sender and the receiver of the message of thanks.

APPROPRIATE USES OF ASSERTIVENESS TECHNIQUES

As discussed earlier, few people are completely nonassertive (passive) or aggressive. Most people vary in assertiveness from situation to situation, and the degree of intimacy shared with others accounts for some of this variation as well. It is possible to be appropriately assertive with one's spouse and to become quite passive with one's mother-in-law. Alternately, being assertive with strangers may be easy, and canceling a date with a friend because of a whim to stay home may seem out of the question. Even at work, people may have a range of responses like being direct with a supervisor and being unable to give followers explicit directions on assignments.

One of the more common differences in assertiveness within rather than between individuals has to do with "managing up" versus "managing down." In the workplace, this is often compounded when authority figures are male and subordinates are female. When the component of unequal training or education is added, one may see how being assertive can be potentially confusing and difficult.

Being Assertive with Authority Figures

Many people have been raised to respect their elders and obey their parents. Although unchallenged in childhood when dependent on parents and teachers, those attitudes are not appropriate dicta for self-directed adults who bear sole responsibility for their lives. It is unlikely that parents, for instance, can rescue a subordinate from a tyrannical superior; further, it is unlikely that the authority figure's attitudes will change simply because a subordinate wants them to. Subordinates need to help the supervisor to understand that they are not doormats or children or passive troops, ready to blindly follow orders. Although most supervisors know this, some are not as adept as others in interpersonal skills. Being assertive with supervisors may be the only way that subordinates express the right to be treated as adults, even though supervisors have position power—more responsibility and authority. Of course, tact and understanding of the supervisor's role responsibilities are essential in asserting oneself.

Being Assertive with Followers

People learn how to be managers and parents by watching role models. If fate looked kindly and provided such modeling by assertive leaders, managers, parents, and helping professionals, effective interpersonal skills would be perpetuated. Fate is not always so benevolent, however, and in moments of stress, it is easy to "pass on" the aggressive or manipulative behaviors that were learned in the past. If people can be assertive with superiors, there is less angry residue that can spill onto contacts with supervisees, patients, and children; moreover, there is less likelihood of forgetting that others less powerful have a right to determine their own responses also. An illustration of this "domino theory" of aggression can be seen in the following example:

> Mrs. Roy is perceived by some as a whining, complaining patient. She has been calling with various complaints and requests every ten minutes since the shift began. Responding to her for the fourth time, you feel annoyed that other responsibilities are not being carried out. Your supervisor, meeting you on your way

out of Mrs. Roy's room, snaps at you because a second-year resident snapped at her because another patient was neglected. You remain silent with your supervisor, secretly cursing Mrs. Roy and the resident. The next time Mrs. Roy calls for attention, it takes you 20 minutes to respond, and when in her room, you seem gruff, uncaring, and irritated.

The irony in the above situation is that everyone (except perhaps Mrs. Roy) perceives a problem and wants it solved. Assertion in this circumstance is breaking the cycle of smoldering anger and serial accusation. On the fourth response to Mrs. Roy, an assertive statement might be: "I understand that you are uncomfortable and unhappy, but I have other patients to care for, and I will not be back for a while. What is the most important thing that I can do for you right now?" The supervisor might be responded to by saying: "It seems like the staff shortage is getting to all of us. It doesn't help when you snap at me." By being assertive, considerably more control over both the situation and personal feelings can be exercised without resentment of the supervisor or of the patient. Each of them is also given a chance to respond further.

MONITORING ONE'S OWN ASSERTIVENESS

Two mechanisms give feedback about assertiveness: internal and external feedback mechanisms.

Internal Feedback Mechanisms

Nonassertion (passivity) can be felt in the body and is usually experienced as tension in the stomach, chest, throat, shoulders, and/or neck. There may also be a sense of shame attached. There may be a wish to strike back, with an equal sense that to do so is too risky. Aggressive anger is often felt as internal rage with a wish to overpower the target of aggression.

External Feedback Mechanisms

The receiver of nonassertive or aggressive messages provides feedback to the sender. Senders who act like victims are likely to be either attacked or ignored. Victims of aggression, however, probably respond by withdrawal and passive resistance; occasionally the response is a counterassault. No one is assertive all of the time. If one has the feeling of losing contact with another through aggression, that person might say something like: "I think I just ignored your feelings—I'm sorry. Can we talk about what just happened?" Alternatively, if hindsight makes one aware of nonassertion in an encounter, one can respond assertively later. For example, "I was really upset yesterday when you yelled at me. I understand that you were frustrated, but I'd rather talk out our difficulties than be shouted at."

ASSESSING AND APPLYING ASSERTIVENESS TECHNIQUES

Because assertiveness training has been so popular for so long, there are many assessment devices to help you determine whether or in what domains you could benefit from assertion training. Good general sources for that purpose can be found throughout *The Assertive Woman* (Phelps & Austin, 1987) and *Your Perfect Right* (Alberti & Emmons, 1986). One of the best ways to improve your skills is to practice through role playing in groups. You can find practice situations anywhere, of course, but there are some particularly useful vignettes reproduced in the experiential exercises, Part III of this book. Practicing these with colleagues is a practical way to get feedback about your strengths and weaknesses in assertive communication.

A FINAL NOTE

Although assertiveness can be taught and can be seen as simply another skill to be learned, the ramifications of not being assertive go much deeper than simply choosing not to use a new technique. Nursing is a demanding profession, one in which others such as patients, physicians, administrators, and families often assume that they have the right to define nursing's professional identity. Not only are patients and their families likely to misunderstand the nurse's role because of their societally reinforced notion of the nurse as an obedient handservant to the physician, but patients are also likely to be at their most anxious and least level-headed conditions when faced with serious illness. Most nurses and nursing students believe that effective interpersonal relationships are an important aspect of nursing responsibility and individual career satisfaction (Everly & Falcione, 1976; Lyon & Iranevich, 1974). Although no one can control the responses of others, and it is impossible to educate all of those who misperceive the nurse's role, one can exert control over one's own behavior. Despite difficult and trying working conditions, frustration can at least be reduced if nurses express feelings and thoughts directly, adequately, responsibly, and with accountability.

SUMMARY

Assertiveness in an interaction between two people means that both express their needs, wants, and concerns; both people listen and respond to the other nondefensively. An assertive message is different from a passive or an aggressive communication. Assertive behaviors have verbal and nonverbal components. Nonverbal components include loudness of voice, fluency of spoken words, eye contact, facial and body expressions, and spatial relations between interactors. Verbal aspects include saying no, asking favors, expressing feelings, asserting rights, and taking a stand on an issue.

REFERENCES

Alberti, R.E., & Emmons, M.L. (1986). *Your perfect right: A guide to assertive living* (5th rev. ed.). San Luis Obispo, CA: Impact.

Angel, G., & Petronko, D.K. (1983). *Developing the new assertive nurse: Essential for advancement*. New York: Springer.

Clark, C. (1978). *Assertive skills for nurses*. Wakefield, MA: Contemporary Publishing.

Clark, C. (1979). Assertiveness issues for nursing administrators and managers. *Journal of Nursing Administration, 9,* 20–24.

Cooley, M., & Hollandsworth, J. (1977). A strategy for teaching verbal content of assertive responses. In Alberti, R.E. (Ed.) *Assertiveness: Innovations, applications, issues*. San Luis Obispo, CA: Impact.

Everly, G., & Falcione, R. (1976). Perceived dimensions of job satisfaction for staff registered nurses. *Nursing Research, 25,* 346–348.

Hayes, S., & Patterson, M. (1975). Interaction between students in multidisciplinary health teams. *Journal of Medical Education, 50,* 473–475.

Jakubowski-Spector, P. (1973). Facilitating the growth of women through assertive training. *The Counseling Psychologist, 4,* 75–86.

Keller, N. (1973). The nurse's role: Is it expanding or shrinking? *Nursing Outlook, 21,* 236–240.

Kilkus, S.P. (1986). Adding assertiveness to the nursing profession. *Nursing Success Today, 3*(8), 17–19.

Kinney, C.K.D. (1985). A reexamination of nursing role conceptions. *Nursing Research, 34*(3), 170–176.

Klein, C.P., & Klein, S. (1984). Emerging independence in nursing graduates: An analysis of traditional-nontraditional value patterns. *Sex Roles, 10*(11/12), 993–1002.

Lyon, H., & Iranevich, J. (1974). An exploratory investigation of organizational climate and job satisfaction in a hospital. *Academy of Management Journal, 17*, 635–648.

MacDonald, J. (1986). Time for a change. *International Nursing Review, 33*(6), 187.

Marriner, A. (1979). Assertive behavior for nursing leaders. *Nursing Leadership, 2*, 14–20.

McIntyre, T.J., Jeffrey, D.B., & McIntyre, S.L. (1984). Assertion training: The effectiveness of a comprehensive cognitive-behavioral treatment package with professional nurses. *Behavioral Research and Therapy, 22*(3), 311–318.

Milauskas, J. (1985). Will nursing assert itself? *Nursing Administration Quarterly, 9*(3), 1–15.

Pardue, S. (1980). Assertiveness for nursing. *Supervisor Nurse, 11*, 47–50.

Percell, L. (1977). Assertive behavior training and the enhancement of self-esteem. In Alberti, R.E. (Ed.) *Assertiveness: Innovations, applications, issues.* San Luis Obispo, CA: Impact.

Phelps, S., & Austin, N. (1987). *The assertive woman: A new look.* (2nd ed.). San Luis Obispo, CA: Impact.

Salter, A. (1961). *Conditioned reflex therapy* (2nd ed.). New York: Capricorn.

Serber, M. (1977). Teaching the nonverbal components of assertiveness training. In Alberti, R.E. (Ed.) *Assertiveness: Innovations, applications, issues.* San Luis Obispo, CA: Impact.

Shoemaker, M., & Satterfield, D. (1977). Assertion training: An identity crisis that's coming on strong. In Alberti, R.E. (Ed.) *Assertiveness: Innovations, applications, issues.* San Luis Obispo, CA: Impact.

Sommer, R. (1969). Studies in personal space. *Sociometry, 22*, 247–260.

Spiegel, D.A., Smolen, R.C., & Jones, C.K. (1985). Interpersonal conflicts involving students in clinical medical education. *Journal of Medical Education, 60*, 819–829.

Super, D.E. (1957). *The psychology of careers.* New York: Harper & Row.

Valiga, T.M.G. (1982). *The cognitive development of and perceptions about nursing as a profession of baccalaureate nursing students.* Unpublished doctoral dissertation. New York: Teachers College, Columbia University.

Wolpe, J.E. (1958). *Psychotherapy by reciprocal inhibition.* Stanford, CA: Stanford University Press.

Group Dynamics

Group dynamics involves the study and analysis of how people interact and communicate with each other in face-to-face small groups. The study of group dynamics provides a vehicle to analyze group communications with the intent of rendering the groups more effective (Davis & Newstrom, 1985; La Monica, 1985).

Chapter 15 begins with a discussion of the purposes for studying group dynamics, followed by details of what can be observed in groups. One area for observation, group roles, is presented in a separate section. Processing group behaviors is then discussed, with common nursing groups concluding the chapter.

PURPOSES FOR STUDYING GROUP DYNAMICS

According to general system theory (von Bertalanffy, 1968, 1975), a system is more than a sum of its parts. It involves pooling the energy of a group of human and material resources toward goal accomplishment. (Refer back to Chapter 2 for a thorough discussion of general system theory.) Contemporary management practices apply this theory. It follows, therefore, that a manager's best bet is to motivate the group to work together toward goal accomplishment. The more effectively a group works as a team, the higher the probability for cost-effective services. Because fostering teamwork is one of the purposes of a manager's communications, studying group dynamics is an important facet of organizational work (Baker, 1980; Weeks, Barrett, & Snead, 1985). What a system (group) accomplishes has as much to do with the goal as it does with how well the group works as a team.

Lippitt and Seashore (1980) delineated more specific purposes for studying group dynamics. The manager's goal is to develop an effective team by facilitating:

1. A clear understanding of purposes and goals;
2. Flexibility in how a group accomplishes goals;
3. Effective communication and understanding among members—on personal feelings and attitudes as well as task-related ideas and issues;
4. Effective decision-making strategies that secure commitment of members to important decisions;
5. An appropriate balance between group productivity and individual satisfaction;
6. Group maturation so that leader responsibilities can be shared according to the group's ability and willingness;
7. Group cohesiveness while maintaining the needed measure of individual freedom;
8. Use of members' different abilities;
9. How a group is solving its own problems; and
10. A balance between emotional and rational behavior—steering emotions into productive teamwork.

WHAT TO OBSERVE IN GROUPS

The literature contains discussions of many aspects in group behavior that can be studied (Charrier, 1980; Clark, 1987; Lippitt & Seashore, 1980; Marram, 1978; Sampson & Marthas, 1981). The labels attached to these aspects differ. Dimensions of group behavior that are discussed in this chapter are: goals, background, participation, communication patterns, cohesion and membership, climate, norms, and decision-making procedures. Group roles will be discussed in the section that follows the present one.

Group Goals

It has been stated repeatedly in this book that groups must have a goal. Sometimes the goal is formal, and sometimes it is informal, such as having a bull session to let off steam. These goals represent the tasks of the group. How the group as a team accomplishes these tasks is group behavior.

Group Background

The history and traditions of the group bear directly on the life of the group as it seeks to accomplish its immediate task (Lippitt & Seashore, 1980). Traditions, norms, procedures, and activities should be studied in terms of how they affect the present. Positive aspects of past group behavior (aspects that a manager considers as having the probability to facilitate task accomplishment) should be fostered. Strategies to counteract previous negative dimensions must be specified and implemented.

Group Participation

A manager's goal should be to facilitate the fullest possible participation of the system's human resources. Recalling von Bertalanffy's (1968) assumption of an open system—a group is more than a sum of its parts (Chapter 2)—the more energy that members put into teamwork, the more output will result from the group. The manager has to apply motivation theory to accomplish this most important aspect of group behavior.

Communication Patterns

This area involves the social organization of the group. The primary reasons for studying communication patterns are to draw out member issues and focus on task issues more effectively. Areas that should be discussed are: who is talking with whom, what is said, how it is said, nonverbal behavior, and who is listening to whom (La Monica, 1985; Lippitt & Seashore, 1980).

Communication Networks. Various communication networks have effects on variables such as speed of performance, accuracy, job satisfaction, flexibility, and so forth. Figure 15.1 shows three classic communication networks. Obviously many other patterns can exist.

Bavelas and Barrett (1951) and Leavitt (1951) suggested that the circle network resulted in slow group speed, poor accuracy, no informal leader, very good job satisfaction, and fast flexibility to change. The chain resulted in speedy performance, good accuracy, increased likelihood that a leader would emerge, poor job satisfaction, and slow flexibility to change. The wheel, called such because all communications are channeled through the center person, obviously has a pronounced leader. Performance is speedy and accuracy is good with this network; however, job satisfaction tends to be poor and flexibility to change is slow. Even though the initial research on communication networks was done early, more recent studies corroborated the findings presented (Cohen, 1962; Mears, 1974; Shaw, 1954a, 1954b). It was underscored by Davis and Newstrom (1985) that groups naturally solve their assigned problem as efficiently as possible using networks that are necessary. One network, therefore, is as good as another, depending on the system.

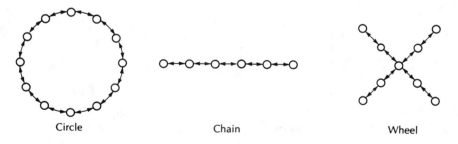

Circle   Chain   Wheel

Figure 15.1 Classic communication networks.

Transactional Analysis (TA). Transactional analysis is another method that can be used to study behavior between and among people. It was developed by Berne (1972, 1978) and led into popularity by Harris (1982), James and Jongeward (1971, 1978), and Jongeward (1976).

According to TA, people have three ego states—parent, child, and adult. The parent state is the evaluative part of us all. It is our conscience, which provides the home for values, rules, standards, and so forth. The two kinds of parent states are nurturing parent and critical parent.

The child ego state is emotion-laden and contains the "natural" impulses and attitudes that are usually identified in children. The child ego state can be categorized as happy and destructive.

The adult is the rational, reality-oriented ego state. The adult solves problems and makes decisions by balancing the child ego state and the parent ego state against the realities of the environment at a specific time and place. Figure 15.2 shows the three ego states with subcategories.

All three ego states exist in people at different times. A problem occurs when one or two of the ego states dominate. Parent-dominated people tend to believe that their answers are right; they know what is right and wrong: Adult dominated people are always working. Child-dominated individuals are often selfish in a group and not inclined to be rational and to think outside of self.

Transactions can be complementary or crossed, as seen in Figure 15.3. A principle in complementary styles is that responses can be expected. Crossed transactions result in communication breakdowns because responses are usually inappropriate and confusing. Figure 15.4 shows various transactions with examples of each.

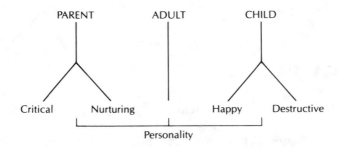

Figure 15.2 Transactional analysis: Ego states.

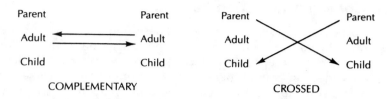

Figure 15.3 Types of transactions.

PARENT-TO-PARENT COMPLEMENTARY

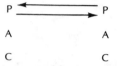

Coordinator to head nurse:
"Primary nursing is the best
model of nursing care delivery."
Response: "I certainly agree."

CHILD-TO-CHILD COMPLEMENTARY

Associate to associate: "I'm tired
of always being interrupted by you!"
Response: "Well, next time don't
talk so much!"

PARENT-TO-CHILD COMPLEMENTARY

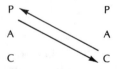

Supervisor to staff nurse: "Come
to my office at 9 AM tomorrow."
Response: "Yes. [Silence] Did I do
something wrong?"

CROSSED TRANSACTION

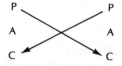

Supervisor to nurse's aide: "You
should not be doing this
procedure by yourself."
Response: "I have been doing this
for five years, and I am in a
hurry at the moment. *I* have
work to do."

ADULT-TO-ADULT COMPLEMENTARY

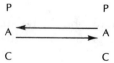

Head nurse to orderly: "Would you
please turn Mr. Robinson in Room 246."
Response: "Yes, as soon as I get
Mr. Jones back in bed."

Figure 15.4 Examples of crossed and complementary transactions.

Group Cohesion and Membership

Lippitt and Seashore (1980) saw group cohesion as the "attractiveness of the group to its members" (p. 4). Cohesion involves the willingness of members to accept group decisions and whether group activities are grounded on commitment to a common goal or on likes and dislikes of persons for each other. Subgroups may form in groups (often called "cliques"). They are usually based on friendship or common needs. If group desires are split among members, two or more factions within a group may develop. Ideally, a group should work together while members maintain their individuality (Lippitt & Seashore, 1980).

Group Climate

The climate of the group refers to the tone and atmosphere that is created by the group. Are members competitive, tense, polite, friendly, flat, energetic, and/or enthusiastic, for example? Creating a positive group climate is important because enthusiasm and energy are catching and tend to snowball in growth. Unfortunately, the converse—a negative climate—also is catching and grows (La Monica, 1985).

Group Norms

Group norms involve standards or ground rules. The beliefs of the group's majority usually set the norms—"what behavior should or should not take place in the group" (Pfeiffer & Jones, 1972, p. 24). Norms may be explicit, implicit, or operating outside of the members' awareness. A manager should seek to facilitate awareness and frequent examination of group norms.

Group Decision-Making Procedures

The procedures used by a group to make decisions should be studied. Schein (1969) discussed six ways in which groups make decisions:

1. *Decision by lack of response (the "plop")*. This occurs when members suggest decisions without due discussion of issues and alternatives; the group simply bypasses the ideas. Then one idea is suggested, and the group immediately decides that it is the best.

There are usually hidden attitudes operating, which are often a lack of commitment to the goal and/or feelings of powerlessness on the part of members. Results of this type of group decision-making procedure are negative feelings about self and other group members.

2. *Decision by authority rule.* Authority is delegated to someone in a position of power—the leader. This type of group decision making is fine if the leader communicates that she or he will make the decision but needs advice. If the leader, however, communicates that the group can decide on a course of action and then concludes the session by ignoring the group's suggestions, then the group may feel duped—rightfully so. Such action results in many negative feelings toward the leader, with harmful long-range effects.

3. *Decision by majority rule.* One or more people use pressure tactics to railroad a decision in this decision-making style. The balance of members are left feeling impotent, helpless, and "out-of-breath." They may wonder what happened.

4. *Decision by majority rule: voting and/or polling.* This is the most common style of group decision making. The position of each group member on the issue is requested either formally (by voting) or informally (by polling). A member can be for or against an issue or resolution or can abstain from making a decision. The best group procedure is to state the issue and then facilitate group discussion on all sides of the issue; decision by voting and/or polling follows. If the group must implement the decision—that is, they must individually do something in order for the goal to be attained—then group decision by majority rule is not best. Decision by consensus would be better than a majority ruling, because it is more probable that group members will be committed to the decision and less probable that the decision or task will be undermined during implementation.

5. *Decision by consensus.* This is a psychological state in which group members see rationale in the decision and agree to support it. This operates even though some members may be more or less committed than others; there even may be a minority vote.

6. *Decision by unanimous vote.* This method, though desirable, is rarely attained in organizations. It is demanded in jury trials but consensus is usually sufficient in management situations.

The roles that the leader and members play in a group also bear observation. They are discussed in the following section.

GROUP ROLES

Understanding the roles that members play in a group can increase effectiveness in group endeavors. Equally important is members' awareness of how they perceive their roles, juxtaposed or consonant with how others perceive their roles. The role of the formal leader is discussed first, followed by a list of common roles that all group members (including the formal and informal leader[s]) can play. It should be noted that members may be observed in one or more roles during a particular group session.

Role of the Formal Leader

The formal leader's behavior in a group can range from almost complete control to delegation, or almost complete control by the group. It follows that the functions required to propel a group toward its goal can be assumed by the leader or can become the responsibility of the members.

The precise dimensions of the formal leader's role are decided after the system is diagnosed (see Chapter 4), and an appropriate leader behavior is selected based on the system's diagnosis (see Chapter 5). Recalling that a leader can behave in any of four styles, the roles that a leader plays in group decision making fit into these same four Ohio State leadership styles (Stogdill & Coons, 1957):

- High structure and low consideration   (LB1)
- High structure and high consideration   (LB2)
- High consideration and low structure   (LB3)
- Low structure and low consideration   (LB4)

Group decision making should only be a leader's option in LB2, LB3, and LB4. In other words, a system that is immature (requiring LB1) should not be involved in group problem solving because the group requires knowledge and experience first—discussion about the issue comes later. Group problem solving is a consideration intervention because it involves two-way communication: leader to followers and followers to leader.

When LB2 is required, given the system's diagnosis, consideration and structure should be high. When LB2 is required, however, the system is only beginning to move toward maturity. The leader should not, therefore, relinquish too much control to the group. In

LB3, greater control should be shifted from the leader to the group, and in LB4, when the group is mature in relation to carrying out the task, the leader can delegate to the group and leave the group alone to solve problems and make decisions.

The types of management decision styles discussed in Chapter 6 (Vroom, 1973; Vroom & Jago, 1988; Vroom & Yetton, 1973) can be applied to make more precise how a leader should behave in a group. The reader can refer back to Table 6.1 and Figure 6.1 for a refresher on these styles.

Roles of Group Members

In order for group goals to be accomplished, two categories of functions must be performed in the group: task functions and maintenance functions. Task functions relate to what the group must accomplish, while maintenance functions are concerned with how the group carries out its task. These activities can be controlled variously by the leader in accordance with the requirements of the group for leader behavior. Given that, members can assume different roles. Figure 15.5 portrays the relationship between leader behavior and group roles.

Benne and Sheats (1948) identified three major categories of group roles. Although different labels may be used in current literature, the basics remain the same. A partial list of the roles is provided (La Monica, 1979, pp. 280–281*), and a complete list can be obtained from the original source.

Task Roles. These relate to the task with which the group is involved:

1. *Initiator*—Introduces new ideas or procedures; tries to establish movement toward the goal.
2. *Information seeker*—Tries to obtain needed information or opinions; points out gaps in information; asks for opinions; responds to suggestions.
3. *Evaluator*—Tries to determine where the group stands on an issue; tests for consensus; evaluates progress.
4. *Coordinator*—Points out relationships among ideas or

---

*Reprinted by permission from La Monica, Elaine L., *The Nursing Process: A Humanistic Approach*, pp. 280–281. Copyright © 1979 by Addison-Wesley Publishing Company, Inc., Menlo Park, Calif.

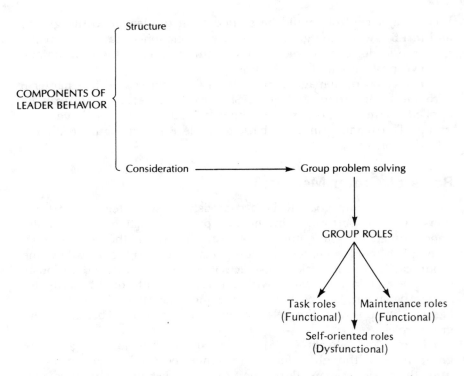

Figure 15.5 Relationship between leader behavior and group roles.

procedures; pulls ideas together and builds on the contributions of others; takes things one step further.

5. *Procedural technician*—Expedites group work by performing routine tasks, distributing material, and so forth.

6. *Recorder*—Writes down ideas, decisions, and recommendations; keeps minutes.

Maintenance Roles. These are oriented toward the functioning of the group as a whole unit, building group-centered attitudes, and strengthening productivity:

1. *Encourager*—Offers warmth and support to another's contribution; accepts what each member says.

2. *Harmonizer*—Mediates the differences between and among members; attempts to reconcile disagreements.

3. *Compromiser*—Seeks a middle position between opposing viewpoints.

4. *Standard setter*—Tries to bring to awareness the norms and standards of the group.

5. *Gatekeeper*—Keeps communication channels open; facilitates participation of all members; keeps track of time.

Self-oriented Roles. These roles involve attempts by members to satisfy their own needs through the group and are usually not directed toward effective group work. Self-oriented roles are often seen as dysfunctional.

1. *Aggressor*—Deflates the status of others; attacks the group, its individual members, or the task; displays envy toward the contributions by taking credit for them.

2. *Blocker*—Negative, stubborn opposer who reintroduces issues that have been previously decided upon.

3. *Recognition seeker*—Works in myriad ways to call attention to self; boastful and self-centered.

4. *Playboy*—Displays lack of interest by being cynical or humorous on important issues.

5. *Dominator*—Asserts authority or superiority over others by manipulating the group; flatters, interrupts, or gives authoritative directions.

6. *Help seeker*—Calls attention to self and seeks a sympathetic response from the group.

PROCESSING GROUP BEHAVIOR

Processing group behavior involves giving feedback to the group on how it functioned. The intent is to increase shared understanding about the behavior, feelings, and motivations of individuals; to facilitate development of a growth relationship by building trust and fostering openness among members; and to increase awareness of how people affect others. Criteria for feedback are found in Chapter 9. The criteria should be applied both to one-to-one and group interactions.

Time should be allotted at the conclusion of meetings to process how the group worked on its task. Group process observation sheets are provided for this purpose in the experiential exercises at the conclusion of Part III. These forms are arranged from simple to complex, and they should be used for learning in that order as group members mature in processing their group behavior.

COMMON NURSING GROUPS

There are numerous situations in which a nurse manager must facilitate group problem solving. This portion of the chapter includes discussion of the common nursing groups: staff support groups, teaching conferences, procedure conferences, patient conferences, directive conferences, and self-help groups.

Staff Support Groups

Scully (1981) described the purpose of staff support groups as helping nurses to help themselves. It has been documented that helpers who are aware of and accepting toward their own feelings will more probably be able to form a helping relationship with another than helpers who are unaware (Rogers, 1961). A ladder effect is operative: if a manager is satisfied with self, there is greater likelihood that the manager will be open to establishing a productive relationship with followers. If followers are then satisfied with their work responsibilities, there is greater chance that they will be more open to giving to their clients.

Nurses need support. Since nursing is a profession of human service, it mandates constant giving—thinking about others. Moreover, by the nature of nursing practice, nurses must give to many people in a short span of time. They must listen to others, feel with others, and respond to others' needs. This is giving, and nurses must be replenished. Otherwise the human tendency is to withdraw when drained, which is counterproductive to nursing's goal. Peer support is the best type of help that managers can engender among the staff members. Conferences can be in areas of stress management, conflict resolution, team building, and/or any issue that is a priority in the group.

Teaching Conferences

A teaching conference involves a skill or a process that is taught to staff members. This type of conference is analogous to a staff development or a continuing education program, but is generally on a smaller scale.

A head nurse who wishes to apprise followers of the outcome of primary nursing on an experimental unit would use a teaching conference. Another example is Marram's (1978) referral to a group dynamics session whose purpose is to increase skill and knowledge in group decision making. Facilitating group leadership experiences for students by having them co-lead a conference (Browne, 1980) would also be considered a teaching conference even though two purposes for the conference would probably exist.

Procedure Conferences

A procedure conference is similar to a teaching conference, but the teaching conference is concerned with skill and knowledge (content) from the domain of helping, which includes nursing, and the procedure conference usually refers to topics of policies and procedures in a specific organization. Alerting staff to a revised informed consent procedure for a hospital is one example of a topic for this type of conference.

Patient Conferences

Problem-oriented care of a patient is discussed and evaluated in a patient conference (Douglass & Bevis, 1979). All persons (the team) involved in the care of the patient and family discuss the care plan, solve problems, explain, gain confidence, or evaluate (La Monica, 1985). The leader of this conference should facilitate multidisciplinary sharing of expertise and perceptions concerning nursing diagnoses. Decisions that result from a patient conference are generally more patient-centered, valid, and creative than decisions of one professional.

Directive Conferences

Directive conferences most often occur at the beginning and end of shifts; occasionally a midshift direction conference is called. The overall purposes of this type of conference are to make assignments and receive reports.

Assigning. Assignments are made at a shift's beginning for communicating job assignments, specifying areas of responsibility, and giving pertinent information regarding patient care. A manager may make general announcements during this conference.

Assignments generally are made according to one of four basic methods for delivering nursing care: the case method, the functional method, team nursing, or primary nursing. "Case management" is a combination of the original case method model and primary nursing. Table 15.1 contains descriptions of the basic methods with the values and disadvantages of each.

TABLE 15.1 Nursing Care Delivery Models: Descriptions, Values, and Disadvantages

Description	Values	Disadvantages
Case Method/Management		
The complete care of one or more clients is assigned to a nurse for a period of time. In the early case method, care was for a shift. In typical case management, the nurse may carry the assigned clients for the entire length of stay and and maybe, even in the home care agency	1. The nurse can better see and attend to the total needs of clients due to the time and proximity of interactors. Coordination of all aspects of care is the responsibility of the nurse: physical, emotional, medical regimen, teaching, and all other aspects. 2. Continuity of care can be facilitated with ease. 3. Client/nurse interaction/ rapport can be developed due to the intensity of time and proximity of those involved. 4. Client may feel more secure	1. Many clients do not require the intensity of care inherent in this type of service. 2. The method must be modified if nonprofessional health workers are to be used effectively. 3. There are not enough nurses to fill the demand of this model; cost-effectiveness must be considered. 4. It is difficult for all levels of professional and technical nurses to share expertise in the process of planning care.

TABLE 15.1 (*continued*)

Description	Values	Disadvantages
	knowing that one person is thoroughly familiar with the needs and the course of treatment. 5. Educational needs of clients can be closely monitored. 6. Family and friends may become better known by nurses and more involved in the care of the client. 7. Work load can be equally divided among available staff. 8. Nurses' accountability for their functions is built-in.	
Functional Method Selected functions (vital signs, medications, and so forth) are assigned to staff members who are qualified to carry out these functions for patients on a unit for a given period of time.	1. One person can become particularly skilled in performing assigned tasks; this method can be efficient and economical. 2. The best utilization may be made of a person's aptitudes, experience, and desires.	1. Client care may become impersonal, compartmentalized, and fragmented. 2. There is a tremendous risk for diminishing continuity of care. 3. Staff may become bored and have little motivation to develop self and

(*continued*)

TABLE 15.1 (*continued*)

Description	Values	Disadvantages
		others. Work may become monotonous.
	3. Less equipment is needed, and what is available is usually better cared for when used only by a few personnel.	4. The staff members are accountable for the task; only the nurse in change of the unit has accountability for the individual, whole client.
	4. This method saves time because it lends itself to strict organizational protocol.	5. There is little avenue for staff development, except as it relates to tasks.
	5. The potential for development of technical skills is amplified.	6. Clients may tend to feel insecure, not knowing who is their own nurse.
	6. There is a sense of productivity for the task-oriented nurse.	7. Only parts of the nursing care plan may be known to personnel.
	7. It is easy to organize the work of the unit and staff.	8. It is difficult to establish client priorities and operationalize the care plan reflecting same.
		9. It is only safe when the head nurse can coordinate the activities of all members of the staff and make certain that nothing essential in client care is overlooked or forgotten. This

TABLE 15.1 (*continued*)

Description	Values	Disadvantages
		is a tremendous responsibility for one person who probably has to think of approximately 30 or more clients, plus the staff.
Team Nursing Total care of a group of patients is the responsibility of a team of professionals and nonprofessionals who work together to give comprehensive, quality, individualized nursing care. There is no protocol for how the work gets assigned; the team leader assigns the care of patients to those qualified to carry out specific tasks.	1. It includes all health-care personnel in the group's functioning and goals. 2. Feelings of participation and belonging are facilitated with team members. 3. Work load can be balanced and shared. 4. Division of labor allows members the opportunity to develop leadership skills. 5. Every team member has the opportunity to learn from and teach colleagues. 6. There is a variety in the daily assignments. 7. Interest in clients' well-being and care is shared by several people; reliability of decisions is increased.	1. Establishing the team concept takes time, effort, and constancy of personnel. Merely assigning people to a group does not make them a "group" or "team." 2. Unstable staffing patterns make team nursing difficult. 3. All personnel must be educated in client-centered nursing care. 4. The team leader must have complex skills and knowledge: communication, leadership, organization, nursing care, motivation, and other skills. 5. There is less individual responsibility and independence regarding nursing functions.

(*continued*)

TABLE 15.1 (*continued*)

Description	Values	Disadvantages
	8. Nursing care hours are usually cost-effective.	
	9. The client is able to identify personnel who are responsible for his or her care.	
	10. All care is directed by a registered nurse.	
	11. Continuity of care is facilitated, especially if teams are constant.	
	12. Barriers between professional and nonprofessional workers can be minimized; the group effort prevails.	
	13. Everyone has the opportunity to contribute to the care plan.	
Primary Nursing*		
A professional nurse has 24-hour responsibility for the care of assigned patients [or cases] —all aspects of the nursing process are directed by the primary nurse.	1. There is opportunity for the nurse to see the client and family as one system. 2. Nursing accountability, responsibility, and independence are increased. 3. The nurse is able to use a wide range of	1. The nurse may be isolated from colleagues. 2. There is little avenue for group planning of client care. 3. Nurses must be mature and independently competent. 4. It may be cost-ineffective even though recent

TABLE 15.1 (*continued*)

Description	Values	Disadvantages
	skills, knowledge, and expertise.	articles indicate otherwise.
	4. The method potentiates creativity by the nurse; work satisfaction may increase significantly.	5. Staffing patterns may necessitate a heavy client load.
	5. The scene is set for increased trust and satisfaction in the client and nurse.	

*The usual procedures of the case method of nursing care delivery and primary nursing overlap into what in currently identified as case management.
Source: Reprinted and adapted by permission from La Monica, Elaine L., *The Nursing Process: A Humanistic Approach,* pp. 369–373. Copyright © 1979 by Addison-Wesley Publishing Company, Inc., Menlo Park, Calif.

Remember, there is no best model of nursing care delivery, even though nursing literature currently abounds with announcements that boast the benefits of primary nursing and case management (Deiman, Noble, & Russell, 1984; Kasch, 1986; McClure, 1984; Mutchner, 1986; Zander, 1985, 1987, 1988). Though these models definitely enhance the professional base for nursing practice, in essence, any model for delivering nursing care is *only* as effective as is the competency of the nursing staff who function within the model. This point was recently documented by Shukla (1981) in a study comparing primary and team nursing.

The needs and care of patients are priority considerations when making out assignments: what is involved; how long it takes; and what skills, knowledge, and experience are required in order to meet the needs. Then the abilities of the staff must be matched to the requirements of the patients so that members of the team are functioning according to their qualifications. Members who need to learn a particular treatment or skill should be assigned to work with another person who has that expertise.

Mechanically, assignments should be written out so that members have copies during the conference and can make notes. Responsibilities should be explicit.

Reporting. Verbal reports are made at the end of work shifts; in some agencies, these reports are tape-recorded. Pertinent information about the patients is communicated to those continuing patient care in inpatient facilities and to those in charge of outpatient facilities. Listening is the most important function of the leader in this type of conference. Douglass and Bevis (1979, p. 163) further stated that report conferences have four goals: (1) to report information about patients, (2) to give reactions to situations, (3) to evaluate care, and (4) to update care plans.

Self-Help Groups

Self-help groups are generally composed of nonprofessionals who organize and operate themselves around specific topics. These groups range from informal ones to organized ones such as Alcoholics Anonymous and Parents Without Partners. Self-help groups are concerned with self-care and self-improvement (Maloney, 1979). The principal force behind self-help groups is peer support. People with common problems pool their resources to help and receive help from one another. In one sense, staff support groups discussed earlier can be thought of as self-help groups—only composed of members who are professional.

Professional nurses, as well as other helpers, are often involved in self-help groups. Marram (1978, p. 39) saw the role of the nurse as: (1) verifying the success of individuals and the group, (2) identifying and referring people to the groups, and (3) providing knowledge to the group as a resource person and a teacher. Self-help groups are also often organized and led by agency staff around particular needs of their clientele.

SUMMARY

Group dynamics involves the study of how people interact with each other in small groups. The goal of study is to render the groups more effective. The more effectively a group works as a team, the higher is the probability for cost-effectiveness of the services. Studying group dynamics is, therefore, an essential aspect of the manager's responsibilities—fostering team maturity. Areas of group behavior that require observation and study include the following: goals, background, participation, communication patterns, cohesion and membership, climate, norms, and decision-making procedures. Group roles are other important areas in group dynamics. The formal leader's behavior can range from almost complete control to delegation or almost complete control by the group. How a manager behaves specifically is governed by the maturity level of the system in relation to the system's ability to carry out the task.

Task functions and maintenance functions are performed in group problem-solving activities. Group members can assume various functional and dysfunctional roles in each of these categories. Processing group behavior involves giving the group feedback on how it functioned.

Nurses must facilitate group problem solving in a variety of informal and formal situations. Among the most common formal situations are the following groups: staff support groups; teaching conferences; procedure conferences; patient conferences; directive conferences—assigning and reporting; and self-help groups.

REFERENCES

Baker, K. (1980). Application of group theory in nursing practice. *Supervisor Nurse, 11,* 22–24.

Bavelas, A., & Barrett D. (1951). An experimental approach to organizational communication. *Personnel, 27,* 366–371.

Benne, K., & Sheats, P. (1948). Functional roles of group members. *Journal of Social Issues, 4,* 41–49.

Berne, E. (1972). *What do you say after you say hello?* New York: Bantam Books.

Berne, E. (1978). *Games people play.* New York: Ballantine.

Browne, S. (1980). Group leadership experiences for students. *Nursing Outlook, 28,* 166–169.

Charrier, G. (1980). Cog's ladder: A model of group growth. In M. Berger, D. Elhart, S. Firsich, S. Jordan, & S. Stone (Eds.). *Management for nurses: A multidisciplinary approach* (2nd ed.). St. Louis: Mosby.

Clark, C. (1987). *The nurse as group leader* (2nd ed.). New York: Springer.

Cohen, A. (1962). Changing small-group communication networks. *Administrative Science Quarterly, 6,* 443–462.

Davis, K., & Newstrom, J. (1985). *Human behavior at work: Organizational behavior* (7th ed.). New York: McGraw-Hill.

Deiman, P., Noble, E., & Russell, M. (1984). Achieving a professional practice model: How primary nursing can help. *Journal of Nursing Administration,* 14(7), 16–21.

Douglass, L., & Bevis, E. (1979). *Nursing managemnt and leadership in action.* St. Louis: Mosby.

Harris, T. (1982). *I'm OK—You're OK.* New York: Avon.

James, M., & Jongeward, D. (1971). *Born to win: Transactional analysis with gestalt experiments.* Reading, MA: Addison-Wesley.

James, M., & Jongeward, D. (1978). *Born to win.* New York: NAL Pub.

Jongeward, D. (1976). *Women as winners: Transactional analysis for personal growth.* Reading, MA: Addison-Wesley.

Kasch, C. (1986). Establishing a collaborative nurse-patient relationship: A distinct focus of nursing action in primary care. *Image, 18*(2), 44–47.

La Monica, E. (1979). *The nursing process: A humanistic approach.* Menlo Park, CA: Addison-Wesley.

La Monica, E. (1985). *The humanistic nursing process.* Boston: Jones and Bartlett.

Leavitt, H. (1951). Some effects of certain communication patterns on group performance. *The Journal of Abnormal and Social Psychology, 46,* 38–50.

Lippitt, G., & Seashore, E. (1980). *Group effectiveness: A looking-into-leadership monograph.* Fairfax, VA: Leadership Resources.

Maloney, E. (1979). A perspective on groups in the health field in the 1980s. In E. La Monica. *The nursing process: A humanistic approach.* Menlo Park, CA: Addison-Wesley.

Marram, G. (1978). *The group approach in nursing practice.* St. Louis: Mosby.

McClure, M. (1984). Managing the professional nurse: Part II. Applying management theory to the challenges. *Journal of Nursing Administration, 14*(3), 11–17.

Mears, P. (1974). Structuring communication in a working group. *The Journal of Communication, 24,* 71–79.

Mutchner, L. (1986). How well are we practicing primary nursing? *Journal of Nursing Administration, 16*(9), 8–13.

Pfeiffer, J., & Jones, J. (Eds.). (1972). *The 1972 annual handbook for group facilitators.* La Jolla, CA: University Associates.

Rogers, C. (1961). *On becoming a person.* Boston: Houghton Mifflin.

Sampson, E., & Marthas, M. (1981). *Group process for the health professions.* New York: Wiley.

Schein, E. (1969). *Process consultation: Its role in organization development.* Reading. MA: Addison-Wesley.

Scully, R. (1981). Staff support groups: Helping nurses to help themselves. *Journal of Nursing Administration, 11,* 48–51.

Shaw, M. (1954a). Some effects of problem complexity upon problem solution efficiency in different communication nets. *Journal of Experimental Psychology, 48,* 211–217.

Shaw, M. (1954b). Some effects of unequal distribution of information upon group performance in various communication nets. *The Journal of Abnormal and Social Psychology, 49,* 547–553.

Shukla, R. (1981). Structure vs. people in primary nursing: An inquiry. *Nursing Research, 30,* 236–241.

Stogdill, R., & Coons, A. (Eds.). (1957). *Leader behavior: Its description and measurement.* Research Monograph No. 88, Columbus, Bureau of Business Research, Ohio State University.

von Bertalanffy, L. (1968). *General system theory.* New York: Braziller.

von Bertalanffy, L. (1975). *Perspectives on general system theory: Scientific-philosophical studies.* New York: Braziller.

Vroom, V. (1973). A new look at managerial decision-making. *Organizational Dynamics, 1*, 66–80.

Vroom, V., & Yetton, P. (1973). *Leadership and decision-making.* Pittsburgh: University of Pittsburgh Press.

Vroom, M., & Jago, A. (1988). *The new leadership: Managing participation in organizations.* Englewood Cliffs, NJ: Prentice-Hall.

Weeks, L., Barrett, M., & Snead, C. (1985). Primary nursing: Teamwork is the answer. *Journal of Nursing Administration, 15*(9), 21–26, 34.

Zander, K. (1985). Second generation primary nursing: A new agenda. *Journal of Nursing Administration, 15*(3), 18–24.

Zander, K. (1987). Nursing case management: A classic. *Definition, 2*(2), 1–3.

Zander, K. (1988). Managed care within acute care settings: Design and implementation via nursing case management. *Health Care Supervisor, 6*(2), 24–43.

Conflict Resolution

Every human being has a unique set of drives, goals, and needs that are constantly seeking satisfaction. Earth contains all of these individuals who move in various directions across time and space on their journeys. If these journeys could be thought of as self-contained capsules that floated around other capsules, then each would be autonomous, and humans could not be considered sociologically; general system theory would not be viable.

In a sense, people are capsules, but needs are met by being dependent and interpendent on other capsules and independent of other capsules. If all people and their capsules desired complementary things, that is, what one wanted to obtain the other wished to give, and what one wanted to keep the other did not want, then systems could exist with total integration. Such harmony, however, does not exist in reality. Conflict exists in the absence of harmonious total integration. Conflict always exists, therefore, even though it may be suppressed. People simply do not think, believe, and desire the same things.

Conflict is an absolute; a manager must learn to effectively facilitate the resolution of conflict among people in order to accomplish goals, which is the content of this chapter. The chapter begins with definitions of conflict, followed by discussion of the types and causes of conflict. These content areas set the stage for the conflict process and strategies for resolving conflict. Productive and destructive outcomes of conflict are the final topics.

DEFINITIONS OF CONFLICT

Deutsch (1969) defined conflict as a clash or a struggle that occurs when one's balance among feelings, thoughts, desires, and behavior is threatened. This disturbance results in incompatible behavior that interferes with goals. Douglass and Bevis (1979) stated that conflict is a struggle between interdependent forces. This struggle can be within an individual (intrapersonal conflict) or within a group (intragroup conflict) (Nielsen, 1977).

Since conflicts exist, a manager has the power to move the conflict to a constructive or a destructive resolution. In the constructive approach, the outcomes of an encounter result in individual and/or group growth, heightened awareness and understanding of self and others, and positive feelings toward the outcomes of the interaction. Destructive resolutions result in an expansion of the conflict and negative feelings toward self and/or others.

TYPES OF CONFLICT

Conflict arises within, between, and among people out of differences in facts, definitions, views, authority, goals, values, and controls. Conflict in an organization can be structurally categorized as vertical or horizontal (Marriner, 1979a). Vertical conflict involves differences between superiors and followers. It often results from poor communication and a lack of shared perceptions regarding expectations of appropriate behavior for one's own role and/or that of others. Horizontal conflict is line-staff conflict and has to do with domains of practice, expertise, authority, and so forth. It is often interdepartmental strife.

Conflict can be further broken down into types as shown in Table 16.1. Examples are provided for each type of conflict.

TABLE 16.1 Types of Conflict

Conflict*	Description*	Example
Intrasender	Same sender, conflicting messages	The same supervisor demands high-quality care, refuses to fire incompetent staff members, and refuses to recruit additional staff.
Intersender	Conflicting messages from two or more senders	Top nursing management stresses the need to adopt primary nursing as the nursing care model; followers believe that they can achieve individualized, quality nursing care using the team method.
Interrole	Same person belonging to conflicting groups	Nursing director belongs to a community-based consumer group seeking to consolidate obstetrical and pediatric services in a geographic locality by having all obstetrics shared between two of four hospitals and all pediatrics shared between the other two hospitals. The same nurse is also an employee of one hospital that is fighting to keep both services.
Person-role	Same person, conflicting values (cognitive dissonance)	A nurse believes that patients should receive individual attention in a clinic by one nurse who follows them from visit to visit. Requirements of the position and the system for delivering care make achieving such a goal infrequent if not impossible.
Interperson	Two or more people acting as protagonists for different groups	The director of nursing competes with other directors for new positions.
Intragroup	New values from outside	Continuing education

TABLE 16.1 (*continued*)

Conflict*	Description*	Example
	are imposed on an existing group	(CE) is mandated by the state for continuing nursing licensure. The rural healthcare agency has no funds to send staff nurses to CE programs, and staff nurses, who are under-paid but satisfied, cannot afford to support their own CE.
Intergroup	Two or more groups with conflicting goals	The nursing department demands that the operat-ing and recovery room nurses organizationally come under nursing. The surgery department, composed of physicians, believes that they should control nurses in these areas.
Role ambiguity	A person is not aware of the expectations others have for a particular role	A newly hired nursing supervisor has no position description and has no previous experi-ence as a supervisor.
Role overload	A person cannot meet the expectations of others for a role	A new baccalaureate graduate is expected by a nursing director to be in charge of a 40 bed acute-and-chronic-medical unit on the night shift.

*Source: Columns 1 and 2 from Marriner, A., Conflict theory. *Supervisor Nurse, 10*, 12–16. Copyright 1979 by S-N Publications, Inc. Reprinted by permission.

CAUSES OF CONFLICT

Nursing and health care literature is replete with discussions of the predisposing factors of conflict (Coombs, 1987; Douglass & Bevis, 1979; Filley, 1980; Marriner, 1982; Nielsen, 1977; Silber, 1984). Ed-munds (1979) cited the following nine general factors that seem to account for all possible causes:

Specialization—A group that assumes responsibility for a

particular set of tasks or area of service sets itself apart from other groups. Intergroup conflict often results.

Multitask Roles—The nursing role requires that one be a manager, a skilled care giver, a human relations expert, a negotiator, an advocate, and so forth. Each subrole with its tasks requires different orientations that can cause conflict.

Role Interdependence—A role of nurse practitioner in private practice would not be as complicated as one being a part of a multidisciplinary health-care team. In the latter, the individual domains of practice have to be discussed with others who may compete for certain areas.

Task Blurring—This results from role ambiguity and failure to designate responsibility and accountability for a task to one individual or group.

Differentiation—A group of people may occupy the same role but the attitudinal, emotional, and cognitive behaviors of these people toward their role differs. This engenders conflict, especially in problem-solving and decision-making activities.

Scarcity of Resources—Competition for money, patients, and positions are an absolute source of interperson and intergroup conflict.

Change—Whenever change occurs, conflict is not far behind. As change becomes more apparent and/or threatening, the probability and depth of conflict increases proportionately.

Conflict Over Rewards—When people are differentially rewarded, conflict is often a result unless they were involved in developing the reward system.

Communication Problems—Ambiguities, perceptual distortions, language failures, and incorrectly used communication channels all can cause conflict.

Conflict exists within people and within groups; the causes of conflict, though stated generally, are unique. The next portion of the chapter contains a discussion of the conflict process.

THE CONFLICT PROCESS

Filley (1980), drawing from the early works of Corwin (1969), Fink (1968), Pondy (1967, 1969), Walton and Dutton (1969), and Schmidt

(1973) depicted the following six steps to the conflict process, shown in Figure 16.1:

1. *Antecedent conditions* are causes of conflict and were discussed in the previous section of this chapter.
2. *Perceived conflict* is the recognition of conditions that exist between parties or within self that can cause conflict. Perceived conflict is logical, impersonal, and objective.
3. *Felt conflict* is subjective because people feel the conflict relationship. These feelings are often described as threat, hostility, fear, and/or mistrust.
4. *Manifest behavior* can take the forms of aggression, nonassertion, assertion, competition, debate, or problem solving. Perceived and/or felt conflict generally result in action—actual overt behavior.

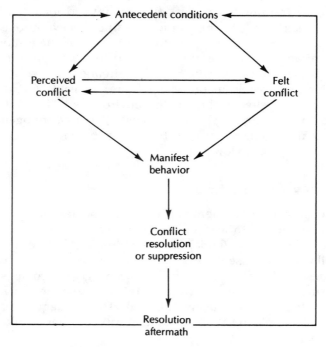

Figure 16.1 The conflict process.

Source: From *Interpersonal Conflict Resolution* by Alan C Filley. Copyright © 1975 Scott, Foresman and Company. Reprinted by permission.

5. *Conflict resolution or suppression*, the next step in the conflict process, brings the conflict to an end either by
   agreement among those involved or through the defeat
   of one party. In competitive conflict, rules specify the
   outcome.

6. *Resolution aftermath* is the legacy left at the end of this
   cycle—feelings, beliefs, awards, and so forth. Sometimes these leftovers are called consequences. Since conflict is experienced, learning takes place within an
   individual and both negative and positive learning can
   become antecedent conditions for conflict in another
   time and place.

RESOLVING CONFLICT

Now that one has an understanding of how conflict works, what can
a manager do to facilitate positive conflict resolution? Authors within
and outside of the nursing profession offer myriad ideas on helping
groups to resolve conflict. This author does not believe in one or two
best ways to resolve or prevent conflict. An array of suggestions from
the literature and experience are offered so that learners can choose
what they believe to be best in a unique situation. All strategies are
useful to have accessible in one's repertoire, available for use given
diagnosis of the system including the environment. Two formal approaches to preventing conflict are discussed first—contingency contracting and management by objectives. A subsection of less formal
approaches will then follow.

Contingency Contracting

Contingency contracting (Homme, 1970) is one leadership strategy
that can be employed to lead followers developmentally toward self-
management. This has potential for preventing conflict between leaders and followers because control will be given to followers based on
their abilities to handle it effectively toward goal accomplishment.
Control issues, as almost everyone is aware, can range in strength
from relatively benign to positively lethal. This strategy is based on
theory—what people need to reach maturity as they work toward
goal accomplishment.

     According to Homme (1970), a manager controls (1) what fol-
lowers are supposed to do (the task) and (2) what reward(s) followers

will receive for doing it (the reinforcement). Five types of contingency contracts are delineated, and an application in nursing for each is provided.

Leader Control. The task and the reinforcement are determined by the manager. The manager presents the contract; the follower accepts the contract and performs.

> Example: The nursing director formulates a policy, prepares a memorandum or directive, and presents it to the supervisors.

Partial Control by Follower. The follower assumes joint control over the reinforcement, and the manager retains full control over the task, or the follower assumes joint control over the task, and the manager retains full control over the reinforcement.

> Example: A head nurse prepares a survey questionnaire on which there are two alternative procedures. The nursing staff is requested to elect their procedure of choice. Upon tabulation of the responses, the procedure of choice is apparent. A directive is then sent to all staff stipulating the procedure that will become policy.

Equal Control by Leader and Follower. The manager and follower assume equal control over the task and reinforcement, or the manager retains control over one of the two areas, and the follower assumes control over the other area.

> Example: A nursing director requests that the nursing administrative staff develop a policy on a specific issue. The policy is formulated by a subgroup within the administrative staff. It is then taken back to the administrative conference, which is composed of all members in nursing administration, and voted upon.

Partial Control by Leader. The follower has full control over the task or reinforcement and shares joint control with the manager over the other.

> Example: In order to resolve a specific patient care problem, the team nurses, the head nurses, and the charge nurses brainstorm and list all possible procedures that could resolve the situation at hand. The list is sent to all patient care staff on the unit; each staff member is asked to select the procedure that she or he believes is best. The procedure that becomes policy is based on a majority vote.

Follower Control. Both the task and the reinforcement are determined by the follower.

> Example: Followers are aware of the required holiday coverage on a unit. They meet by themselves and jointly decide the staffing schedule. It is then given to the head nurse.

Hersey and Blanchard (1988) integrated contingency contracting into situational leadership theory. This author adds the Ohio State model

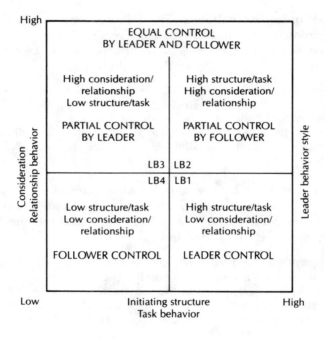

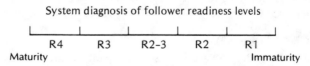

Figure 16.2 Contingency contracting, situational leadership theory, and the Ohio State model of leadership.

Source: This figure was adapted from one presented by Paul Hersey, & Kenneth H. Blanchard, *Management of Organizational Behavior: Utilizing Human Resources*, (5th ed.), © 1988, p. 443. Reprinted by permission of Prentice Hall, Inc, Englewood Cliffs, NJ.

of leadership (Stogdill & Coons, 1957). Figure 16.2 presents this integration. Given the relationships shown in Figure 16.2, the following suggestions can be made (Hersey & Blanchard, 1988):

1. *Leader-control contracting* is appropriate when the system is at R1 level of maturity (low maturity), and LB1 (high structure/task and low consideration/relationship) is indicated.

2. *Partial-control-by-follower contracting* would be used by a leader when the system is at R2 (moderate maturity), and LB2 (high structure/task and high consideration/relationship) is required.

3. *Equal-control-by-leader-and-follower contracting* should be used when a system is at R2-3 (moderate maturity), and the leader behavior style is consistent with LB2 and LB3 (high structure/task and high consideration/relationship or high consideration/relationship and low structure/task).

4. *Partial-control-by-leader contracting* parallels with R3 (moderate maturity) and LB3 (high consideration/relationship and low structure/task).

5. *Follower-control contracting* should be used with a highly mature system (R4) when LB4 (low structure/task and low consideration/ relationship) is indicated.

A manager can now employ contingency contracts in strategies for accomplishing goals. These should be based on the system diagnosis and resultant identification of a leader behavior style that has the highest probability for motivating a system to accomplish a goal.

Management by Objectives

Management by objectives (MBO) is a participative approach for developing and sharing performance expectations among staff members at all levels in an organization. The concept was developed by Drucker (1954, 1985a, 1985b, 1985c) and also advanced by Odiorne (1965, 1979) and Humble (1967). The concept has received a wealth of attention in the literature, both in the disciplines of business and nursing (Cain & Luchsinger, 1978; Golightly, 1979; Odiorne, 1975; Palmer, 1973; Skarupa, 1971).

MBO is defined by Odiorne (1965, 1979) as a process whereby

superiors and their followers jointly identify and set goals, define individual areas of responsibility, plan strategies and designate tasks for achieving goals, and measure and evaluate success. The MBO approach, when effectively implemented, enables expectations between followers and superiors to be public. Potential conflict is thereby reduced because goals are negotiated between involved parties, and then a contract is set; mutual commitment is, therefore, gained. MBO can provide a framework for achieving organizational goals and employee satisfaction (Olsson, 1968). Odiorne (1965) graphically portrayed the entire cycle of MBO, as shown in Figure 16.3.

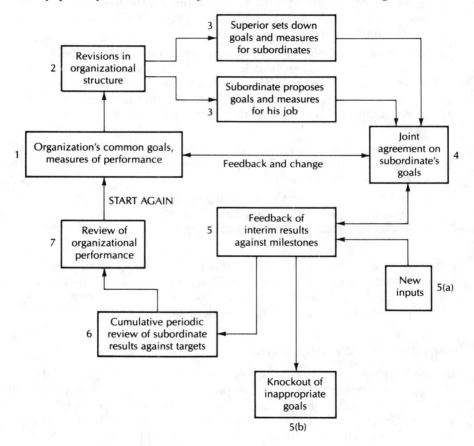

Figure 16.3 Cycle of management by objectives.
Source: Odiorne, G., *Management by Objectives: A System of Managerial Leadership*. Copyright © 1965 by Pitman Publishing Corporation. Reprinted by permission of Pitman Learning, Inc, Belmont, Calif.

Even though the attention MBO has received in the literature might lead someone to suggest that MBO is a managerial plus, the concept has received major criticisms (Ford, 1979; Hersey & Blanchard, 1988; Levinson, 1970). MBO is participatory in nature—equal control by superiors and followers. Not all followers are mature enough in their position to be able to set realistic objectives for themselves. Hersey and Blanchard (1988) pointed out that the role a superior will play in helping the follower to accomplish the set objectives is not clearly defined in MBO. Further, if a leader behavior style is in the contract, it can tie a manager to one way of behaving, which may not be appropriate for all tasks. Ford (1979) asserted, among other important issues, that companies using MBO may overlook opportunities that develop after objectives were set.

Given the positive and negative points regarding MBO, it should be employed by the leader if appropriate given the needs of the system or the individual follower.

Other Ways to Resolve Conflict

Nielsen (1977) suggested an approach called creative conflict resolution that is composed of six phases, similar to the problem-solving method:

1. Problem recognition with desire to solve it.
2. Concentrated effort to solve the problem through routine behavior.
3. A period of frustration due to failure of customary actions, resulting in withdrawal.
4. An incubation period to reformulate the problem into a new perspective—redefinition.
5. Tentative solution to the newly defined problem.
6. A final solution.

One of the benefits of the creative approach is that conflict is given time to breathe and change. Forcing conflict resolution often has the effect of heightening the energy in the direction of greater conflict.

Marriner (1979b) suggested three ways of dealing with conflict. Win-lose methods include use of position power, mental or physical power, silence, majority rule, and railroading. Lose-lose strategies include compromise, bribes for accomplishing unpleasant tasks, arbitration, and use of general rules instead of looking at issues qualitatively. Win-win strategies focus on goals, emphasizing consensus and integrative approaches to decision making. The steps to win-win strategies follow the problem-solving method.

Edmunds (1979) underscored what Marriner (1979b) suggested and added that the most constructive way to handle conflict involves verbal rather than nonverbal communication—talking out rather than acting out. This author believes that both behaviors are important; verbal communication is often best when it precedes nonverbal communication—talk it out and then act on the basis of what has been discussed.

Assertive confrontation as a way to resolve conflict is discussed by Hughes (1979), Haw (1980), and Nichols (1979). Express opinions, feelings, and ideas directly and honestly in a way that does not insult, degrade, or humiliate others. Group processing activities and giving and receiving feedback are other useful ways for resolving potential and present conflict. Davis and Newstrom (1985) suggested employee counseling as another way to resolve conflict, especially individual conflict. Thomas and Kilmann (1977) identified five conflict resolution modes: accommodating, avoiding, competing, compromising, and collaborating.

OUTCOMES OF CONFLICT

Conflicts result in outcomes that can be productive to the growth of an individual or an organization. Conversely, conflict can be extremely destructive (Kramer & Schmalenberg, 1978; Lewis, 1976; Myrtle & Glogow, 1978; Nielsen, 1977).

Deutsch (1969, 1973) identified four primary factors that determine the outcome of conflict: the issue, power, responsivity to needs, and communication. The discussion follows that provided by Kramer and Schmalenberg (1978).

The Issue

In destructive conflict, the issue is amplified, broadly defined with the addition of tangential items, and emotionally charged. In constructive conflict, the issue is focused and kept to a manageable size. Only peripheral issues that relate to the main point are discussed, and the process of choice is action rather than reaction.

Power

In destructive power, situations are maintained or changed through threats and coercion. Competition is the climate with a resultant winner and loser. Constructive power involves finding an acceptable solution that may be a compromise or a new one; personal needs and views are not imposed on others.

Responsivity to Needs

Only one's own needs are considered in destructive conflict. As time goes on, one becomes surer that one's beliefs and behaviors are right. Constructive conflict resolution is characterized by solutions that respond to the needs of all participants in the conflict.

Communication

Mutual distrust, misperception, and escalated emotional charges make up a destructive conflict course. Constructive resolution involves open and honest dialogue, sharing individual concerns, and listening with the desire to understand others. The intent is to get the problem out in the open so that it can be dealt with effectively.

Conflict is beneficial in an organization, providing that the leader is skilled in facilitating constructive conflict resolution. When different opinions on an issue are voiced and when problems are aired, it shows that people are involved and care. The opposite of love is not hate; the opposite is indifference. With both love and hate there is energy—those about whom one cares have the power to engender hate. Indifference is empty. Energy derived through effective conflict resolution can be used positively toward goal accomplishment. Nielsen (1977) said that conflict is "the root of personal and social change" (p. 153). It stimulates problem solving and the resultant creative solutions, it can be enjoyable, and it permits the development of a personal identity.

SUMMARY

Conflict is a clash or a struggle that occurs when one's balance among feelings, thoughts, desires, and behavior is threatened. The struggle can be within an individual or within a group. Leaders can move the conflict to destructive or constructive outcomes.

Structurally, conflict can be vertical, involving differences between superiors and followers, or it can be horizontal as in line-staff relationships. Nine types of conflict are noted in the literature: intrasender, intersender, interrole, person-role, interperson, intragroup, intergroup, role ambiguity, and role overload.

Causes of conflict are unique and compounded. General causes, however, are cited and discussed. These refer to areas such as specialization, multitask roles, role interdependence, task blurring, differentiation, scarcity of resources, change, rewards, and communication. The process of conflict starts with antecedent conditions that move to perceived and/or felt conflict. Behavior follows with the conflict either being resolved or suppressed.

Constructive conflict resolution is an important aspect of managerial responsibility. An array of approaches, including contingency contracting and management by objectives, is discussed. There is no best method for facilitating conflict resolution. A manager must have knowledge of possible strategies together with knowledge of the processes of managing and leading people; the best strategy given the unique environment must then be chosen and implemented.

REFERENCES

Cain, C., Luchsinger, V. (1978). Management by objectives: Applications to nursing. *Journal of Nursing Administration, 8,* 35–38.

Coombs, C. (1987). The structure of conflict. *American Psychologist, 42*(4), 355–363.

Corwin, R. (1969). Patterns of organizational conflict. *Administration Science Quarterly, 14,* 507–521.

Davis, K., & Newstrom, J. (1985). *Human behavior at work: Organizational behavior* (7th ed.). New York: McGraw-Hill.

Deutsch, M. (1969). Conflict: Productive and destructive. *Journal of Social Issues, 25,* 7–41.

Deutsch, M. (1973). *The resolution of conflict: Constructive and destructive processes.* New Haven: Yale University Press.

Douglass, L., & Bevis, E. (1979). *Nursing management and leadership in action.* St. Louis: Mosby.

Drucker, P. (1954). *The practice of management.* New York: Harper & Row.

Drucker, P. (1985a). The discipline of innovation. *Harvard Business Review, 64,* 67–72.

Drucker, P. (1985b). *Effective executive.* New York: Harper & Row.

Drucker, P. (1985c). *Managing in turbulent times.* New York: Harper & Row.

Edmunds, M.(1979). Conflict. *Nurse Practitioner, 4,* 42, 47–48.

Filley, A. (1975). *Interpersonal conflict resolution.* Morristown, NJ: Scott, Foresman.

Filley, A. (1980). Types and sources of conflict. In M. Berger, D. Elhart, S. Firsich, S. Jordan, & S. Stone (Eds.). *Management for nurses: A multidisciplinary approach* (2nd ed). St. Louis: Mosby.

Fink, C. (1968). Some conceptual difficulties in the theory of social conflict. *Journal of Conflict Resolution, 13,* 413–458.

Ford, C. (1979). MBO: An idea whose time has gone? *Business Horizons, 22,* 48–55.

Golightly, C. (1979). MBO and performance appraisal. *Journal of Nursing Administration, 9,* 11–20.

Haw, M. (1980). Conflict resolution and the communication myth. *Nursing Outlook, 28,* 566–570.

Hersey, P., & Blanchard, K. (1988). *Management of organizational behavior: Utilizing human resources* (5th ed.). Englewood Cliffs, NJ: Prentice-Hall.

Homme, L. (1970). *How to use contingency contracting in the classroom.* Champaign, IL: Research Press.

Hughes, E. (1979). Helping staff to manage conflict well. *Hospital Progess, 60,* 68–71, 83.

Humble, J. (1967). *Management by objectives.* London: Industrial Education and Research Foundation.

Kramer, M., & Schmalenberg, C. (1978). Conflict: The cutting edge of growth. *Nursing Digest, 5,* 59–65.

Levinson, H. (1970). Management by whose objectives? *Harvard Business Review, 48,* 125–134.

Lewis, J. (1976). Conflict management. *Journal of Nursing Administration, 6,* 18–22.

Marriner, A. (1979a). Conflict theory. *Supervisor Nurse, 10,* 12–16.

Marriner, A. (1979b). Conflict resolution. *Supervisor Nurse, 10,* 46, 49, 52–54.

Marriner, A. (1982). Comparing strategies and their use: Managing conflict. *Nursing Management, 6,* 29–31.

Myrtle, R., & Glogow, E. (1978). How nursing administrators view conflict. *Nursing Research, 27,* 103–106.

Nichols, B. (1979). Dealing with conflict. *The Journal of Continuing Education in Nursing, 10,* 24–27.

Nielsen, J. (1977). Resolving conflict. In K. Claus, & J. Bailey, *Power and influence in health care.* St. Louis; Mosby.

Odiorne, G. (1965). *Management by objectives: A system of managerial leadership.* Belmont, CA: Pitman.

Odiorne, G. (1975). Management by objectives: Antidote to future shock. *Journal of Nursing Administration, 5,* 27–30.

Odiorne, G. (1979). *MBO II: A system of managerial leadership for the 80s.* Belmont, CA: D.S. Lake Pub.

Olsson, D. (1968). *Management by objectives.* Palo Alto, CA: Pacific Books.

Palmer, J. (1973). Management by objectives. *Journal of Nursing Administration, 3,* 55–60.

Pondy, L. (1967). Organizational conflict: Concepts and models. *Administrative Science Quarterly, 12,* 296–320.

Pondy, L. (1969). Variances of organizational conflict. *Administration Science Quarterly, 14,* 449–506.

Schmidt, S. (1973). *Lateral conflict within employment service district offices.* Unpublished doctoral dissertation. University of Wisconsin, Madison.

Silber, M. (1984). Managing confrontations: Once more into the breach. *Nursing Management, 15*(4), 54–58.

Skarupa, J. (1971). Management by objectives: A systematic way to manage change. *Journal of Nursing Administration, 1,* 52–56.

Stogdill, R., & Coons, A. (Eds.). (1957). *Leader behavior: Its description and measurement* (Research Monograph No. 88). Columbus: Bureau of Business Research, Ohio State University.

Thomas, K., & Kilmann, R. (1977). Developing a forced-choice measure of conflict-handling behavior: The "MODE" instrument. *Education and Psychological Measurement, 37,* 309–325.

Walton, R., & Dutton, J. (1969). The management of interdepartmental conflict: A model and review. *Administrative Science Quarterly, 14,* 73–84.

Time Management

People plan within a boundary of time, look on the past over a span of time, and set goals for the future that are to be met within a period of time. Time can facilitate goal accomplishment, and it can be an oppressive force in finishing tasks. It can make people nervous in one context and can relax those same people in another context. Life is run on a time schedule—in some instances the schedule is philosophical, and in other instances it is concrete. For example, one has six months to live or one has a whole lifetime. Is there any philosophical difference in these statements? Clocks, calendars, watches, seasons, holidays, birthdays, and so forth, all point to time—the unidirectional process of growth.

Managers should attend particularly to time because it costs money to an organization—efficiency pays off. Life without wasted time is impossible. A manager, however, can increase the probability that time will be used efficiently by following some general guidelines that have been primarily developed by Cooper (1971), Dayton (1983), Drucker (1967), Lakein (1973), Mackenzie (1972), McCay (1959), Oncken and Wass (1974), and Webber (1981). Applications of the time management concept have recently been observed in literature from the helping professions (Brown, 1980; Byrd, 1977, 1980; Eliopoulos, 1984; Ferri, 1987, McGee-Cooper, 1986a, 1986b, 1986c, 1986d; Marriner, 1979; Rutkowski, 1984; Schwartz & Mackenzie, 1979; Smith & Besnette, 1978; Volk-Tebbitt, 1978; Wiley, 1978).

Every person has all the time there is, yet few people have enough time (Mackenzie, 1972). Since no manager is going to get more time, the time one has must be used more efficiently. Believe it or not, this is possible. The philosophy of time will be discussed first in this chapter followed by the time management process. Time-managing techniques are discussed in the concluding part of the chapter. The intent is to help managers to learn how to get "a little more" out of the time given.

PHILOSOPHY OF TIME

Time has been defined by Arnold (cited in Volk-Tebbitt, 1978) as a system of references for understanding and describing the occurrence and sequence of events. It is also a resource (Mackenzie, 1972) that cannot be stockpiled or accumulated— it cannot be turned on or off. According to Drucker (1967), time is so important that unless it is managed, nothing else can be managed.

Classifying Activities

Activities are either time wasters or time consumers. The Health Care Management Team of the Minnesota Hospital Association (Volk-Tebbitt, 1978) said that a time waster is an activity that has a lower payoff than an alternate activity that could be done during a particular time period. Drop-in visitors, unproductive meetings, telephone interruptions, and so forth, are examples of time wasters.

Lakein (1973) viewed a time-consumer activity as complex and/or difficult with high payoffs. He classified activities as As, Bs, and Cs. Cs are activities that no one asks about; they are trivial and have little or no payoff. If a memo is received, then the activity is a B—moderately important with moderate payoff. Activities receiving an A are important—calls get received on them, and people come to visit and inquire about them. As have a high payoff. Lakein (1973) claimed that people spend 80% of their time doing C activities and only 20% doing As. Yet A priorities make the difference. This factual philosophy leads into the Pareto Principle.

The Pareto Principle

The Pareto Principle, named after the 19th century Italian economist and sociologist Vilfredo Pareto, stated that a relatively small number of items, tasks, or behaviors in a group are significant ones (Mackenzie, 1972). Juran (1964) labeled these items as the "vital few" and the balance of items as the "trivial many." The Pareto Principle is a way of explaining that normally the trivial many situational problems use 80% of the group's time in producing 20% of the positive results. In contrast, the vital few situations or problems use 20% of the expended time to produce 80% of the positive results.

Applying the principle to nursing, suppose the goal of increasing patient satisfaction with nursing care were sought. The nursing system, above average in readiness on this task, required LB3—high consideration and low structure. They identified 20 interventions that could be made to increase patient satisfaction. When the Pareto Principle is applied, 4 of the 20 would generally account for 80% of the change in patients when the interventions were implemented and evaluated. The rest of the interventions would reap little payoff in terms of cost effectiveness. The time used in low-payoff activities—time wasters—could be channeled into higher-payoff interventions connected to solving another problem, which is also of high priority but on a different level. Figure 17.1 portrays this priority process.

The primary goal of time management is to make activities count, to the degree that is possible. This goal is achieved by controlling time so that the least amount of effort produces the greatest positive outcomes—making the 1:4 (effort:payoff) ratio shown in Figure 17.1 even better with less effort and better results.

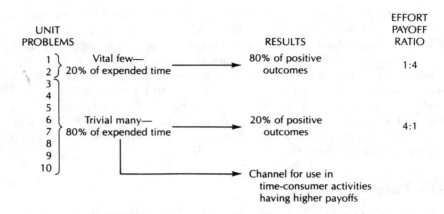

Figure 17.1 Priority process using the Pareto Principle.

Kinds of Time

A manager has two categories of time: specialty time and managerial time (Graf, 1979; Mackenzie, 1972). Specialty time involves those responsibilities which are accomplished alone. This does not exclude the need of input from others, as required by the task. It simply means that when the activity is to be done, it is usually done by the manager. A nurse supervisor might see staffing, mapping out long-term goals, and/or preparing the agenda for the next head nurses' meeting as specialty items. Keep in mind that the inclusion of activities into either category is relative to the unique system and its particular needs.

Managerial time is time that is shared with or given to others in a system— it involves some level of interaction between or among people. Managerial time can be subdivided into response time and discretionary time. Response time generally involves such activities as speaking on the telephone to a caller or returning a call, having office visits, attending meetings, and making rounds. Discretionary time has to do with activities that suggest or ask for a response but the leader has the option of deciding whether or not to actually behave in accordance with the request. Time may be better used in another activity.

Specialty and managerial time contain activities that can be prioritized according to Lakein's (1973) ABC system, described earlier in this chapter. There is no formula for the ratio of managerial time to specialty time in a manager's position. This is purely according to the environment that includes the unique manager, system, and tasks. One general rule of thumb, however, is that the more generally mature the system is, the greater opportunity the manager has to corner specialty time. Obviously, the opposite is also true—the more generally immature the system is, the fewer options the manager has to corner specialty time.

THE TIME MANAGEMENT PROCESS

The time management process is another extension of the problem-solving method, as shown in Table 17.1. Perusing Table 17.1 and thinking about the focus of this chapter can lead to the conclusion that the problem-solving method pertains to managing others toward cost effectiveness, whereas the time management process focuses on managing the self so that the ratio of effort to payoff is high. The

TABLE 17.1 The Time Management Process and the Problem-Solving Method

Time Management Process*	Problem-Solving Method
Analyzing the present situation (Where I am now?)	Problem identification
Developing relevant assumptions (What conditions will most likely exist within the time span of the plan?)	Point of view
Establishing objectives (What do I want to achieve?)	Problem definition and/or goal statement / Problem analysis
Developing alternatives (What ways might I attain objectives?)	Alternative solutions
Making a decision	Recommended action
Implementing the decision	
Establishing review and control procedures	

*Source: Column 1 is taken from Mackenzie R: *The Time Trap: Managing Your Way Out*, New York, McGraw-Hill, 1972, pp. 44–45.

processes are parallel while the content and subjects differ. All the previously discussed principles of managing, goal setting, motivation, and so forth apply in this chapter also.

A person must first look at his or her present situation (the actual) on personal and professional (specialty and managerial) grounds. One should pose and answer the question of where one is on important areas. Then, given reasonable projections of what environmental conditions will exist at different slices of time—one month, one year, five years, and whenever—ask where would one like to be on those same areas. What comes out of this thinking, as the reader of this book already knows, is the problem/goal. The objectives, which flow from the goal, describe the desired outcome. (Refer to Chapter 12 on teaching for further discussion on goals and objectives.)

Once objectives have been designated, they must be arranged on the basis of priorities. One useful way of doing this is according to Lakein's (1973) ABCs. Or ponder each objective with the questions: "How much effort will be involved in fulfilling this objective, and what is the expected payoff?" Then assign priorities according to least effort/most payoff (high priority) down to most effort/least payoff (low priority). A scale of one to five (low to high) can be used if finer quantification in this process is sought. Then attack the top priorities—just two or three.

Develop alternative strategies for accomplishing these objectives. These strategies are concerned with how the objectives will be attained. The goals and objectives themselves are what is to be attained. Again, develop an effort/payoff ratio for each solution and pinpoint the best strategy for action. Implement it and evaluate it by comparing intent with results. Evaluation can range from completely subjective to very objective. The need for formality of the evaluation phase can be assessed by looking at the effort against the possible payoff. As a side note, formal evaluations are costly in terms of effort. They may, however, be worth it. Consult a book on evaluation procedures and evaluation research such as Thorndike and Hagen (1977) should formal evaluation controls be indicated.

Now, does all of this seem simple? Do not be fooled. Parasites eat and piranhas nip away at our time, and the concept called time management is most useful because readers on the topic can receive myriad helpful hints on controlling parasites and piranhas. The next portion of this chapter is devoted to discussing these techniques. The content is not inclusive—many more tips are available in time management literature and from personal experiences.

TIME MANAGEMENT TECHNIQUES

This section presents an array of techniques for attacking parasites and piranhas (Lakein, 1973; Mackenzie, 1972). Each topic is discussed separately.

Personal Commitment to Improving

How many psychiatrists does it take to change one 60-watt light bulb? The answer is "only one, but the light bulb has to be willing"—corny but true. Brown (1980) termed personal commitment to time saving as the sine qua non. So examine yourself. Those who care should read on. Those who discover unwillingness should try to discern why it exists and work on changing from unwillingness to willingness—then read on. McConnell (1983) underscored that in order to become an effective manager of others, a leader must first become an effective manager of self—through personal effort.

Deciding What Not to Do

A requisite for success, according to Nunlist (cited in Mackenzie, 1972) is refusing to do the unimportant. "They must learn to forget the unnecessary and to ignore the irrelevant" (p. 55). Then do a fantastic job on the essentials.

Learning to Say No

Read the book entitled *When I Say No, I Feel Guilty* by Smith (1985). Someone always has a priority—essential—that another must do. In a hospital, the "someones" abound. The manager must sort out the important from the unimportant, or high-payoff tasks from low-payoff tasks, and say no to the latter tasks and yes to the former ones—without feeling and probably communicating guilt or some other self-defeating emotion.

Recording How Time Is Used

The "Time Analysis Worksheet" (Brown, 1980) that is found in the exercises at the conclusion of this chapter is one way to find out how time is used—where it goes. This raises consciousness of one's own behavior by making the abstract concrete. The "Time Log," also found in the exercises, can be used for the same purpose.

Planning Use of Time

List responsibilities, choose priorities, and schedule for their accomplishment. Develop a daily, weekly, and/or monthly "to do" list. Check off progress; this is self-reinforcement for further accomplishment. Do not let minutia intrude on the list but also allow for some flexibility, especially in the longer-term lists.

Fire Fighting Versus Fire Prevention

Graf (1979) explained fire fighting as responding to whatever comes up, like applying oil to the squeaky wheel. It is necessary when planning is poor. Fire prevention involves contingency planning—looking ahead and asking, "What can be done today to avoid problems in the future?" Of course, preventing fires can become a parasite in and of itself. So invest enough energy in this area to make the payoff worthwhile.

Prime Time

Most people have a certain portion of a day that they know is their "prime time." During this period, people are at their best, and work is usually easiest to accomplish. Find out what this block of time is and use it—hang a "do not disturb" sign outside the door, refuse calls, do not schedule meetings, and so forth. This is probably the time when 80% of work gets accomplished, so protect it.

Programming Blocks of Time

Graf (1979) pointed out that "one of the best ways to complete big projects is to program large blocks of time for the effort" (p. 17). Otherwise, the task will be broken up into smaller pieces and much time will be wasted getting oriented to where one was at the end of the last session.

Organizing the Workspace

Arrange the environment to make life easier. Make the office space fit your individual personality—from the color of the walls to the arrangement of furniture or addition of plants to anything else that is pleasing. Keep the desk uncluttered; keep only the project in immediate focus on it. Any other material on the desk may become a distractor. Have tools such as pencil sharpeners, staplers, and so forth handy. Eliminate the need to get up and wander around—time gets wasted both from the short journey and from reentry.

Memoitis

Oh, the memoranda that infest American offices! Mackenzie (1972) reported an estimate that puts the paperwork cost of running the United States economy at a sum equal to about one-seventh of the total yearly output of goods and services. Memos are part of this mountain.

Memos are to remind, to clarify, and to confirm (Mackenzie, 1972). They involve one-way communication. Use them only when essential. In many instances, a phone call is the better bet.

Learn to scan memos received for a quick assessment of their importance. If it passes the test of "reading worthiness," then read it fully. If not, throw it immediately in a conveniently placed wastebasket. Take a speed-reading course if possible.

Blocking Interruptions

Common courtesy is always necessary but it should not be confused with a need to extend carte blanche to telephone calls or to visits (Mackenzie, 1972). A manager can extend the "open door policy" when it is decided that the door should be opened—definitely not during one's prime time.

Drop-in visitors should be discouraged. Simply say once,"I would like to talk with you at a time when I am not involved in a project. We can schedule an appointment at. . . .:" A drop-in-type person usually gets the message after the first or second such interchange. Confer with drop-in visitors standing up and outside one's office, if possible. This is a barrier to the visitor's discourteous intrusion. Consider the intruder who "knows it is not regular office hours but just needs one minute for a 'quick' question." The scene might go like this.

> That one minute intrusion minimally involves the following, without exaggeration: (1) thinking about what you were doing ends; (2) your mind switches gear to contain anger at the disruption first and then to think about what the intruder is asking; (3) time to respond coherently, masking flaming anger; (4) listening to the almost sure second and third questions and/or comments

of the intruder; (5) responding again when secretly vowing not to
let this situation be repeated, maybe even blaming your secretary;
(6) bidding farewell and emphasizing that it would be a pleasure
to talk again—simply make an appointment or come in during
regular office hours; (7) getting coffee to calm your nerves; and
(8) sitting down trying to recall what you were doing prior to the
intrusion and where you were on the matter. This intrusion costs
at least 30 minutes, ignoring the nonquantifiable cost to your
nervous system.

The telephone is another piranha because it can ring anytime,
and sometimes just the ring is intrusive. If possible, have a secretary
screen calls on the following basis: "immediate response is required"
and "delayed response is required." Handle the immediate calls and
arrange telephone hours to return other calls. When available, have a
secretary place the calls and then transfer them to the caller.

Managing Meetings

"Parkinson's Second Law stated that people tend to devote time and
effort to tasks in inverse relation to their importance" (adapted from
Mackenzie, 1972, p. 107). Mackenzie (1972) offered several pages of
rules for getting more out of meetings; here are a choice few together
with beliefs of this author:

1. Start on time; give warning only the first time.
2. End on time.
3. Develop an agenda and circulate it to the attendees
   prior to the meeting.
4. Only those needed should attend a meeting.
5. Gather information prior to a meeting; summarize it
   during the meeting.
6. Stick to the agenda; avoid interruptions; squelch side-
   trips around or away from the agendas.
7. Limit the amount of time for particular agenda; place
   the meeting so that the intended gets accomplished.
8. Arrange for a comfortable environment but not so
   plush that people would rather be there than some-
   place else.
9. Items that involve one-way communication by their
   nature should be typed and distributed—not verbally
   announced. The latter simply wastes time.

10. Have a secretary take and distribute the minutes of the meeting within one week from the date of the meeting. Minutes should record the issues and the decisions. Brief reports of the points of discussion may be included. When minutes are verbatim accounts of the meetings, the secretary wastes time and so do all the readers.

Managing People

Time management books, such as those in the references at the end of this chapter, include a portion on delegating. The focus is to alert the manager that managers lead people to accomplish goals. Therefore, managers should delegate work to others.

As the reader is aware by now, managers must use a variety of styles to help followers mature in relation to accomplishing a task. Depending on the system's level of maturity at a certain time and place, the manager must appropriately either tell, sell to, participate with, or delegate to followers. Managers must examine themselves in order to discern whether they use different leader behavior styles because the system needs them or because of their own needs. When a system's maturity indicates, the push is always toward delegation because then the manager has freed time for other managerial and/or specialty tasks. It behooves managers to examine themselves and to give followers the leadership they need, pushing them toward maturity. This is a responsibility of managers, and in terms of time management it is a reward of management.

Springing the Time Trap

In *The Time Trap*, Mackenzie (1972) included an appendix on time wasters he has most commonly encountered, their causes, and their possible solutions. The list is not exhaustive but certainly can help. Table 17.2 presents his work.

TABLE 17.2 How to Spring the Time Trap

Time Waster	Possible Causes	Solutions
Lack of planning	Failure to see the benefit	Recognize that planning takes time but saves time in the end.

(continued)

TABLE 17.2 (continued)

Time Waster	Possible Causes	Solutions
	Action orientation	Emphasize results, not activity.
	Success without it	Recognize that success is often in spite of, not because of, methods.
Lack of priorities	Lack of goals and objectives	Write down goals and objectives. Discuss priorities with subordinates.
Overcommitment	Broad interests	Say no.
	Confusion in priorities	Put first things first.
	Failure to set priorities	Develop a personal philosophy of time. Relate priorities to a schedule of events.
Management by crisis	Lack of planning	Apply the same solutions as for lack of planning.
	Unrealistic time estimates	Allow more time. Allow for interruptions.
	Problem orientation	Be opportunity-oriented.
	Reluctance of subordinates to break bad news	Encourage fast transmission of information as essential for timely corrective action.
Haste	Impatience with detail	Take time to get it right. Save the time of doing it over.
	Responding to the urgent	Distinguish between the urgent and the important.
	Lack of planning ahead	Take time to plan. It repays itself many times over.
	Attempting too much in too little time	Attempt less. Delegate more.
Paperwork and reading	Knowledge explosion	Read selectively. Learn speed reading.
	Computeritis	Manage computer data by exception.

TABLE 17.2 (*continued*)

Time Waster	Possible Causes	Solutions
	Failure to screen	Remember the Pareto Principle. Delegate reading to subordinates.
Routine and trivia	Lack of priorities	Set and concentrate on goals. Delegate nonessentials.
	Oversurveillance of subordinates	Delegate; then give subordinates their space. Look to results, not details or methods.
	Refusal to delegate; feeling of greater security dealing with operating detail	Recognize that without delegation it is impossible to get anything done through others.
Visitors	Enjoyment of socializing	Do it elsewhere. Meet visitors outside. Suggest lunch if necessary. Hold stand-up conferences.
	Inability to say no	Screen. Say no. Be unavailable. Modify the open-door policy.
Telephone	Lack of self-discipline	Screen and group calls. Be brief.
	Desire to be informed and involved	Stay uninvolved with all but essentials. Manage by exception.
Meetings	Fear of responsibility for decisions	Make decisions without meetings.
	Indecision	Make decisions even when some facts are missing.
	Overcommunication	Discourage unnecessary meetings. Convene only those needed.
	Poor leadership	Use agendas. Stick to the subject. Prepare concise minutes as soon as possible.

(*continued*)

TABLE 17.2 (continued)

Time Waster	Possible Causes	Solutions
Indecision	Lack of confidence in the facts	Improve fact-finding and validating procedures.
	Insistence on all the facts—paralysis of analysis	Accept risks as inevitable. Decide without all facts.
	Fear of the consequences of a mistake	Delegate the right to be wrong. Use mistakes as a learning process.
	Lack of a rational decision-making process	Get facts, set goals, investigate alternatives and negative consequences, make the decision, and implement it.
Lack of delegation	Fear of subordinates' inadequacy	Train. Allow mistakes. Replace if necessary.
	Fear of subordinates' competence	Delegate fully. Give credit. Ensure corporate growth to maintain challenge.
	Work overload on subordinates	Balance the work load. Staff up. Reorder priorities.

Source: Reprinted, by permission of the publisher, from *The time trap: Managing your way out*, by R. Alec Mackenzie, © 1972 by AMACOM, a division of American Management Associations, pp. 173–176. This list is adapted from "Troubleshooting Chart for Time Wasters," in R. Alec Mackenzie, *Managing time at the top*. New York, The President's Association, 1970.

SUMMARY

The concept of time is a constant phenomenon. Each person has all the time there is, and no one ever has enough time. The intent of applying time management techniques is to get "a little more" out of the time given.

Time is a system of references for understanding and describing the occurrence and sequence of events. Activities can be classified as time wasters or time consumers, which are relative terms. The Pareto Principle is a way of explaining how 20% of one's time involved in time consumers produces 80% of positive outcomes. Eighty percent of expended time in activities that are time wasters result in 20% of positive outcomes. The trick/goal is to have the least amount of effort produce the greatest positive outcomes.

Managers have specialty time for themselves and managerial time spent interacting in some form with others. The time management process parallels the problem-solving method. It can be used to guide a manager toward goal fulfillment in professional and personal areas.

Time management techniques were discussed in the last part of the chapter. The intent of these techniques is to offer a manager a potpourri of interventions against the parasites and piranhas of time. It is essential that each person recognize his or her inherent potential to waste and to save time—his or her own as well as another's.

REFERENCES

Brown, D., (1980). *The use of time: A looking-into-leadership monograph.* Fairfax, VA: Leadership Resources.

Byrd, E. (1977). Time management. *American Rehabiliation, 2,* 24–26.

Byrd, E. (1980). Irrational ideas in the management of time. *Journal of Applied Rehabilitation Counseling, 11,* 46–49.

Cooper, J. (1971). *How to get more done in less time.* Garden City, NY: Doubleday.

Dayton, E. (1983). *Tools for time management: Time saving tools for managing your life* (rev. ed.). Grand Rapids, MI: Zondervan.

Drucker, P. (1967). *The effective executive.* New York: Harper & Row.

Eliopoulos, C. (1984). Time management: A reminder. *Journal of Nursing Administration, 14*(3), 30–32.

Ferri, R. (1987). In search of the excellent one-minute megatrend...or how to tolerate the five minute burden. *American Journal of Nursing, 87,*(1), 109–110.

Graf, P. (1979). *Ten techniques for improving time management.* Unpublished manuscript.

Juran, J. (1964). *Managerial breakthrough: A new concept of the manager's job.* New York: McGraw-Hill.

Lakein, A. (1973). *How to get control of your time and your life.* New York: Peter H. Wyden.

Mackenzie, R. (1972). *The time trap: Managing your way out.* New York: AMACOM (A Division of the American Management Association).

Marriner, A. (1979). Time. *Journal of Nursing Administration, 9,* 16–18.

McCay, J. (1959). *The management of time.* Englewood Cliffs, NJ: Prentice-Hall.

McConnell, C. (1983). Supervisor, manage yourself. *The Health Care Supervisor, 1*(3), 57–68.

McGee-Cooper, A. (1986a). Time management—Part II: Rewriting obsolete work rules. *AORN Journal, 44,* 409–414.

McGee-Cooper, A. (1986b). Time management—Part III: Making the time for joy. *AORN Journal, 44,* 599–602.

McGee-Cooper, A. (1986c). Time management—Part IV: Decontaminating work and play time. *AORN Journal, 44,* 809–813.

McGee-Cooper, A. (1986d). Time management—Part V: Energy engineering. *AORN Journal, 44,* 977–982.

Oncken, W., & Wass, D. (1974). Management time: Who's got the monkey? *Harvard Business Review, 52,* 75–80.

Rutkowski, B.(1984). The nursing approach to better time management. *Nursing Life, 4*(5), 54–57.

Schwartz, E., & Mackenzie, R. (1979). Time-management strategy for women. *Journal of Nursing Administration, 9,* 22–26.

Smith, H., & Besnette, F. (1978). Effective time management: The forgotten administrative and nursing supervisor art. *Hospital Topics, 56,* 32–37.

Smith, M. (1985) *When I say no, I feel quilty.* New York: Bantam.

Thorndike, R., & Hagen, E. (1977). *Measurement and evaluation in psychology and education* (4th ed.). New York: Wiley.

Volk-Tebbitt, B. (1978). Time: Who controls yours? *Supervisor Nurse, 9,* 17–22.

Webber, R. (1981). *Time and management.* Nutley, NJ: Moffat.

Wiley, L. (1978). The ABCs of time management. *Nursing 78, 8,* 105–112.

Performance Evaluation

Performance evaluation is one method for a manager to control what is occurring in the organization. It is a way to compare the outcomes of individual and group behaviors toward goal accomplishment with the initiatives that were planned. Further, it is the way most managers formally and informally guide employees in their professional development within an organization.

The literature is replete with articles on the topic of performance appraisal and evaluation. There are authors who have developed objective performance-evaluation systems (Ganong & Ganong, 1983; Richards, 1984; Stalker, Kornblith, Lewis, & Parker, 1986); others have studied the process for conducting the performance evaluation

(Meyer, 1984; Rothwell, 1984; Stull, 1986); and investigators have studied the effects of feedback and other processes on employee development (Lachman, 1984; Pearce & Porter, 1986). There is literature on the factors that should be included in various criterion-referenced performance appraisals (Johnson & Luciano, 1988; Lampe, 1986; McCloskey & McCain, 1988) and then there is discussion about whether performance evaluations **really** work in producing the desired outcomes (Momeyer, 1986; Zemke, 1985).

Even though discussions about performance evaluations from both managers and followers always involve some degree of hesitation, anxiety, and even pain, the performance evaluation seems here to stay—in one form or another. The purpose of this chapter, therefore, is to discuss the general reasons for the performance evaluation, principles of evaluation, tactics for appraising, and classic methods used in conducting the performance evaluation.

PURPOSES OF THE PERFORMANCE EVALUATION

There are two general purposes for the performance evaluation: judgmental purposes and developmental purposes (Ivancevich, Donnelly, & Gibson, 1989).

Judgmental Purposes

When performance appraisals are accomplished for the purposes of determining salary standards and salary increases and/or awarding merit increases, then it is being carried out for judgmental purposes. Other reasons in this area include selecting qualified individuals for promotions and/or transfers and demoting or terminating employees due to unsatisfactory performance (Rowland & Rowland, 1985). Performance evaluations that are done for judgmental purposes carry the highest stakes and necessarily result in the most anxiety from both the rater and the ratee.

Developmental Purposes

Developmental purposes are predominantly educative and involve coaching the employee to gain professionally through working within organizational goals. Self-learning and personal growth both are involved (Ivancevich, Donnelly, & Gibson, 1989). Rowland and

Rowland (1985) described specific examples such as the following: identifying talent in the organization; determining training and development needs of individuals or groups; improving interpersonal relationships among group members; establishing standards of performance and gaining acceptance of those standards; providing employee recognition; discovering employee aspirations and reconciling them with the goals of the organization; team building; and giving employees feedback.

PRINCIPLES OF PERFORMANCE EVALUATION

There are certain principles of performance evaluation that must be met in order for an evaluation to be useful in any purpose.

First, the evaluation must contain content that is *relevant* to the individual being evaluated in a particular setting (Ivancevich, Donnelly, & Gibson, 1989). This answers the question, What is to be evaluated? In other words, the content of the evaluation must encompass a valid sample of the behaviors or traits that are seen as important in a specified position. The affective, the cognitive, and the psychomotor areas involved in carrying out specified responsibilities in a position must be represented. Therefore, the evaluation should be based on a position analysis and a resultant position description for a given level of expertise. In typical clinical career ladders, for example, there are different position descriptions for the role of staff nurse with two years of experience, then from two to five years of experience, and so forth. At each level of experience, an employee ought to be able to achieve excellence.

Second, the *criteria* that will be used to evaluate performance should be stated and *standards* should be specified whenever possible. The criteria may be stated in a paper-and-pencil rating scale by a follower or maybe a paper-and-pencil self-report or a test, for example. The standard is the minimally acceptable level of performance, such as 90% passing rate on a test or writing care plans on all patients within 24 hours of their admission. It is important that the criterion method be reliable, that is, that it be stable over time and between/among raters. If two raters rated the same person and had the same information, would their ratings be very similar? If a criterion method is said to be reliable, both raters would have similar scores. This same principle applies when the same rater is rating at two different intervals. If no change has occurred, then the score should be similar; in contrast, if the employee has grown or learned, then the score on the criterion should show improvement.

Third, a performance evaluation should be able to *discriminate* between excellent, good, and poor performance (Ivancevich, Donnelly, & Gibson, 1989). Any purpose for which an evaluation is done should involve identification of areas requiring further development and areas that just need to continue in the effective vein with possibly some enrichment.

Last, any performance evaluation must be *practical* (Ivancevich, Donnelly, & Gibson, 1989) or in measurement terminology, it must have *utility*. There are many organizations and people in those organizations that spend tremendous amounts of time developing, testing, and implementing extremely lengthy performance evaluations. In contemporary nursing practice, one must evaluate the effort/payoff ratio in such an endeavor. Sometimes people develop a criterion-referenced evaluation over such a long period of time that the content is no longer valid given the requirements of the position—which seem to change quickly in current practice. Further, the longer the evaluation forms, the less likely managers are going to find time to complete them.

TACTICS OF PERFORMANCE EVALUATION

The process of the performance evaluation can be paralleled with the problem-solving method that was presented, discussed, and applied in Part I of this book. Table 18–1 contains a comparison of these processes. The performance evaluation process noted is a blend by this author of information contained from many sources. Operationally, it identifies the steps for planning, conducting, and following up on the evaluation.

Who Should Evaluate?

Ivancevich, Donnelly, & Gibson (1989) identified five possible parties who could evaluate or rate another person: a supervisor, peers, the ratee, subordinates of the ratee, or raters outside of the organizational environment. In most cases, employees should be rated by their immediate supervisors, since this person has the greatest opportunity to observe the individual's behavior against organizational objectives.

TABLE 18.1 Comparisons of Processes: Problem-Solving and Performance Appraisal

Problem-Solving Process	Performance Appraisal Process
1. Identify the problem	Define the job requirements—expectations
	Define the standards (benchmarks) of performance for a particular role
2. Designate the system	Specify the employee qualifications
3. Diagnose the system (self and others)	Review the objectives set by manager and employee
	Review the performance records
	Tentatively complete the appraisal form
4. Choose leader behavior	Conduct the appraisal
5. Specify alternative solutions	Co-develop a performance improvement plan using Management by Objectives or goal-setting
6. Recommend an action	Agree on a plan of action
7. Implement the plan	Provide on-the-job coaching or daily reinforcement and development activities
8. Evaluate the results	Provide ongoing feedback on performance

Who Should be Evaluated?

Most organizations evaluate employees at all levels of the organization—from the bottom of the organizational chart right to the top managerial levels. Education and development can occur anyplace and people require feedback as a stimulus to develop further in specified directions.

When Should Evaluations Occur?

There is no rule; however, most organizations evaluate older or tenured employees about once or twice a year. New employees are evaluated about six weeks to two months after being hired and employees at various stages of development may be evaluated more or less often than twice a year, depending on the objectives set during the previous evaluation. Progressive discipline procedures are examples of evaluations that may occur as often as every two weeks. An evaluation should contain a progress note at the bottom that is written by the evaluator; it should designate when the next evaluation will occur and the objectives for the period of time until that date.

The Evaluation Interview

The evaluation interview is a way of providing formal feedback to the employee. This author recommends that both rater and ratee complete the evaluation form or make notes relative to each criterion. Following discussion in the interview, a record can be made by the evaluator that reflects information from all involved.

In addition to the principles and discussion in Chapter 13 on interviewing, Ivancevich, Donnelly, and Gibson (1989) provided

---

TABLE 18.2 Guidelines for Preparing and Conducting an Appraisal Interview

---

Preparing for the interview:

---

1. Hold a group discussion with employees to be evaluated and describe the broad standards for their appraisals.
2. Discuss your employees with your own manager and several of your peers.
3. Clarify any differences in language between the formal written appraisal and the interview.
4. If you are angry with an employee, talk about it before the interview, not during the interview.
5. Be aware of your own biases in judging people.
6. Review the employee's compensation plan and be knowledgeable about his or her salary history.
7. If you already have given the employee a number of negative appraisals, be prepared to take action.

Conducting the interview:

---

1. Focus on positive work performance.
2. Remember that strengths and weaknesses usually spring from the same general characteristics.
3. Admit that your judgment of performance contains some subjectivity.
4. Make it clear that responsibility for development lies with the employee, not with you (the rater).
5. Be specific when citing examples.

Source: Ivancevich, J., Donnelly, J. Jr., & Gibson, J. (1989). *Management: Principles and functions* (4th ed.). Homewood, IL: Irwin, p. 534.

guidelines for preparing and conducting an appraisal interview. Their thoughts are found in Table 18–2.

Research Findings on Performance Evaluation

The following insights regarding performance evaluation seem important for the evaluator and the evaluatee to keep in mind. With the exception of the first finding presented, Kreitner and Kinicki (1989) synthesized these results from several sources including Hedge and Kavangh (1988) and Landy and Farr (1980).

- Kraiger and Ford (1985) found that appraisers typically rate same-race appraisees higher. In a meta-analysis involving 74 studies and 17,159 individuals, white supervisors favored white subordinates. Similarly, in a meta-analysis of 14 studies and 2,248 people, black supervisors favored black subordinates. These findings support the findings of Hornstein (1976) in his research on prosocial and antisocial behavior in similar and dissimilar groups
- No consistent gender bias was found
- The more experienced rater and the higher performance manager tended to result in higher-quality appraisals. Training and development had positive effects of appraisal quality.
- Peer ratings and self-evaluations tended toward leniency when compared with ratings from a supervisor.

PERFORMANCE EVALUATION METHODS

There are many methods that can be used to evaluate a person. The ones used predominantly in health care systems will be presented and discussed.

Graphic Rating Scales

This is the most widely used method of evaluating performance and involves having behavior statements or traits each rated on a continuum that may be quantitative or qualitative. The Likert-type scale that moves from 1 (poor) to 5 (excellent), for example, is a quantitative scale. Occasionally, qualitative adjectives may be used such as poor, average, and excellent to describe numbers. Graphic rating scales can be used by superiors in rating subordinates, or they may be used in self-reports or ratings by peers. When the quantitative scale is used, an overall evaluation score can be derived by adding all the individual scores and dividing it by the number of items.

In graphic rating scales, it is important to understand that the greater the number of quantitative intervals, the greater the chance that the intervals will not be stable across raters. In other words, if two raters are observing the same person in the same context and have been given the same information, their ratings will be more similar as the number of rating possibilities decreases.

Critical Incidents

These are examples of good and bad performances that are written down soon after occurring. In a sense, they are a diary of significant events in the work performance of an employee. Critical incidents should focus on work-related behavior and not personality traits (Kreitner & Kinicki, 1989).

Written Essays

This is a narrative description of one's perception of another's work-related performance or it may actually be written as a self-report. This is the most subjective of the evaluation techniques since something liked (the halo effect) or something disliked (the horn effect) often runs through and flavors the entire essay. Furthermore, they are usually written long after the actual behavior has been observed; hence, they are subject to the distortion caused by time.

Goal Setting

This method employs Drucker's (1954, 1985a, 1985b, 1985c). Management by Objectives or modifications of the method. In Management by Objectives, results are emphasized rather than activities. Objectives are mutually set between supervisor and follower and a time period during which the goals are to be met are specified. When the date is reached, then another discussion takes place in which actual results are compared with expected outcomes and a new set of objectives is formulated.

In practice, a manager can also designate activities into the plan so that the follower will have a map on how to attain the stated goals. This author recommends that goal setting be included in any of the other types of performance evaluations. In a sense, there should be a portion of the appraisal report that is open for writing objectives that are expected to be met within a given period of time. All unsatisfactory performances should have at least one objective that is intended for alleviating the unsatisfactory performance. Enrichment activities and areas of talent should be amplified in this section also.

Rankings

This technique involves ranking employees on a particular dimension of work performance (Kreitner & Kinicki, 1989). If there are several dimensions on which employees are to be ranked, then their rankings can be summed to provide an overall ranking for each employee. In health care systems, this type of evaluation is usually not evident formally. However, many supervisors have this ranking system readily available in their own thought processes.

Behaviorally Anchored Rating Scales

This type of rating scale is similar to the graphic scale, only at each point there are behavioral statements that define what each ranking represents. This method usually results in greater rater interreliability of the evaluation.

A NURSE'S NOTE

It is possible to spend a lifetime developing a rating scale that is both reliable and valid. This is, the scale rates consistently across raters and among items (reliability), and measures a sample of behaviors that adequately represents the responsibilities in a given position (validity). Both of these concepts must be evaluated—a judgment is made that the reliability and validity of an appraisal form are adequate given the purposes for which the appraisal is used.

The amount of time that a nurse has in a health care organization for the purposes of conducting performance appraisals varies greatly. However, it is safe to say that the process of appraisal is among many equally important responsibilities. It therefore should not be a totally time consuming activity, expending a great amount of effort for an important but moderate payoff.

This author always suggests that the time spent in developing the performance appraisal form and establishing reliability and validity of the instrument should be a careful and planned consideration. It has been observed that such a great amount of time is spent on developing reliability and validity tests that by the time the developer/researcher concludes that it should be implemented, the behaviors of nursing practice have changed—which renders the instrument invalid.

Make performance appraisals short and specific. Develop the part of the appraisal that points people in directions for growth. The end of the appraisal should have room for the appraiser's notes— goals for the next appraisal time period with specific ways that the goals will be attained. Then comments could be made in a continuous record, thereby documenting growth. Be clear on what is acceptable and unacceptable behavior—and then, what is exceptional or distinguished. So often, nurses use a rating scale that moves from 1 (poor) to 5 (excellent). It is difficult to know the differentiation between a rating of 2 or 3 and 3 or 4. And furthermore, is such a fine discrimination really important in charting the growth of an individual over the next six months or a year? This author's advice is to keep the appraisal short, simple, educative, and positive—for both the appraisor and the employee being appraised.

SUMMARY

Performance evaluation was presented as a process that may have both judgmental and development/educative purposes. Principles of performance evaluation were presented followed by specific tactics that the appraiser should understand. The performance evaluation process was compared with the problem-solving method. The chapter concluded with various methods that are used in performance evaluation programs, especially in health care environments.

REFERENCES

Drucker, P. (1954). *The practice of management*. New York: Harper & Row.
Drucker, P. (1985a). The discipline of innovation. *Harvard Business Review, 64,* 67–72.

Drucker, P. (1985b). *Effective executive*. New York: Harper & Row.

Drucker, P. (1985c). *Managing in turbulent times*. New York: Harper & Row.

Ganong, J. & Ganong, W. (1983). *Performance approasal for productivity: The nurse manager's handbook*. Rockville, MD: Aspen.

Hedge, J., & Kavangh, M. (1988). Improving the accuracy of performance evaluations: Comparisons of three methods of performance appraiser training. *Journal of Applied Psychology, 73*(1), 68–73.

Hornstein, H. (1976) *Cruelty and kindness*. Englewood Cliffs, NJ: Prentice-Hall.

Ivancevich, J., Donnelly, J. Jr. & Gibson, J. (1989). *Management: Principles and functions* (4th ed.). Homewood, IL: Irwin.

Johnson, J. & Luciano, K. (1988). Managing by behavior and results— Linking supervisory accountability to effective organizational control. *Readings from JONA: Readings in nursing administration*. Philadelphia: Lippincott.

Kraiger, K., & Ford, J.K. (1985). A meta-analysis of ratee race effects in performance ratings. *Journal of Applied Psychology, 70*(1), 56–65.

Kreitner, R., & Kinicki, A. (1989). *Organizational behavior*. Homewood, IL: Irwin.

Lachman, V. (1984). Increasing productivity through performance evaluation. *Journal of Nursing Administration, 14*(12), 7–14.

Lampe, S. (1986). Getting the most out of needs assessments. *Training, 23*(10), 101–104.

Landy, F., & Farr, J. (1980). Performance rating. *Psychological Bulletin, 87*(1), 72–107.

McCloskey, J., & McCain, B. (1988). Variables related to nurse performance. *Image: Journal of Nursing Scholarship, 20*(4), 203–207.

Meyer, A. L. (1984). A framework for assessing performance problems. *Journal of Nursing Administration, 14*(5), 40–43.

Momeyer, A. (1986). Why no one likes your performance appraisal system. *Training, 23*(10), 95–98.

Pearce, J., & Porter, L. (1986). Employees responses to formal performance appraisal feedback. *Journal of Applied Psychology, 71*(2), 211–218.

Richards, R. C. (1984). How to design an objective performance-evaluation system. *Training, 21*(3), 38–43.

Rothwell, W. (1984). How to conduct a real performance audit. *Training, 21*(6), 45–49.

Rowland, H., & Rowland, B. (1985). *Nursing administration handbook* (2nd ed.). Germantown, MD: Aspen.

Stalker, M., Kornblith, A., Lewis, P., & Parker, R. (1986). Measurement technology application in performance appraisal. *Journal of Nursing Administration, 16*(4), 12–16.

Stull, M. (1986). Staff nurse performance: Effects of goal-setting and performance feedback. *Journal of Nursing Administration, 16*(7 & 8), 26–30.

Zemke, R. (1985). Is performance appraisal a paper tiger? *Training, 22*(12), 24–32.

Part III

Management Skills: Experiential Exercises

EXERCISE 1   **Communication—Are You Good at Following Directions?**

Purposes
1. To diagnose reading comprehension.
2. To find out how well one follows directions.

Facility
A classroom large enough to accommodate participants.

Materials
Worksheet A: Following Directions.
Pencil or pen.

Time Required
30 minutes.

Group Size
Unlimited.

Design
1. Instruct group members to proceed to Worksheet A and follow the directions.

2. State that members who complete the worksheet should sit quietly until the entire class is finished.

3. When the entire group is done, discuss the experience in the large group. The following questions may form the basis of discussion: Are members good at following directions? Can members scan written messages and still comprehend? If not, why not and can comprehension be learned? If yes, why and how?

(continued)

EXERCISE 1 *(continued)*
WORKSHEET A: Following Directions

The following test is designed to find out how well you read and how well you can follow directions. It has been used by a California teacher with junior high school students. It should not take longer than three minutes to complete if you concentrate.

1. Read everything before you do anything.
2. Put your name in the upper right-hand corner of this paper.
3. Circle the word *name* in Step 2.
4. Draw five small squares in the upper left-hand corner of this paper.
5. Put an *x* in each square.
6. Put a circle around each square.
7. Sign your name under the title.
8. After the title write *yes, yes, yes.*
9. Put an *x* in the lower left-hand corner of this paper.
10. Put a circle around each word in Step 7.
11. Draw a triangle around the x in Step 9.
12. On the reverse side of this paper, multiply 703 by 1805.
13. Draw a rectangle around the word *paper* in Step 4.
14. Call out your first name when you get to this point in the test.
15. If you think you have followed directions up to this point, call out "I have."
16. On the reverse side of this paper, add 8950 and 9850.
17. Put a circle around your answer. Put a square around the circle.
18. Count out loud in your normal speaking voice backward from ten to one.
19. Now that you have finished reading carefully, do only Steps 1 and 2.

Source: This material was received by this author at the School of Nursing, University of Massachusetts, 1972. Author unknown.

EXERCISE 2   Communication—Observation

Purposes

1. To sharpen observational skills.

2. To increase perception of nonverbal behavior.

Facility

A classroom large enough to accommodate participants.

Materials

None

Time Required

Twenty minutes.

Group Size

Unlimited pairs.

Design

1. Members should form pairs.

2. Pairs should sit facing one another for two minutes, each person observing everything about his/her partner. If necessary, it can be suggested that certain items be noted, such as: posture, eye contact, placement of hands and feet, facial expressions, dress, jewelry, and so forth.

3. Then members of each pair should turn back-to-back with the agreed-upon partner changing five things about herself or himself.

4. When changes have been accomplished, members should once again face each other. The observing partner should verbalize the noticed changes.

5. Roles are reversed

6. Discuss the experience.

(continued)

Source: Reprinted by permission from La Monica, Elaine L., *The Nursing Process: A Humanistic Approach*, p. 294. Copyright © 1979 by Addison-Wesley Publishing Company, Inc, Menlo Park, Calif. The idea for this exercise came from Kenneth Blanchard, School of Education, University of Massachusetts, 1973.

EXERCISE 2 *(continued)*

Variation   The exercise can be lengthened by using the
                       same pairs and requesting members to change
                       five more things about themselves. This occa-
                       sionally poses a problem and people often do
                       not know what to change further. During dis-
                       cussion, ask participants if they thought of ask-
                       ing for help from another close member of a
                       pair who was also searching for changes. If
                       they did, how did they feel about needing help
                       on a seemingly simple task? If they did not re-
                       quest assistance, why not?

EXERCISE 3   Communication—Interpreting Nonverbal Behavior

Purposes

1. To increase awareness of how emotions can be expressed nonverbally.

2. To interpret perceptions of nonverbally expressed emotions.

3. To validate perceptions of nonverbal behaviors.

Facility

Large enough room to accommodate participants sitting around table or on the floor in a circle.

Materials

Small pieces of paper. Two hats or baskets.

Time Required

Thirty minutes or more, depending on group size.

Group Size

Twelve to 15 is ideal; two or more groups may be formed if the group is large.

Design

1. In a large group, ask participants to verbalize emotions/ feelings. Write one each on a slip of paper, fold the paper and place in a hat.

2. Repeat Step 1, except this time ask that participants verbalize parts of the body that can be used to express emotions/feelings.

3. A person from the group should then distribute or have participants pick a slip of paper from each hat.

4. Request each participant who has picked an emotion and body part to role play the emo-

(continued)

Source: Adapted by permission from La Monica, Elaine L., *The Nursing Process: A Humanistic Approach*, p. 295. Copyright © 1979 by Addison-Wesley Publishing Company, Inc, Menlo Park, Calif.

EXERCISE 3 *(continued)*

tion nonverbally, primarily using the designated body part.

5. Group participants should then try to guess what feeling is being expressed.

6. Discussion follows.

7. Role players should place papers back in each respective hat, and Steps 3 through 6 should be repeated. This should be done so that all members have a chance to role play.

Variation

If two or more groups of 12 are possible, equalize the number of emotions and body parts for both groups and time how long it takes for groups to carry out the task. Then have groups work against one another; all role plays should result in the group accurately diagnosing the emotion and body part used in expression. Only then may they proceed to the next role play. The group finishing first has the sharpest observational skills, given those present.

EXERCISE 4   Communication—Perceiving

Purposes	1. To increase awareness of the variety of perceptions that can be elicited from a given situation.
	2. To raise self-awareness regarding individual perceptual fields.
Facility	Room to accommodate the class size in groups of six.
Materials	Worksheet A: Scenarios Paper and pencils.
Time Required	One hour.
Group Size	Unlimited groups of six.
Design	1. Have participants individually read Scenario 1 and write down their perceptions and reactions concerning what happened, their feelings in the situation, and what conclusions they reach.
	2. Ask that participants share these notations with their small group.
	3. Observe and discuss perceptual differences, possible reasons for such, and rationale for conclusions. Dichotomous differences between members should be studied more fully.
	4. Repeat the design with Scenario 2.
Variation	Participants can develop their own scenarios based on actual or hypothetical experiences. They can then share them with their small group and follow the design for as many scenarios as time permits.

(continued)

Source: Adapted by permission from La Monica, Elaine L., *The Nursing Process: A Humanistic Approach*, pp 296–297. Copyright © 1979 by Addison-Wesley Publishing Company, Inc, Menlo Park, Calif.

EXERCISE 4 (continued)
WORKSHEET A: Scenarios

Scenario 1: It is 11:15 A.M. Ms. Blue, a supervisor, is making rounds on a surgical unit. She observes a patient with traction of the right leg, a basin of water on the bedside table, the bed stripped, a gown placed over patient's chest, and the patient, Ms. Green, reading a book. As the supervisor enters the room, the patient explains that the student nurse assigned to assist her with a bath had struck his head against the crossbar of the traction frame at 10:30 A.M. The nursing instructor had taken him to the emergency room. On the way to the nurse's station, the supervisor notices several nursing personnel, including the head nurse, drinking coffee in the utility room. As she begins calling the Nursing School office to report that a nursing student and instructor had left a patient unattended, the head nurse comes in to tell her about the accident.

Scenario 2*: The setting is a general hospital unit in an urban city. Three people are involved: Ms. King, the new head nurse of the medical unit; Ms. James, the director of Nursing Services; and Ms. Carmichael, the day supervisor of the building. Ms. King gives the patients' nursing care file a last-minute check to be sure all patients' activities, treatments, medications, and so forth, are taken care of or are in process. Then she checks the patients, going from room to room. "It's going pretty well," she thinks—she is particularly satisfied with the way Ms. Garcia is responding to the care plan now. She has spent a great deal of time working with Ms. Garcia. Certainly, Ms. King thinks, Ms. James can find nothing wrong here; the patients are all receiving excellent care. Ms. King has heard a lot about these "spontaneous rounds" by Ms. James. Shortly therefore, Ms. James and Ms. Carmichael arrive on the unit by the backstairs, so it is some time before Ms. King even knows they are there.

During the "rounds" with Ms. James and Ms. Carmichael, Ms. King makes several attempts to comment on certain patients and their progress. Ms. James ignores the attempts and starts to jot down notes on her clipboard. Ms. James and Ms. Carmichael

---

*Source: This scenario was received by this author at the College of Nursing, University of Florida, 1966. Author unknown.

maintain a general conversation about the unit while they finish the rounds. No attempt is made to draw Ms. King into the conversation. After rounds are completed on the unit, Ms. King asks if there is any additional information they need. Ms. James says, "No, however there are a few small items I would like to call to your attention, Ms. King. The shelves in the medicine cupboard are rather dusty, and the utility room is very cluttered. Will you please see that these things are taken care of?" With that Ms. James and Ms. Carmichael leave the unit.

On the way to the next unit Ms. James remarks to Ms. Carmichael, "On the whole, I think Ms. King is doing a good job with her unit. She should make a fine head nurse."

EXERCISE 5   **Communication—Leader/Follower**
                    Interactions

Purposes   1. To focus on verbal and nonverbal messages
                    that may be emitted in interactions between
                    a manager and a follower.

                    2. To validate messages received with mes-
                    sages sent.

Facility   Large enough room to accommodate group
                    members seated around tables or in circles on
                    the floor.

Materials   None.

Time Required   One hour or more, depending on group size
                    and number of volunteers.

Group Size   Unlimited groups of 12.

Design   1. Paired volunteers should be given a couple
                    of minutes to develop a hypothetical leader/
                    follower interaction. They should decide
                    which of them is to be the leader and which
                    is to be the follower. A hypothetical leader/
                    follower interaction is a made-up interchange
                    in which the leader is functioning in one of
                    the four leader behavior styles: (1) high
                    structure, low consideration—telling; (2) high
                    structure, high consideration—selling; (3)
                    high   consideration,   low   structure—
                    participating; and (4) low structure, low
                    consideration—delegating.

                    2. The pair should then role play the situation
                    with direction being given to the leader that
                    she or he should decide whether to be effec-
                    tive or ineffective in the role. Only the leader
                    should be aware of what is decided.

3. Following the role play, players and the group members should give feedback on their reactions and perceptions of what was nonverbally and verbally communicated. Players should reveal their intent after group members give feedback.

4. Discuss the experience.

Variations

1. The instructor can prepare the scenes to be role played prior to class.

2. Learners may be given a homework assignment to prepare a scene prior to the class in which the exercise will take place.

EXERCISE 6   Communication—Verbal Directions

Purposes	1. To practice giving verbal directions.
	2. To validate messages received with messages sent.
Facility	A classroom large enough to accommodate participants.
Materials	Plain paper or construction paper. Pencils, crayons, or magic markers.
Time Required	Thirty to 45 minutes.
Group Size	Unlimited pairs.
Design	1. Members should form into pairs and sit back-to-back.
	2. One member of each pair should take paper and a pencil/crayon and draw a geometric design. An example of a design is as follows:

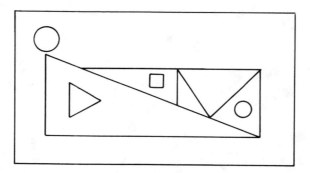

Source: This exercise is an adaptation of one developed by Hewitt, F. (1981). Introduction to communication. *Nursing Times*, 77, center pages.

3. Provide partner with paper and pencil. Partners should not be able to see each other's work. The member who has drawn a design should verbally describe to the partner, step-by-step, what was drawn. Each step should be one clear statement (for example, put a circle on the top corner of the triangle). Descriptions should not be expressed again or revised. No questions should be asked or answered.

4. The member receiving directions should draw the geometric design as perceived.

5. Upon completion, compare the design that was verbally directed with the original. How good were the directions?

Variation

The design can be repeated with the same partners, only two-way communication is allowed—the receiver can ask the sender questions and receive answers. Discuss the differences between one-way and two-way communication in this experience.

EXERCISE 7   **Change—Force Field Analysis for Self-Directed Growth***

Purposes

1. To learn the process of force field analysis.

2. To develop an awareness of one's needs.

3. To analyze the need area using a force field approach.

4. To develop a strategy for meeting one's need.

Facility

None—this exercise is a self-study homework assignment.

Materials

Worksheet A: Problem Areas.

Worksheet B: Force Field.

Worksheet C: The Strategy.

Pen or pencil.

Time Required

One hour.

Group Size

Unlimited—homework assignment.

Design

Explain to participants the purpose of the exercise and then the design of the exercise. Participants can be instructed to do the exercise individually as a home assignment.

1. Using Worksheet A, have participants jot down 10 problems in personal and/or professional aspects of self. Then rank order them from one (low priority) to ten (top priority).

2. Choose the top-priority problem and identify the actual and the optimal situation. Write the resulting problem area statement in the

---

*Every aspect of this book is directed toward changing people. When a manager leads, it is for the purpose of changing others—moving them from actual to optimal.

space provided on the top of Worksheet B. Fill in the optimal and actual statement on Worksheet B also. Continue to use Worksheet B for Steps 3 through 6.

3. List the forces that are pushing or driving to solve, eliminate, or overcome the problem.

4. List the forces that are blocking, impeding, or restraining the change.

5. Weigh each of the driving and restraining forces from one (low-energy force) to ten (high-energy force). How does the situation look? Are driving and restraining forces equal?

6. Examine both sets of forces. Can any restraining forces be reduced or eliminated? Can any driving forces be amplified or increased?

7. Focus on the three driving and the three restraining forces that have the highest energy. Develop a step-by-step strategy for increasing each driving force and decreasing each restraining force. Use Worksheet C.

Variation

This exercise can be done in class and shared in small groups at the end of Steps 4, 6, and/or 7. The amount of time to do the exercises, of course, increases with group involvement.

(continued)

EXERCISE 7 (continued)
WORKSHEET A: Problem Areas

	Rank Order
Problems:	
_____	_____
_____	_____
_____	_____
_____	_____
_____	_____
_____	_____
_____	_____
_____	_____
_____	_____
_____	_____
_____	_____
_____	_____
_____	_____

Top priority problem: _____

_____

_____

Actual situation: _____

_____

_____

_____

Optimal situation: _____

_____

_____

_____

EXERCISE 7
WORKSHEET B: Force Field

Problem: _____

Actual Situation: _____

Optimal situation: _____

Driving Forces (+)	Weight	Restraining Forces (−)	Weight
_____	____	_____	____
_____	____	_____	____
_____	____	_____	____
_____	____	_____	____
_____	____	_____	____
_____	____	_____	____
_____	____	_____	____
_____	____	_____	____
_____	____	_____	____
_____	____	_____	____
_____	____	_____	____
_____	____	_____	____

(*continued*)

EXERCISE 7 (*continued*)
WORKSHEET C: The Strategy

Force (+ or −)	Action
1.	A.
	B.
	C.
	D.
	E.
2.	A.
	B.
	C.
	D.
	E.
3.	A.
	B.
	C.
	D.
	E.

Force (+ or −)	Action
4.	A.
	B.
	C.
	D.
	E.
5.	A.
	B.
	C.
	D.
	E.
6.	A.
	B.
	C.
	D.
	E.

EXERCISE 8   Power—The New Car Dilemma

Purposes

1. To further develop group decision-making abilities.

2. To experience potential and actual power struggles.

3. To practice the roles of superior, follower, or process observer.

Facility

A classroom large enough to accommodate unlimited groups of six.

Materials

Magic markers for name tags.

For each participant—a name tag for the name of the character to be played. Process observers are called "pros." Worksheet A: General Instructions.

For each character player—Worksheet B containing further information only on the role to be played. (These descriptions should be individually typed on separate sheets of paper and distributed after members have selected their roles.) *Information from Worksheet B should not be common knowledge to all participants*.

For each process observer—Worksheet C: Processing the New Car Dilemma.

Time Required

One hour for the exercise and 30 minutes for processing.

Group Size

Unlimited groups of six.

Source: This simulation was adapted into health care from a business exercise. The original material is presented by Maier, N.R., Solem, A.R., & Maier, A.A. (1957). The new truck dilemma. *Supervisory and Executive Development: A Manual for Role Playing*. New York: John Wiley, pp. 20–37.

Design

1. Pairs of teams will work together. One team of six will be players sitting in an inside circle and the other team will be process observers sitting around the players in an outside circle.

2. The team of players should choose the characters to be role played by each player. If the role-play team only contains five players, discard the role of Eileen.

3. After the roles have been selected, players should fill out their name tags and then should receive only the part of Worksheet B that describes their particular character. Instruct players not to discuss roles with anyone else and not to read about other roles. Players should not receive Worksheet B prior to role selection because its contents should not be known by everyone.

4. Process observers should not communicate verbally with the role players. They should use Worksheet C to assist them in observing the players' group dynamics.

5. When all members are ready, the instructor should signal for the role plays to begin. All groups should start role playing at the same time. The role-play should last 45 minutes.

6. At the end of the role play, the process observers should report their observations to the group they observed. Group members should also join in the process observations. Were they satisfied with the decision? They should be able to provide rationale for their satisfaction and/or dissatisfaction. A general class discussion should conclude the experience—who received the new car in each group and why? Processes used by groups to make decisions may be shared.

(continued)

EXERCISE 8 *(continued)*
WORKSHEET A: General Instructions

You work for a state-supported community agency that investigates reports of child abuse. One of you will be the director, and the others will be members of the professional interdisciplinary team. Each team member has a case load; responsibilities include making home visits, collaborating with professionals in hospitals, meeting physicians in their offices, visiting teachers in schools, and participating in various nonprofit health organizations. The director is usually a promoted staff member, which is true in this case. She has a small case load in comparison with others, spending a great deal of time at the main office in administrative detail and writing grant reports and proposals. She accompanies other team members on various cases as needed; on the average this amounts to two days' time out of five. Of course, this time is spread out over the entire week. Each team member works alone and ordinarily is involved in several cases or assignments in a day.

The team members drive to various locations in the district to do their work. The agency is located in a major New England city, but cases are referred in from a 50-mile radius of the city. Members drive compact cars that are assigned to them for as long as they work for the agency. The car is used only during working hours. Members drive their personal cars to and from the main office in the morning and in the evening. Members seem to take pride in keeping their business cars looking good; they have a possessive feeling about their cars since other people seldom if ever drive them. Maintenance is requested by the individual team members and is carried out when the members have a block of work to accomplish in the home office.

Here are some facts about the team members and their cars:

EILEEN JONES, BS, RN, a psychiatric nurse, has been with the agency for 17 years and has a 2-year-old Ford.

BILL SMITH, PhD, a state licensed psychologist, has been with the agency for 11 years and has a 5-year-old Dodge.

JOHN ALLEN, MS, a psychiatric social worker, has been with the agency for 10 years and has a 4-year-old Ford.

CHARLIE GOLD, MSN, RN, a psychiatric and pediatric nurse specialist, has been with the agency for 5 years and has a 3-year-old Ford.

MARY HERTZ, MD, a child psychiatrist, has been with the agency for 3 years and has a 5-year-old Chevrolet.

JANICE MARSHALL, EdD, the director, has been with the agency 8 years and has no car assigned to her. She is a psychiatric nurse with a doctorate in human relations and counseling. Generally, she rides places with others.

Most of the team members do all of their driving in the city; John and Charlie cover most of the cases in the suburbs.

In role playing your part, accept the facts as given, as well as assuming the attitude supplied in your specific role. From this point on, let your feelings develop in accordance with the events that transpire in the role-playing process. When facts or events arise that are not covered by the roles, make up things that are consistent with the way it might be in a real-life situation.

(*continued*)

EXERCISE 8 *(continued)*
WORKSHEET B: Character Information

EILEEN JONES: When a new Chevrolet becomes available, you think you should get it because you have seniority, and you do not like your present car. Your own car is a Chevrolet, and you prefer a Chevrolet for business, too. You had one assigned to you before you got the Ford.

BILL SMITH: You feel you deserve a new car. Since the more senior team member has a fairly new car, you feel you should get the next one. You have taken excellent care of your present Dodge and have kept it looking like new. A man deserves to be rewarded if he treats a company car like his own.

JOHN ALLEN: You have to do more driving than most of the other team members because you work in the suburbs. You have a fairly old car and feel you should have a new one because you do so much driving.

CHARLIE GOLD: The heater in your present car is inadequate. Furthermore, since Mary backed into the door of your car, it has never been repaired to fit right. You attribute your frequent colds to the cold air that the door lets in. You want a warm car since you have a good deal of driving to do. As long as it has good tires, brakes, and is comfortable, you do not care about its make.

MARY HERTZ: You have the poorest car in the crew. It is five years old, had been in a bad wreck before you got it, and has never been mechanically sound. You have put up with it for three years and feel the next new car should be yours. You have a good safety record. The only accident you have had was when you sprung the door of Charlie's car when he opened it as you backed out of the garage. You hope the new car is a Ford since you prefer to drive that make.

JANICE MARSHALL: You are the director of the team, each of whom drives a compact car to and from various case assignments. Every so often you get a new car to exchange for an old one, and you have the problem of deciding which of the team members should receive the new car. There are often hard feelings because each member seems to feel she or he is entitled to the new car. You have a tough time being fair—as a matter of fact, most people usually disagree with whatever you decide. You now have to face the issue again because a new car has just been allocated to you for assignment. The new car is a Chevrolet.

In order to handle this problem, you have decided to put the decision up to the team members themselves. You will tell them about the car and pose the problem in terms of what would be the fairest way to assign the car. Do not take a position yourself, because you want to do what the members think is most fair. Your leadership style will be high consideration and low task.

(*continued*)

EXERCISE 8 (*continued*)
WORKSHEET C: Processing the New Car Dilemma

The following items are furnished as a guide for observing what the leader did and how the team reacted:

1. How did the director present the problem?

   A. In presenting the problem, did the director's attitude convey asking for help?

   B. Was the director's presentation of the problem brief and to the point?

   C. Did the director scrupulously avoid suggesting a solution?

2. What occurred in the discussion?

   A. Did all group members participate?

   B. Was there free exchange of feelings between/among group members?

   C. Did the group use social pressure to influence any of its members?

   D. On which member(s) of the team was social pressure used?

   E. Was the director permissive?

   F. Did the director avoid taking sides or favoring any person?

   G. What were the points of disagreement in the group?

3. What did the director do to facilitate problem solving?

   A. Did the director ask questions to help the group explore ideas?

   B. Did the leader and others accept all ideas equally?

C. Did the director avoid hurrying the group to develop a solution?

D. Did the director avoid favoring any solution?

E. Who supplied the final solution?

F. What, if anything, did the director do to get unanimous agreement on the final solution?

G. What were the bases of the final solution (for example, seniority)?

H. How effective was the leader?

EXERCISE 9   **Teaching—A Beginning**

Purposes   1. To begin the experience of teaching.

2. To gain experience in using different instructional modes and media to teach a content area.

3. To experience a variety of teaching strategies.

Facility   Large room to accommodate class.

Materials   Specified by the students in their teaching module.

Time Required   Ten minutes per member.

Group Size   Under 25

Design   1. As a homework assignment, ask learners to think of anything (skill, philosophy, belief, and so on) that they know or do well.

2. Then have them prepare a five- to seven-minute teaching module on the area chosen. The module should include objectives and teaching modes and media.

3. Request that preparation be made for a class presentation.

4. At a subsequent class, have students teach the module to small groups of peers.

5. Encourage group discussion of the experience, focusing on the teacher's experience as well as that of the learner.

Variation   Nursing skills or competencies as well as theory can be substituted for the content in the original design.

Source: Adapted by permission from La Monica, Elaine L., *The Nursing Process: A Humanistic Approach*, p. 302. Copyright © 1979 by Addison-Wesley Publishing Company, Inc., Menlo Park, Calif.

EXERCISE 10   Teaching—Applying the Process

Purposes	1. To apply the teaching process.
	2. To broaden experience in diagnosing the teaching needs of clients and colleagues in a health environment.
	3. To increase awareness of the teaching diagnoses that others perceive in the same situation.
	4. To identify appropriate objectives and the most effective teaching strategies to accomplish them.
	5. To evaluate a teaching intervention.
Facility	Large room to accommodate participants seated in groups of six.
Materials	Worksheet A: Scenarios
	Worksheet B: Instructional Analysis.
	Paper and pencils.
Time Required	One to two hours.
Group Size	Unlimited groups of six.
Design	1. Participants should consider themselves as head nurses. Using all or any combination of the scenarios, ask participants to individually respond to the following in each situation:
	A. Is there a teaching need? If the answer is *yes,* use Worksheet B to complete Step 1. (Worksheet B may have to be duplicated.)
	B. If there is a teaching need, what needs to be taught and to whom? Give rationale for response.

(continued)

Source: Adapted by permission from La Monica, Elaine L., *The Nursing Process: A Humanistic Approach*, p. 302. Copyright © 1979 by Addison-Wesley Publishing Company, Inc., Menlo Park, Calif.

EXERCISE 10 *(continued)*

C. Identify objective(s) for teaching.

D. Specify teaching strategy: mode(s) and medium (media).

E. Delineate how the accomplishment of objectives would be evaluated.

2. In groups of six, participants should share and discuss their responses. Different perceptions between/among learners should receive particular attention.

Variations

1. Step 1 may be done as a homework assignment.

2. Individuals or small groups can develop and actually carry out the teaching strategy with their peers, as in Exercise 9.

3. The students' actual clinical placement can be the scene for identifying a learning need and carrying out the process, even to the point of teaching the staff and having them evaluate the program.

EXERCISE 10
WORKSHEET A: Scenarios

1. Three times in the past two days you've found that elderly patients who have been gotten out of bed rather early in the morning have stayed up sitting in chairs for the rest of the morning. In each case when you noted this, the patient's respiration was either labored or rapid. The pulse was rapid, and the patient appeared tired and said that he or she was tired.

2. A patient on your unit has been on a Stryker frame for two weeks. You have been told that tomorrow a newly employed graduate nurse and two senior nursing students will be with you for the first time.

3. A patient on your unit has been on a Stryker frame for two weeks. Today when you go in to help turn her, two beginning sophomore students ask if they may come with you to see what you are doing.

4. During afternoon conference, a patient was mentioned who had just returned from the operating room following "repair of a fractured hip." A nurse said, "We'll have to be careful of his back since he'll have to stay on it for some time."

5. When making rounds on your unit after lunch, you notice that although many patients are in their beds, most of the beds are elevated, and in many cases the linen is rumpled. A TV set is audible through most of the area, and three of your staff members are talking rather loudly in the corridor.

6. On Monday, Mr. Smith tells you that his doctor told him he might be going home in a couple of days. Mr. Smith has congestive heart failure, has been on digitalis and a diuretic, still has some peripheral edema, and is on a low-sodium diet. He lives alone.

7. Ms. Jones has asked for and received a prescribed narcotic for pain for several days prior to and following her surgery. The nurse assigned to give medications and the one assigned to care for her yesterday both questioned "if she really needed it." The doctor was told of this and gave permission for a PRN placebo. Today it is discussed by others on the team. Ms. Jones responded well the first time the placebo was given but then seemed to "want the other medicine" (she recognized

(*continued*)

EXERCISE 10
WORKSHEET A *(continued)*

that a different injection had been given). The medicine nurse today said she felt Ms. Jones had no real need for the narcotic, but another nurse said he thought Ms. Jones acted as if she really had pain.

8. When an aide attempting to change a patient's position was experiencing evident difficulty, a graduate nurse came over to the aide, assisted, and then explained the procedure to the aide and patient.

9. You observe a patient walking down the corridor in a coat and hat, carrying a suitcase—an aide is walking beside the patient. A graduate nurse leaves the nurse's station, greets the patient, takes the suitcase, and hands it to the aide. The nurse discusses the patient's plans for discharge as they walk down the hall. The situation was discussed with the aide after the aide returned from taking the patient to the hospital lobby.

10. A team leader asked an aide to do a sugar and acetone test for a patient and reminded the aide not to obtain the urine for testing from the patient's tube (indwelling Foley catheter). The aide took a sample from the drainage bottle and reported the test to the team leader, who then recorded the results.

11. A patient is shaking the side rails and is stating in a loud voice that he wants to go to the bathroom. The aide and practical nurse remove the side rails, explaining to the patient why side rails are necessary. (He had slipped getting out of bed yesterday.) The practical nurse escorts the patient to the bathroom and waits to escort him back to bed.

12. A graduate nurse wheels a patient into the solarium, places the wheelchair close to another patient, and introduces them to each other. The nurse then asks each patient to demonstrate active and passive exercises of their arms. As the nurse leaves the room, the patients continue the exercises and discuss each other's progress.

Source: Scenarios were received by this author at the College of Nursing, University of Florida, 1966. Author unknown.

EXERCISE 10
WORKSHEET B: Instructional Analysis

Scenario No. _____

What needs to be taught and to whom?

Program objectives:

(*continued*)

EXERCISE 10
WORKSHEET B (*continued*)

Teaching strategy—mode(s) and medium (media):

Evaluation procedure:

EXERCISE 11   Teaching—Course Evaluations

Purpose	To provide feedback to the course planner/instructor.
Facility	Regular classroom setting.
Materials	Evaluations A, B, and/or C.
Time Required	Approximately 10 minutes.
Group Size	Unlimited.
Design	The course evaluations may be used when the instructor desires feedback from the learners. Each can be administered in class or taken home for completion.

1. Evaluation A: Usable at any point during the semester in which the class is given. It provides a means for evaluating the needs of students midway through the semester in order for adjustments to be made as indicated by the responses. Instructors must list in the left hand column the broad content areas covered to date of the evaluation.

2. Evaluation B: This is a short, end-of-course evaluation.

3. Evaluation C: A more descriptive end-of-course report. All evaluations can be either anonymous or identified with the students. They can be openly discussed or not, with relevant participants or the entire group.

(continued)

EXERCISE 11 (*continued*)
EVALUATION A: Course Content Evaluation

Circle the number that best describes each content area.

Course Content Areas	Too Little 1	Just Right 2	Too Much 3
	1	2	3
	1	2	3
	1	2	3
	1	2	3
	1	2	3
	1	2	3
	1	2	3
	1	2	3
	1	2	3
	1	2	3
	1	2	3
	1	2	3
	1	2	3
	1	2	3
	1	2	3
	1	2	3
	1	2	3
	1	2	3
	1	2	3
	1	2	3
	1	2	3
	1	2	3

EXERCISE 11
EVALUATION B: End-of-Course Evaluation

For each item, circle the number that best represents your evaluation.

	Poor			*Average*			*Excellent*		
A. Subject content									
Interesting in terms of new knowledge	1	2	3	4	5	6	7	8	9
Valuable in terms of daily activities	1	2	3	4	5	6	7	8	9
Up-to-date in terms of current trends, issues, and problems	1	2	3	4	5	6	7	8	9
B. Program leader									
Attitude toward participants	1	2	3	4	5	6	7	8	9
Command of subject matter	1	2	3	4	5	6	7	8	9
Ability to hold participants' interest	1	2	3	4	5	6	7	8	9
Organized presentation of material	1	2	3	4	5	6	7	8	9
Coverage of material	1	2	3	4	5	6	7	8	9
Use of handouts	1	2	3	4	5	6	7	8	9
C. Overall evaluation of program	1	2	3	4	5	6	7	8	9

D. Program comments

1. What was of most value to you in the course/program? ___

_____

_____

_____

2. What was of least value? _____

_____

_____

_____

3. Do you have any specific suggestions about how to improve this course/program? _____

_____

_____

_____

(*continued*)

EXERCISE 11 (continued)
EVALUATION C: End-of-Course Evaluation

Course number and title:

Professor:

Date:

Using the scale provided, rate each item on its overall idea rather than on specific parts.

CONTENT:

1. The objectives are appropriate for the course content.   1 2 3 4 5 6
2. The objectives were met through class seminars, clinical practicum, and course design.   1 2 3 4 5 6
3. The course has provided me with extensive knowledge in the content area and is applicable in my professional practice.   1 2 3 4 5 6
4. Course requirements cover essential aspects of the course and have learning value.   1 2 3 4 5 6
5. This course has increased my learning, given me new viewpoints and appreciation, and increased my capacity to think and to formulate questions. 1 2 3 4 5 6
6. Contrasting viewpoints, current developments, and related theory were integrated into class topics.   1 2 3 4 5 6

Scale:
Strongly disagree / Moderately disagree / Slightly disagree / Slightly agree / Moderately agree / Strongly agree

PROCESS:

1. The instructor is clear, states objectives, summa-
rizes major points, presents material in an organized manner, and has extensive knowledge of
subject.   1 2 3 4 5 6
2. The instructor is sensitive to the response of the
class, encourages student participation, and facil-
itates questions and discussion.   1 2 3 4 5 6
3. The instructor is available to students, conveys a
genuine interest in students, and recognizes their
individuality in learning.   1 2 3 4 5 6
4. The instructor enjoys teaching, is enthusiastic,
and makes the course content stimulating and
alive.   1 2 3 4 5 6
5. The instructor has provided a class environment
that increases my motivation to do my best and
acquire knowledge independently.   1 2 3 4 5 6
6. This course, as taught by this instructor, is one
that I would recommend. On the whole, the
course was excellent.   1 2 3 4 5 6

What was of most value in the course?

What was of least value in the course?

Other suggestions/comments.

Source: Adapted from a faculty evaluation form used at the University of Massachusetts, 1975.

EXERCISE 12   **Teaching—Self-Diagnosis of Learning Needs**

Purposes   1. To diagnose one's own strengths and weaknesses in leading and managing.

                    2. To diagnose one's own learning needs in relation to management skills.

                    3. To develop strategies for meeting one's own learning needs.

Facility   Large room to accommodate groups of six to eight.

Materials   Worksheet A: Self-Diagnosis Form.
                    Pen or pencil.

Time Required   One and one-half hours.

Group Size   Unlimited groups of six to eight.

Design   1. Request that individual learners respond to the Self-Diagnosis Form in class.

                    2. Request that learners share with the group their learning needs along with strategies for meeting them. Peers should offer alternative strategies to each other.

Variations   1. Step 1 can be done as a homework assignment.

                    2. This exercise can be used midway through the course to identify learning needs of the majority of the class. Strategies for filling these needs can be developed, and content for meeting the needs can become part of the course substance.

3. The self-diagnosis can be used by in-service and human resource educators to pinpoint areas requiring staff development programs.

4. The self-diagnosis can form the basis for teacher/learner evaluation conferences.

(*continued*)

EXERCISE 12 (*continued*)
WORKSHEET A: Self-Diagnosis Form

DIRECTIONS: Select the three areas in which you feel you perform
the best. Then select the three areas in which you perform the
poorest. This is an evaluation of your comparative strengths and
weaknesses, not one comparing you with others. Put comments
regarding your choices in the right-hand column. Also comment
on as many other areas as are important to you.

Area of Competency	Best	Poorest	Comment
Problem-Solving Method:			
Problem identification	_____	_____	_____
Problem definition	_____	_____	_____
Problem analysis	_____	_____	_____
Diagnosing self	_____	_____	_____
Diagnosing the system	_____	_____	_____
Diagnosing the task	_____	_____	_____
Determining leader behavior	_____	_____	_____
Developing alternative solutions	_____	_____	_____
Choosing an action	_____	_____	_____
Management Skills:			
Communication	_____	_____	_____
Change	_____	_____	_____
Power	_____	_____	_____
Teaching	_____	_____	_____
Interviewing	_____	_____	_____
Assertiveness	_____	_____	_____
Group dynamics	_____	_____	_____

Conflict resolution   _____   _____   _____

Time management   _____   _____   _____

Performance
  evaluation   _____   _____   _____

Ethics   _____   _____   _____

Other comments/goals

_____

_____

_____

_____

_____

_____

_____

_____

_____

_____

_____

_____

_____

_____

(*continued*)

EXERCISE 12
WORKSHEET A *(continued)*

Learning Needs	Strategies for Meeting Them
1.	
2.	
3.	
4.	
5.	

EXERCISE 13   Interviewing—Role Plays

Purposes

1. To develop personal interview formats based on one's individual philosophy of practice.

2. To experience using these formats in role plays with peers.

Facility

A large room where participants can form dyads and interview one another.

Materials

Paper and other writing materials.

Time Required

One hour or more

Group Size

Unlimited dyads

Design

1. As a homework assignment, have participants read Chapters 13 and 18, and other related articles and written materials on the topic.

2. With the information, request each learner to bring to class a structured script for one of the following interview purposes:
   Hiring
   Promotion
   Planning individualized nursing care
   Describing an event

3. Request that members form into dyads and use their scripts on each other. The student being interviewed should then provide feedback on the process, if requested by the interviewer. Roles should reverse.

4. Personal reactions of the interviewer and interviewee may be shared.

5. Interview formats can then be reevaluated and changed by the interviewer, based on the results of this experience.

(*continued*)

EXERCISE 13 (*continued*)

6. Reform into a total group and discuss the experience.

Variations

1. This exercise may be done completely as a homework assignment.

2. Participants may repeat the experience using different purposes for the interview and/or different types of interviews such as the semi-structured and unstructured interview.

EXERCISE 14   Assertiveness—The Compassion Trap

Purpose   To gauge the extent to which one is the Com-
                          passion Trap: existing to serve others and pro-
                          viding tenderness and compassion to all at all
                          times.

Facility   A classroom large enough to accommodate
                          participants.

Materials   Worksheet A: The Compassion Trap Quiz.
                          Worksheet B: Scoring Key.
                          Pen or pencil.

Time Required   Thirty minutes.

Group Size   Unlimited

Design   1. Instruct members to respond individually to
                             the items in Worksheet A, following direc-
                             tions on the instrument.

                          2. After completing Step 1, go to Worksheet B
                             to score responses and to read interpreta-
                             tions.

                          3. Discuss findings in small groups.

Variation   This can be a self-study assignment.

(continued)

EXERCISE 14 (continued)
WORKSHEET A: The Compassion Trap Quiz

DIRECTIONS: Gauge the extent to which you are in the Compassion Trap by taking the quiz below. Answer each question honestly. If you have not personally experienced some situations, choose the response that most closely approximates the way you think you would respond. After you have finished, go to Worksheet B and add up your score according to the key. The interpretation of your score will tell you how "trapped" you really are.

1. You have been seeing this man socially for several weeks, but you are beginning to feel bored and uninterested in continuing the relationship. He likes you very much and would like to see you more often. Do you:
   A. Tell him you'd prefer not to see him, feeling you've been honest with yourself?
   B. Feel a sudden attack of the Hong-Kong flu coming on?
   C. Continue to be the object of his affections, because leaving would really hurt his ego?
   D. Tell him that he bores you to tears, and that even if you were both marooned on a desert island, you would camp out on the opposite shore?
2. You invited a friend of yours who lives out of the state to spend her/his two-week vacation with you at your home. It is now one month later, and your friend shows no intention of leaving, or reimbursing you for food and telephone bills. You would like your friend to leave. Do you:
   A. Not mention anything about your expenses or feelings, because you don't want to damage the friendship?
   B. Leave a note saying that you're terribly sorry, but your mother has decided to live with you, and you'll need the room?
   C. Tell your friend that you really value your friendship, and that her/his extended visit is putting a strain on it. You ask that your friend make plans to leave?
   D. Put all of your friend's belongings out on the doorstep with a note: "Don't call me; I'll call you"?
3. You are enjoying one of your rare visits to San Francisco, and you are staying with your brother and sister-in-law. One of your favorite things to do in San Francisco is to sample the fine restaurants. Your brother and sister-in-law are terrible cooks,

but they insist on "treating" you by cooking for you themselves. You would much prefer going out to eat. Do you:

A. Decide to have dinner at your brother and sister-in-law's home because you don't want to disappoint them by refusing their offer?

B. Tell them that you appreciate their thoughtfulness, and explain that one of the reasons you come to San Francisco is to enjoy the restaurants? You suggest that all of you go out to eat instead.

C. Loudly tell them that you're not there for their food?

D. Call and claim that you are unavoidably detained, tell them not to wait dinner for you, and then sneak out and eat by yourself?

4. You are working on a project that is very important to you. Some friends drop by unexpectedly. You'd really like to continue working on your project. Do you:

A. Shelve your project, prepare hors d'oeuvres, and apologize for your cluttered living room?

B. Loudly berate your friends for not having called first?

C. Explain that you're in the middle of an important project and arrange to see them at a mutually convenient time?

D. Ignore your friends and continue working on your project while they are there, hoping they'll get the message?

5. Your 10-year-old daughter customarily walks to school, but today she wants you to drive her. You have driven her on rainy days, but it is not raining today. She continues to ask you to drive her, adding, "Besides, everyone else's mother drives them." Do you:

A. Tell your daughter she can walk to school today, as usual?

B. Begin by telling your daughter that you won't drive her to school but after a short time you give in and drive her, feeling guilty that you hesitated?

C. Reply "Oh, okay, I'll drive you," thinking of all the other children whose mothers faithfully drive them? You will feel like a neglectful mother if you don't drive your daughter to school.

D. Threaten to call the truant officer and report on your daughter if she doesn't leave for school immediately?

(continued)

Source: From *The Assertive Woman: A New Look,* © 1987, by Stanlee Phelps and Nancy Austin. Reproduced for Springer Publishing Company, Inc., by permission of Impact Publishers, Inc., P.O. Box 1094, San Luis Obispo, CA 93406. Further reproduction prohibited.

EXERCISE 14 (*continued*)
WORKSHEET B: Scoring Key

1. A. An assertive choice (3)
   B. Honesty is the best policy here. (0)
   C. Don't forget *your* feelings. (0)
   D. Don't forget *his* feelings. (0)
2. A. You'll feel resentful later. You're trapped. (0)
   B. This may get her/him out, but how do you feel
      about trapping yourself with *that* one? (1)
   C. Right. This will also get her/him out, and leave you
      with your self-respect. (3)
   D. This will get your friend out of your life, also. (0)
3. A. This Compassion Trap will result in your disappointment
      and indigestion. (0)
   B. The assertive thing to do. (3)
   C. Better look for a hotel room—your brother and
      sister-in-law won't want to have you as a guest
      for some time. (0)
   D. You'll soon run out of excuses. Then what? (0)
4. A. The Compassion Trap. (0)
   B. Only if you *never* want to see them again. (0)
   C. Ain't it the truth? (3)
   D. You're wasting time; it may take hours for
      them to get the hint! (0)
5. A. You've got it! (3)
   B. A good start—but you're in the Compassion Trap here. (1)
   C. Are you really neglectful? The Compassion Trap again. (0)
   D. You avoided the Compassion Trap, but stepped
      into the Aggression Trap! (0)

Add up your total points and gauge the extent of *your* Compassion Trap.

14+: We couldn't ask for more. You can choose what to do without being trapped. Be on the lookout, though, for other situations that may trap you.

9—13: You can avoid the Compassion Trap most of the time, and you're moving in the right direction. Give some extra attention to the people/situations that continue to trap you, and attempt more assertive ways of handling them.

2—8: Consider the price you are paying when you do things at the expense of your own happiness. With some practice, you can leave the Compassion Trap and enjoy what you choose to do. Be an assertive person and be loved for it.

EXERCISE 15   Assertiveness—Self-Assessment

Purposes   1. To evaluate the frequency of one's asser-
                  tions.

                  2. To identify areas of communication that re-
                  quire further assertiveness training.

Facility   A classroom large enough to accommodate
                  participants.

Materials   Worksheet A: Assertion Self-Assessment Table
                  Worksheet B: Problem Areas
                  Pen or pencil, blackboard, and chalk or news-
                  print and magic markers.

Time Required   One to one and one-half hours.

Group Size   Unlimited

Design   1. Individuals working alone should read Work-
                  sheet A and use the following question with
                  each row and column heading: "Do I (behav-
                  iors) to/from/of with (persons) when it is ap-
                  propriate?" For instance, beginning with the
                  upper left hand cell, form the following ques-
                  tion: Do I give compliments to friends of the
                  same sex when it is appropriate?

                  2. In answering the question for each cell, par-
                  ticipants should write in the word that best
                  describes how often they engage in the be-
                  havior in that situation. Choose *usually,
                  sometimes,* or *seldom.* For example, if one
                  seldom gives compliments to friends of the
                  same sex when appropriate, one would write
                  the word *seldom* in the upper left-hand cell
                  of the Table.

Source: From *Assert Yourself: How to Be Your Own Person*, by J. Galassi and M.
Galassi. Copyright © 1977 by Human Sciences Press, New York. Reprinted by permission.

3. Complete each cell in the Table in the manner described in Steps 1 and 2.

4. After completing the Table, members should find the places where they answered with *seldom* and *sometimes.* Are there one or more behaviors (for example, making requests) for which one has given a number of seldom or sometimes answers? If there are, the behaviors should be listed on Worksheet B under the individual problem areas for behaviors.

5. Participants should again look at the places where the words *seldom* and *sometimes* are written. Are there one or more persons (for example, spouses, boyfriends, girlfriends) for whom one has given a number of seldom or sometimes answers? If there are, list those persons on Worksheet B under the individual problem areas for persons.

6. Inform participants that answers of seldom and sometimes occasionally do not group into any particular behavior or persons. This is not uncommon since people often have difficulty expressing only certain feelings with only certain people.

7. Have participants form into groups of six to eight. Request that they share and discuss their problem areas with each other and specify three problem areas each in "behaviors" and "persons" that are shared by the greatest number of people in the group—the group modes. Jot these in the appropriate area on Worksheet B.

8. Reassemble as a total class and record the problem areas for each group on the blackboard. Modal problem areas for the class can be identified and special attention can be given these areas in assertiveness train-

(continued)

EXERCISE 15 *(continued)*

ing. Individual problem areas can be worked
on in the small-group activities that usually
occur in assertiveness training programs and
classes.

Variations

1. Steps 1 through 6 can be done as a homework assignment.

2. Galassi and Galassi (1986) also present a design for evaluating the presence of anxiety,
   areas of aggression, knowledge of appropriate behavior, and knowledge of personal
   rights, all using the same table. Details can
   be found in the original source and in a
   chapter by Galassi, J. and Galassi, M. (1986).
   Assessment procedures for assertive behaviors. In R. Alberti (Ed.). *Assertiveness: Innovations, applications, issues.* San Luis
   Obispo, CA: Impact.

EXERCISE 15
WORKSHEET A: Assertion Self-Assessment Table

Persons

Behaviors	Friends of the same sex	Friends of the opposite sex	Intimate relations (spouse, boyfriend, girlfriend)	Parents, in-laws, and other family members	Children	Authority figures (bosses, professors, doctors)	Business contacts (sales-persons, waiters)	Coworkers, colleagues, and subordi-nates
Expression of positive feelings								
Give compli-ments								
Receive compli-ments								
Make requests (ask for favors, help)								

(continued)

375

EXERCISE 15
WORKSHEET A: *(continued)*

Persons

Behaviors	Friends of the same sex	Friends of the opposite sex	Intimate relations (spouse, boyfriend, girlfriend)	Parents, in-laws, and other family members	Children	Authority figures (bosses, professors, doctors)	Business contacts (sales-persons, waiters)	Coworkers, colleagues, and subordi-nates
Express liking, love, and affection								
Initiate and maintain conver-sations								
Self-Affirmation								
Stand up for your legitimate rights								

Refuse requests							
Express personal opinions including disagreement							
Expression of negative feelings							
Express justified annoyance and displeasure							
Express justified anger							

(continued)

EXERCISE 15 (continued)
WORKSHEET B: Problem Areas

INDIVIDUAL PROBLEM AREAS:

Behaviors   Persons

_____   _____

_____   _____

_____   _____

_____   _____

_____   _____

_____   _____

_____   _____

_____   _____

_____   _____

GROUP PROBLEM AREAS:

Behaviors   Persons

_____   _____

_____   _____

_____   _____

_____   _____

_____   _____

_____   _____

_____   _____

_____   _____

EXERCISE 16   Assertiveness—Situations to Role Play

Purposes

1. To role play assertiveness in common situations.

2. To receive feedback on one's own assertiveness.

3. To recognize assertiveness in others.

4. To give feedback to others on their assertiveness.

Facility

A classroom large enough to accommodate the class in groups of six to eight.

Materials

Worksheet A: Situations.
Worksheet B: Responses.
Worksheet C: Practice Situations.
Pencil or pen.

Time Required

One to one and one-half hours.

Group Size

Unlimited groups of six to eight.

Design

1. Lecture or discussion on assertion theory should precede this exercise.

2. Have participants individually respond to the situations in Worksheet A, using the space provided following each situation.

3. After completing Step 1, ask participants to form into groups of six to eight and practice role playing the five situations in pairs. Participants not involved in the immediate role play should give feedback to the players on their assertiveness.

4. After group members have completed Steps 2 and 3, hand out Worksheet B and have

(*continued*)

EXERCISE 16 (continued)

them compare their responses with the examples of responses provided. Discuss these results.

5. Worksheet C, Practice Situations, can be used as small groups wish to role-play assertiveness techniques in various situations, according to individual and group needs. The process noted in Step 3 can be applied.

EXERCISE 16
WORKSHEET A: Situations

1. You and Jessica are associates on a patient care unit. Jessica asks you to give her a ride home every afternoon from now on. You don't want to do it. You say:

_____

_____

_____

_____

_____

2. It is your lunch hour. You're waiting for a friend. She breezes in a half-hour late and, without any reference to her lateness, asks, "How are you?" You answer:

_____

_____

_____

_____

_____

3. Just as you're about to leave for the hospital, your cousin George calls you on the telephone. He starts to tell you about a problem he's been having with his parents. You're anxious to get off the phone. You say:

_____

_____

_____

_____

_____

(*continued*)

EXERCISE 16
WORKSHEET A (*continued*)

4. You're standing in line in a restaurant waiting to be seated. The hostess says, "Who's next?" It is your turn. The woman next to you says, "I am" You turn to her and:

_____

_____

_____

_____

_____

5. You're at an agencywide directors' meeting. An associate speaks up and urges members not to appropriate extra funds to the nursing budget. He gives inaccurate information in his attempt to persuade people that there is no need for extra positions. You disagree with his ideas and his data. You:

_____

_____

_____

_____

_____

Source: The situations and responses from Worksheets A and B, Exercise 16, are a slight modification of those presented in *The New Assertive Woman*, by L. Bloom, K. Coburn, and J. Pearlman. Copyright © 1975 by Delacorte Press. Reprinted by permission.

EXERCISE 16
WORKSHEET B: Responses

Responses to Situation 1:

- ◼ "Well. . . uh. . . I guess I could. . . (pause). . . Uh. . . O.K." (*Nonassertive:* pauses with apparent hesitancy)

- ◼ "I'd love to take you, but sometimes I have to stop at the market on the way home. And sometimes I leave late." (*Nonassertive:* excuses)

- ◼ "What's the matter? Haven't you and Norman gotten around to buying that second car yet?" (*Aggressive:* sarcastic)

- ◼ "You've got nerve! Do you think I have nothing better to do than chauffeur you around?" (*Aggressive:* attempt to make the requester feel guilty)

- ◼ "I know it's a pain to wait around for Norman to pick you up, but I'd rather not be tied down to giving you a ride every day. I'd be happy to do it once a week, though." (*Assertive:* compromise)

- ◼ "I understand that you don't like having to wait for Norman to pick you up every day, but I really don't want to be tied down to having to take you." (*Assertive:* direct refusal)

Responses to Situation 2:

- ◼ "Fine, thanks," said with a smile. (*Nonassertive:* denial of actual feelings)
- ◼ "O.K., I guess," said with a frown on your face. (*Nonassertive:* attempt to communicate the real message, but indirectly)

- ◼ "What do you mean, how am I? How do you think I am, sitting here, waiting for you and staring at the ceiling? Do you ever stop to think of anyone but yourself?" (*Aggressive:* attempt to humiliate the latecomer)

(*continued*)

EXERCISE 16
WORKSHEET B (*continued*)

■ "Well, I'd been looking forward to our lunch, but since I've been waiting so long, I've really gotten upset. Now we'll have only a half-hour together." (*Assertive:* a direct statement of feelings)

Responses to Situation 3:

■ You listen. . . and listen. . . and listen. . . . (*Nonassertive:* accommodation of the other's needs at the expense of your own)

■ "Look, I'm too busy to talk to you now. You've always got some little problem, and I have more important things to do. Good-bye." (*Aggressive:* disregard of the other's wishes and feelings)

■ "I'd like to hear more about it later. I was just on my way to work when you called. I'll call you back tonight.' (*Assertive:* direct statement of wishes)

Responses to Situation 4:

■ Smile. (*Nonassertive:* accommodation of the other's needs at the expense of your own)

■ Frown silently. (*Nonassertive:* attempt at indirect communication of your wishes)

■ Mutter under your breath, "Some people are so pushy"— but you say nothing directly to anyone. (*Nonassertive:* repression of your own wishes)

■ "No you're not. I was here first. You can't take advantage of me, lady." (*Aggressive:* hostile overreaction)

■ "I believe I was here before you." (*Assertive:* direct expression of your own wishes)

Responses to Situation 5:

■ Say nothing to anyone. (*Nonassertive:* refrain from expressing your own opinion)

■ Stand up and say, "I don't know much about this. I'm no expert, but. . . ." (*Nonassertive:* self-demeaning and self-deprecating)

■ Whisper to the person sitting next to you about how stupid the speaker is. (*Nonassertive:* indirect, inhibited behavior)

■ Stand up and say, "You're a liar. You don't know what you're talking about." (*Aggressive:* intent to humiliate)

■ Stand up and say, "I've heard what you have to say, and I disagree with you. I would like you to listen to my point of view." (*Assertive:* stand up for legitimate rights without violating the other's rights)

(*continued*)

EXERCISE 16 (continued)
WORKSHEET C: Practice Situations*

Family Situations

Slumber Party. Your 12-year-old daughter is having a slumber party with five other girls. It is past 2 A.M.; the girls should have settled down to sleep by now, but they're still making a lot of noise.

Alternative Responses:

(a) You toss and turn in bed, wishing your spouse would get up and say something to the girls. You're really angry, but just lie there trying to block out the sounds.

(b) Jumping out of bed, you scold the girls angrily, especially your daughter, for their conduct.

(c) Talking to the girls in a firm tone, so they'll know you mean business, you tell them that you've had enough for tonight. You point out that you need to get up early tomorrow, and that everyone needs to get to sleep.

Late for Dinner. Your wife was supposed to be home for dinner right after work. Instead, she returns hours later explaining she was out with the girls for a few drinks. She is obviously drunk.

Alternative Responses:

(a) You say nothing about how thoughtless she has been, but simply start preparing something for her to eat.

(b) Screaming, yelling, and crying, you tell her that she is a drunken fool, doesn't care about your feelings, is a poor example for the children. You ask about what the neighbors will think. You demand that she get her own dinner.

(c) You calmly and firmly let her know that she should have informed you beforehand that she was going out for a few drinks and would likely be late. Telling her that her cold dinner is in the kitchen, you add that you expect to discuss her behavior further tomorrow.

Visiting Relative. Aunt Margaret, with whom you prefer not to spend much time, is on the telephone. She has just told you of her plans to spend three weeks visiting you, beginning next week.

Alternative Responses:

(a) You think, "Oh, no!" but say, "We'd love to have you come and stay as long as you like!"

(b) You tell her the children have just come down with bad colds, and the spare bed has a broken spring and you'll be going to cousin Bill's weekend after next—none of which is true.

(c) You say, "We'll be glad to have you come for the weekend, but we simply can't invite you for longer. A short visit is happier for everyone, and we'll want to see each other again sooner. We have lots of school and community activities which take up most of our evenings after work."

Past Midnight. Your teenage son has just returned from a school party. It is 3 o'clock in the morning, and you have been frantic, concerned primarily for his well-being, since you had expected him home before midnight.

Alternative Responses:

(a) You turn over and go to sleep.

(b) You shout, "Where the hell have you been? Do you have any idea what time it is? You've kept me up all night! You thoughtless, inconsiderate, selfish, no-good bum—I ought to make you sleep in the street!"

(c) You say, "I've been very worried about you, son. You said you'd be home before midnight, and I've been frantic for hours. Are you all right? I wish you'd called me! Tomorrow we'll discuss your arrangements for staying out late."

Consumer Situations

Haircut. At the barber shop, the barber has just finished cutting your hair and turns the chair toward the mirror so you can inspect. You feel that you would like the sides trimmed more.

Alternative Responses:

(a) You nod your head and say, "That's ok."

(b) Abruptly you demand that he do a more thorough job, adding sarcastically, "You sure didn't take much off the sides, did you?"

(c) You tell the barber you would like to have the sides trimmed more.

Short-changed. As you are leaving a store after a small purchase, you discover that you have been short-changed by three dollars.

(*continued*)

EXERCISE 16
WORKSHEET C (continued)

Alternative Responses:

(a) Pausing for a moment, you try to decide if $3 is worth the effort. After a few moments, you decide it is not and go on your way.

(b) You hurry back into the store and loudly demand your money, making a derogatory comment about "cashiers who can't add."

(c) Re-entering the store, you catch the attention of the clerk, saying that you were short-changed by three dollars. In the process of explaining, you display the change you received back.

Waiting in Line. You are standing near a cash register waiting to pay for your purchase and have it wrapped. Others, who have come after you, are being waited on first. You are getting tired of waiting.

Alternative Responses:

(a) You give up and decide not to buy the article.

(b) Shouting, "You sure get poor service in this store!" you slam the intended purchase down on the counter and walk out.

(c) In a voice loud enough to be heard, you tell the clerk you were ahead of people who have already been served. You ask to be waited on now.

Phone Blues. You are at home, hoping for a restful day. The phone rings, and you answer to a voice stating your full name and asking if that is you. The call is long distance, so you feel it might be important. Then you hear, "This is Rocky Road Magazine. We are conducting a readership survey. Have you heard of our magazine?"

Alternative Responses:

(a) you are polite, don't interrupt, and answer all of the caller's questions. Soon you hear a "sales pitch" instead of a readership survey. The call lasts ten minutes.

(b) You yell, "You people are a bunch of vultures! Don't you know anything about telephone privacy? Stick it in your ear!" You slam down the phone.

(c) You state firmly, "I am not interested." The caller replies, "I only want to ask you a few questions." You repeat firmly, "I am not interested." You hang up the phone.

Employment Situations

Working Late. You and your partner have an engagement this evening which has been planned for several weeks. You plan to leave immediately after work. During the day, however, your supervisor asks you to stay late this evening to work on a special assignment.

Alternative Responses:

(a) You say nothing about your important plans and simply agree to stay until the work is finished.

(b) In a nervous, abrupt voice you say, "No, I will not work late tonight!" Adding a brief criticism of the boss for not planning the work schedule better, you then turn back to your work.

(c) In a firm, pleasant voice, explain your important plans and say you will not be able to stay this evening to work on the special assignment, but perhaps you can help find an alternative solution.

Deniable Passion. One of your co-workers has been making sexual overtures toward you. You are not the least bit interested and have begun to feel harassed.

Alternative Responses:

(a) You begin wearing clothing that is less appealing, change your hair style, and start looking down each time the person approaches.

(b) The next time the person makes an overture you state, "I hate your guts! You are scum! You are so ugly that Frankenstein wouldn't have you."

(c) After a recent incident, you sit and talk quietly with the person. You note that you are feeling pursued and do not wish to be, giving examples of what you mean. Finally you say that if the approaches do not stop, you will file a report with your employer.

Below Par. One of your employees has been doing substandard work recently. You decide it is best to deal with the situation before it gets out of control.

Alternative Responses:

(a) "I'm sorry to bring this up, but I know you must have a good reason why your work has seemed to slide a little lately."

(b) "Things between us are not right. You have been making

(*continued*)

EXERCISE 16
WORKSHEET C (*continued*)

me mad lately by doing a lousy job. If you don't shape up pronto,
you will be out of here."

(c) "I am very concerned about your work performance recently. You won't be receiving a pay increase this period. Let's
analyze what's been going on and see what improvements you
can make for the future."

Job Error. You have made a mistake on the job. Your supervisor discovers it and is letting you know rather harshly that you
should not have been so careless.
Alternative Responses:

(a) Overapologizing, you say, "I'm sorry. I was stupid. How
silly of me. I'll never let it happen again!"

(b) You bristle up and say, "You have no business whatsoever
criticizing my work. Leave me alone, and don't bother me in the
future. I'm capable of handling my own job!"

(c) You agree that you made the mistake, saying, "It was my
mistake. I will be more careful next time. However, I feel you are
being somewhat harsh and I see no need for that."

Late to Work. One of your subordinates has been coming in
late consistently for the last three or four days.
Alternative Responses:

(a) You grumble to yourself or to others about the situations,
but say nothing to the person, hoping he will start coming in early.

(b) You tell the worker off, indicating that he has no right to
take advantage of you and that he had better get to work on time
or else you will see that he is fired.

(c) You point out to the worker that you have observed him
coming in late recently and wonder, "Is there an explanation I
should know about? You'll have to start coming to work on time.
You should have come to me and explained the situation, rather
than saying nothing at all, and leaving me up in the air."

School and Community Situations

Quiet Prof. In a lecture with 300 students, the professor speaks
softly and you know that many others are having trouble hearing
him as you are.

Alternative Responses:

(a) You continue to strain to hear, eventually moving closer to the front of the room, but say nothing about his too-soft voice.

(b) You yell out, "Speak up!"

(c) You raise your hand, get the professor's attention, and ask if he would please speak louder.

Clarification. At a Lion's Club meeting, the President is discussing the procedures for the annual high school speech contest. You are puzzled by several of his statements and believe he has incorrectly described the rules.

Alternative Responses:

(a) You say nothing, but continue to puzzle over the question, looking up your notes from last year's contest later in the day.

(b) You interrupt, telling him he is wrong, pointing out the mistake and correcting him from your own knowledge of the contest. Your tone is derisive, and your choice of words obviously makes him ill-at-ease.

(c) You ask the President to further explain the procedures, expressing your confusion and noting the source of your conflicting information.

Morals. You are one of eleven people in a discussion group on human sexuality. The concepts being supported by three or four of the more verbal students are contrary to your personal moral code.

Alternative Responses:

(a) You listen quietly, not disagreeing openly with the other members or describing your own views.

(b) You loudly denounce the views which have been expressed. Your defense of your own beliefs is strong, and you urge others to accept your point of view as the only correct one.

(c) You speak up in support of your own beliefs, identifying yourself with an apparently unpopular position, but not disparaging the beliefs of others in the group.

Know It All. As a member of the community beautification committee, you are dismayed by the continued dominance of group discussion by Ms. Brown, an opinonated member who has "the answer" to every question. She has begun another tirade. As usual, no one has said anything about it after several minutes.

Alternative Responses:

(continued)

EXERCISE 16
WORKSHEET C *(continued)*

(a) Your irritation increases, but you remain silent.

(b) You explode verbally, curse Ms. Brown for "not giving any-one else a chance," and declare her ideas out-of-date and worth-less.

(c) You interrupt, saying, "Excuse me, Ms. Brown." When rec-ognized, you express your personal irritation about Ms. Brown's monopoly on the group's time. Speaking directly to her as well as the other group members, you suggest a discussion procedure which will permit all members an opportunity to take part, and will minimize dominance by a single individual.

Social Situations

Breaking the Ice. At a party where you don't know anyone except the host, you want to circulate and get to know others. You walk up to three people talking.

Alternative Responses:

(a) You stand close to them and smile but say nothing, waiting for them to notice you.

(b) You listen to the subject they are talking about, then break in and disagree with someone's viewpoint.

(c) You break into the conversation and introduce yourself.

(d) You wait for a pause in the conversation, then introduce yourself and ask if you may join in.

Making a Date. You'd like to ask out a person you have met and talked with three or four times recently.

Alternative Responses:

(a) You sit around the telephone going over in your mind what you will say and how your friend will respond. Several times you lift the phone and are almost finished dialing, then hang up.

(b) You phone and as soon as your friend answers, you re-spond by saying, "Hi, baby, we're going out together this week-end!" Seemingly taken aback, your friend asks who is calling.

(c) You call, and when your friend answers, you say who is calling and ask how school (job, etc.) is going. The reply is, "Fine, except I am worried about a test I will be taking soon." Following the lead, you talk for a few minutes about the test. Then you say that you would like to go together to a show on Friday evening.

Smoke Gets in Your Lungs. You are at a public meeting in a large room. A man enters the room and sits down next to you, puffing enthusiastically on a large cigar. The smoke is very offensive to you.

Alternative Responses:

(a) You suffer the offensive smoke in silence, deciding it is the right of the other person to smoke if he wishes.

(b) You become very angry, demand that he move or put out the cigar and loudly assail the evils and health hazards of the smoking habit.

(c) You firmly but politely ask him to refrain from smoking because it is offensive to you.

(d) You ask him to sit in another seat if he prefers to continue smoking, since you were there first.

Family Situation

Holy Terror. Your son's pre-school teacher tells you he is hitting the other children. At home he "runs the show," staying up late, roughing up the pets, not eating properly. In the past you have thought his behavior "cute."

Alternative Responses:

(a) You talk gently to your son about not hitting the other children. He says the other kids are mean, but that he is sorry. He jumps in your lap and you say, "You are such a sweet boy, I love you."

(b) You grab your son roughly and say that if he hits anyone else that you will beat his bottom till it is raw.

(c) After discussing the issue with the teacher and ruling out any physical causes, you sign up the entire family for counseling.

Plastic Money. Finances are tight. When you receive the credit card bill for the month, you are shocked. Your spouse has charges that seem excessive and unnecessary.

Alternative Responses:

(a) You go to the bank and cash a check for an equal amount of money. After spending it, you feel that you have gained your revenge. You don't mention the credit card.

(b) You realize that you also have over-spent before. You still feel upset, but decide to be understanding this time.

(continued)

EXERCISE 16
WORKSHEET C (*continued*)

(c) You arrange an appropriate time to discuss the finances, and tell your partner that when you opened the statement, you were shocked at the charges. Asking your spouse for an explanation, you also express your wish to establish agreeable guidelines for the use of the credit card.

EXERCISE 17   Group Process—Observation Sheets*

Purposes

1. To gain experience in studying small-group processes.

2. To gain experience in communicating with group members on process observations (giving and receiving feedback).

3. To provide feedback on group functioning in relation to task accomplishment.

4. To foster team building.

Facility

Room large enough to accommodate group members seated around tables or in circles on the floor.

Materials

Worksheet A, B, or C: Evaluation of Group Effectiveness.

Time Required

Ten to 30 minutes for each worksheet.

Group Size

Unlimited small groups of six to eight members.

Design

These Worksheets are to be used following any of the exercises in this book when the members of the group wish to study their group process in relation to accomplishment of their group task (how they functioned as a group).

1. At the conclusion of group work, reserve ten minutes or more for group processing. Request members to individually respond to the items in Worksheet A, B, or C.

(continued)

---

*Source: Adapted by permission from La Monica, Elaine L., *The Nursing Process: A Humanistic Approach*, pp. 307–310. Copyright © 1979 by Addison-Wesley Publishing Company, Inc, Menlo Park, Calif.

EXERCISE 17 (*continued*)

2. Instruct the total group to share their responses with one another, amplifying their rationale for choices. Differences in point allocation should be discussed since they point out various group members' perceptions.

Note: Worksheet A is the least complicated instrument, while Worksheet C is the most complicated. The worksheets should be used progressively from A to C as groups move toward above-average maturity in group-processing activities.

EXERCISE 17
WORKSHEET A: Evaluation of Group Effectiveness

Rate the group on each statement below, with 4 representing your greatest agreement and 1 representing your least agreement with the statement. Circle the number that best approximates your rating of the behavior exhibited by the group.

	Disagree		*Agree*	
1. Group members understood the problem under discussion.	1	2	3	4
2. Group members stayed on the topic.	1	2	3	4
3. Group members avoided premature closure on discussion.	1	2	3	4
4. Group members contributed equally to the discussion.	1	2	3	4
5. Group members agreed with group consensus and/or discussions.	1	2	3	4
6. Group members discussed their opinions openly without hiding personal feelings.	1	2	3	4
7. Group members were able to resolve conflict or discontent.	1	2	3	4
8. Group members displayed commitment to the group tasks.	1	2	3	4
9. Group members indicated satisfaction with the group process.	1	2	3	4
10. Group members indicated satisfaction with the group outcomes.	1	2	3	4

(continued)

Source: This instrument was obtained by this author at the School of Education, University of Massachusetts, 1974. Author unknown.

EXERCISE 17 (*continued*)
WORKSHEET B: Evaluation of Group Effectiveness

The following five items will be used to critique work group activity: climate, conflict, communications, decision making, commitment to objectives.

■ *Individual evaluation.* Each person will evaluate the activity of the work group, distributing 100 points among the alternatives for each item.

■ *Work group evaluation.* The group will discuss the point allocation for every item in order to reach consensus on a single distribution that represents member understanding of how work-group activity took place. Any approach that assures that the thinking of each member on each item is heard and considered may be used. Averaging of individual answers to get a single work-group rating is to be avoided. The purpose is to probe for differences in points of view.

CLIMATE:

1. _____ One or more people tried to take over and control the decisions; it was a competitive, tense, win-lose conflict.

2. _____ The discussion was penetrating and challenging—a very rewarding session to which we all were committed.

3. _____ The discussion was polite, easygoing, and pleasant—a very friendly session.

4. _____ The discussion was rather flat and lifeless; comments slid from point to point with little evidence of commitment.

CONFLICT:

1. _____ There was considerable unnecessary and unprofitable disagreement; competitiveness resulted in win-lose conflict.

2. _____ Disagreements were explored to help the group produce the best possible decisions; conflict was confronted and resolved.

3. _____ We were quite polite and pleasant; we took care to avoid conflict.

4. ____ There was very little open disagreement or conflict.

COMMUNICATION:

1. ____ Ideas and opinions were expressed to "win one's own point"; few members listened to conflicting points of view.

2. ____ Ideas and opinions were expressed openly and with candor; close attention was paid to both majority and minority opinions so that we could fully understand all points of view.

3. ____ Ideas and opinions were expressed politely; we listened to all contributions attentively; no feelings were hurt.

4. ____ Ideas and opinions were expressed with little conviction, and people listened with little evidence of concern.

DECISION MAKING:

1. ____ To complete the task, decisions were "railroaded" by one or a few.

2. ____ Once each member understood all points of view, the work group reached a decision to which all were committed.

3. ____ Decisions were made in a way that gave maximum consideration to all people; we did not want to "rock the boat."

4. ____ Compromise was the key to decision making; the traditional decisions resulted from majority rule.

COMMITMENT TO OBJECTIVES:

1. ____ We attempted to stay directly with the problem, and we solved it as quickly and efficiently as possible.

2. ____ There was an attempt to look at the problem as broadly and deeply as possible. Involvement and creativity characterized the discussion.

3. ____ We often seemed to be more interested in harmony than in getting the job done.

(continued)

EXERCISE 17
WORKSHEET B (*continued*)

4. _____ There was little consistent focus on the problem; we solved the problem as rapidly as possible based on precedents.

Source: This instrument was obtained by this author at the School of Education, University of Massachusetts, 1974. Author unknown.

EXERCISE 17
WORKSHEET C: Evaluation of Group Effectiveness

DIRECTIONS: Insert group members' names, including your own, in the diagonal lettered spaces. Place check marks in the column corresponding to the roles played by each group member, again including yourself. Briefly jot down the context in which the roles were played.

	A	B	C	D	E	F	G	H	I	J	K	L
Task Roles												
1. Initiator												
2. Information seeker												
3. Evaluator												
4. Coordinator												
5. Procedural technician												
6. Recorder												
Maintenance Roles												
1. Encourager												
2. Harmonizer												
3. Compromiser												
4. Standard setter												
5. Gatekeeper												
Self-Oriented Roles												
1. Aggressor												
2. Blocker												
3. Recognition seeker												
4. Playboy												
5. Dominator												
6. Help seeker												

Names of Members indicated across top (A B C D E F G H I J K L)

Source: This instrument was obtained by this author at the School of Education, University of Massachusetts, 1974. Author unknown.

EXERCISE 18   Group Process—Self-Diagnosis

Purposes

1. To raise consciousness of one's own behavior in groups.

2. To self-diagnose learning needs regarding small group functioning.

Facility

None—homework assignment.

Materials

Worksheet A: Self-Diagnosis of Small Group Behavior

Time Required

Fifteen to 30 minutes.

Group Size

Unlimited—individual homework assignment.

Design

1. Using Worksheet A, have class members respond to the items in terms of the categories represented.

2. Ask that they consider the following:
   A. Why do they take certain functions most often?
   B. Why are certain functions never or rarely carried out?
   C. How can they experience functions they would like to practice? What assistance, if any, is needed?

Variation

Self-diagnosis can be discussed within small groups; familiar members can offer feedback on their perceptions.

Source: Reprinted by permission from La Monica, Elaine L., *The Nursing Process: A Humanistic Approach*, pp. 311–313. Copyright © 1979 by Addison-Wesley Publishing Company, Inc, Menlo Park, Calif.

EXERCISE 18
WORKSHEET A: Self-Diagnosis of Small-Group Behavior

Listed below are functions that are performed by members of discussion groups. Considering each category, check the columns that apply to you.

Frequency of Behavior(s)

	I perceive myself to use most often	I seldom use	I never use	I would like to practice
Task Roles				
1. Initiator				
2. Information seeker				
3. Evaluator				
4. Coordinator				
5. Procedural technician				
6. Recorder				
Maintenance Roles				
1. Encourager				
2. Harmonizer				
3. Compromiser				
4. Standard setter				
5. Gatekeeper				

(*continued*)

EXERCISE 18
WORKSHEET A (*continued*)

Frequency of Behavior(s)

	I perceive myself to use most often	I seldom use	I never use	I would like to practice
Self-Oriented Roles				
1. Aggressor				
2. Blocker				
3. Recognition seeker				
4. Playboy				
5. Dominator				
6. Help seeker				

Respond to each question explicitly. Use extra paper if necessary.

A. Why do I use certain roles most often?

B. Why are certain roles never or rarely carried out?

C. How can I experience roles that I would like to practice? What assistance, if any, do I need?

EXERCISE 19   **Conflict Resolution—Saturn's First
                      Hospital Station***

Purposes	1. To develop group collaboration and planning.
	2. To experience conflict resolution.
	3. To foster group team building.
	4. To facilitate setting group goals.
Facility	A classroom large enough to accommodate participants.
Materials	Paper and pencil or pen.
	Blackboard and chalk.
Group Sizes	One and one-half to two hours.
Group Size	No more than five groups of six to eight participants.
Design	1. Explain the following to the group: The entire class has been carefully selected to set up the first space hospital station on the planet Saturn. The class will be transported tomorrow on Columbia 6. Members will spend the rest of their lives on Saturn. The shuttle that transports people and equipment will visit Uranus and Mars after stopping at Saturn and then return to Earth. The next visit to Saturn for transporting equipment and personnel is unknown, but it will not be before ten Earth years have passed. The class must decide what is needed to survive and what is needed to equip the hospital. Due to constraints of space on Columbia 6, each person can bring only five specific items on board; these items include personal

---

*Source: The idea for this exercise came from one entitled "Noah's Ark" at the School of Education, University of Massachusetts, 1973.

and hospital needs. Air concentration that is needed to sustain human life is guaranteed as is water. Nothing else is promised.

2. Have members individually write down the five items that they wish to bring. (5 minutes)

3. After completing Step 2, notify the class that you have received word that extra fuel is required on board as a result of a meteor storm that is expected between Saturn and Uranus. The space allocated to the hospital crew has been cut. Class members should therefore form into pairs (have triads if there is an odd number in the group) and select five things out of their combined list of ten items to bring to Saturn. (10 minutes)

4. After step 3 has been completed, a spacegram is received with the following message: "President orders that the intergalactic missile tracking station be housed on Saturn." The effect of this message on the hospital crew is elation. However, all materials for the missile tracking station must be transported in tomorrow's voyage. Space is again decreased and each group of six to eight can only bring five items on board the shuttle to Saturn. After grouping into six to eight members, have each group decide what five items to bring. Pairs (triads) formed in Step 3 should be in the same group. (15 minutes)

5. When groups have selected their five items, announce the following: There is a massive surplus in the country's budget—enough for a sister hospital station in Uranus. The president has selected the crew for Uranus; both crews will be transported together. *Each crew* will bring only five items due to the

(continued)

EXERCISE 19 (*continued*)

shortage of space on the ship. Each group should be instructed to choose a negotiator and plan a strategy for selling other groups on the importance of taking their items (15 minutes). Negotiators from each group will then meet around a table at the head of the class to select the five items that will be brought to Saturn. Negotiations will take place in three rounds within the following time limits: Round 1—meeting of negotiators (15 minutes); Round 2—negotiators consult with their groups (15 minutes); Round 3—meeting of negotiators (15 minutes). The decision on the five items must be made by the end of Round 3. Only the negotiators can talk during Rounds 1 and 3; groups must be quiet.

6. After the five items have been selected, list them on a blackboard and discuss the experience with the class as a whole. Questions that can be asked and areas that usually engender discussion are:
   A. What did the items chosen by individuals represent in comparison with those chosen by groups?
   B. Was their movement from counting on self to counting on others and the interactions between and among others?
   C. Were the resources of the group studied? Could people build things, grow things, and so forth?
   D. Did the final items represent any particular area of Maslow's hierarchy? Explain.
   E. How was the negotiator chosen? Were needed attributes of the negotiator specified?
   F. Was creative problem solving evident as the experience developed?
   G. What was learned from the experience that applies in the present?

EXERCISE 20   Conflict Resolution—Contingency Contracting

Purposes
1. To apply types of contingency contracting to real or hypothetical situations.

2. To role play one type of contingency contract.

3. To receive feedback from peers on the role play.

Facility
A classroom to accommodate participants working in pairs with space between dyads.

Materials
Worksheets A, B, C, D, and E—Types of Contingency Contracts.

Pencil or pen.

Time Required
Forty-five minutes.

Group Size
Unlimited pairs.

Design
1. Instruct participants to individually choose one of the five worksheets and jot down an experienced or hypothetical example that requires the particular contingency contract. If necessary, refer to Chapter 16 for the definitions and examples of each type of contract.

2. Participants should form into pairs and role play the examples. The writer of the example should be the leader first; the other member should be the follower. Members of pairs should provide feedback to each other. If time permits, roles should switch using the same two situations.

3. After dyads have completed Step 2, have two or three dyads volunteer and share their experiences with the group.

(continued)

EXERCISE 20 (*continued*)
WORKSHEET A: Leader-Control Contingency Contract

Example:

_____

_____

_____

_____

_____

_____

_____

_____

_____

_____

_____

_____

_____

_____

_____

_____

_____

_____

_____

_____

_____

_____

_____

_____

_____

EXERCISE 20
WORKSHEET B: Partial-Control-by-Follower Contingency
Contract

Example:

_____

_____

_____

_____

_____

_____

_____

_____

_____

_____

_____

_____

_____

_____

_____

_____

_____

_____

_____

_____

_____

(_continued_)

EXERCISE 20 (*continued*)
**WORKSHEET C: Equal-Control-by-Leader-and-Follower
                 Contingency Contract**

Example:

_____

_____

_____

_____

_____

_____

_____

_____

_____

_____

_____

_____

_____

_____

_____

_____

_____

_____

_____

_____

_____

_____

_____

_____

EXERCISE 20
WORKSHEET D: Partial-Control-by-Leader Contingency
Contract

Example:

_____

_____

_____

_____

_____

_____

_____

_____

_____

_____

_____

_____

_____

_____

_____

_____

_____

_____

_____

_____

_____

_____

_____

_____

(_continued_)

EXERCISE 20 (*continued*)
WORKSHEET E: Follower-Control Contingency Contract

Example:

_____

_____

_____

_____

_____

_____

_____

_____

_____

_____

_____

_____

_____

_____

_____

_____

_____

_____

_____

_____

_____

_____

_____

_____

_____

_____

_____

EXERCISE 21: Time Management—Time Analysis Sheets

Purposes
1. To facilitate identification of time wasters.
2. To analyze time wasters.
3. To use time more effectively.

Facility
None—this exercise is a self-study homework assignment.

Materials
Worksheet A: Time Analysis Worksheet.
Worksheet B: Biggest Time Wasters.
Worksheet C: Time Log.
Pen or pencil.

Time Required
Variable.

Group Size
Unlimited—homework assignment.

Design
Three worksheets are provided for use in individual analysis for professional and/or personal aspects of one's life. It is suggested that they be used in order—Worksheet A through Worksheet C—for the first time. Then they can be reused over and over as one wishes to be in more and more control of time.

Worksheets A and B require simply filling in the blanks.

Worksheet C requires specifying daily goals and keeping a log of activities for the day. The log can then be analyzed using Worksheets A and/or B with new goals set for the next day. Progress can be traced by reviewing these sheets.

Variation
Group members can be encouraged to share analyses with peers. Class time can be allotted for small- and large-group discussion.

(*continued*)

EXERCISE 21 (*continued*)
WORKSHEET A: Time Analysis Worksheet

What items am I spending too much time on?	What am I doing that does not need to be done at all?
What items am I spending too little time on?	What am I doing that could be done better (or more economically, more effectively) by others?
Items in which I can make my most important savings.	Ways by which I can avoid overusing the time of others.
Other ways in which I can make effective savings.	Other suggestions.

Source: Brown, D., *The use of time: A looking-into-leadership monograph*. Fairfax, VA: Leadership Resources, 1980, p. 9. Reproduced by permission.

EXERCISE 21
WORKSHEET B: Biggest Time Wasters

Specifically, my biggest time wasters are:

1. _____
2. _____
3. _____
4. _____
5. _____
6. _____
7. _____
8. _____

Imposed by   Cause   Solution

1. _____   _____   _____

              _____   _____

2. _____   _____   _____

              _____   _____

3. _____   _____   _____

              _____   _____

4. _____   _____   _____

              _____   _____

5. _____   _____   _____

              _____   _____

6. _____   _____   _____

              _____   _____

7. _____   _____   _____

              _____   _____

8. _____   _____   _____

              _____   _____

Source: Graf P. 1979. *Time management*. Unpublished material.

(continued)

EXERCISE 21 (continued)
WORKSHEET C: Time Log

Date _____

Day of the week _____

Goals: 1. _____ 4. _____

2. _____ 5. _____

3. _____ 6. _____

Time	Activity	Priority Rating A, B, or C	Comments
8:00 8:30			
9:00 9:30			
10:00 10:30			
11:00 11:30			
12:00 12:30			
1:00 1:30			
2:00 2:30			

Time	Activity	Priority Rating A, B, or C	Comments
3:00 3:30			
4:00 4:30			
5:00 5:30			
6:00 6:30			
7:00 7:30			
8:00 8:30			
Evening			

Source: Graf P. 1979. Time management. Unpublished material. Reprinted by permission of the author.

EXERCISE 22 **Performance Appraisal—Rating Scale for Clinical Staff Nursing**

Purposes

1. To evaluate the clinical performance of a staff nurse.

2. To practice using a Likert-type rating scale for evaluating performance.

3. To develop strategies for meeting the clinical learning needs of a staff nurse.

Facility

None. This is a clinical assignment.

Materials

Worksheet A: Clinical Nurse Performance Appraisal Form

Pen or pencil

Time Required

One hour or more

Group Size

Unlimited dyads

Design

1. As a homework assignment, have participants read Chapter 18, plus other related articles and written materials on the topic.

2. Ask that participants form into comfortable pairs—teaming with a peer who is seen as nonthreatening and/or is a friend. Using Worksheet A, ask that each pair member observe the other's clinical practice for a period of one to two shifts, trying particularly to assess the areas noted in the performance appraisal form.

3. Using Worksheet A, each pair member should appraise their partner's performance in writing. Following the written appraisal, the pair should meet and role play discussion of the performance appraisals. Each pair member should have the opportunity to be the appraisor and the person being appraised. Together, they should develop an action plan for the next month.

Variation   The pair member being appraised may complete Worksheet A as a self-report prior to the role play discussion. Then both appraisals can be discussed with reference to the appraisee's performance. Also, the period being appraised can be longer than one to two shifts, depending on the available time.

EXERCISE 22
WORKSHEET A: Clinical Nurse Performance Appraisal
Form

Name of Appraisee _____

Name of Appraiser _____

Date of Appraisal _____

	Unacceptable	Acceptable	Distinguished	Not Observed	Not Applicable
Clinical Skills					
Data Collection					
Taking Nursing Histories					
Interviewing					
Interpreting Clinical Data					
Consulting with Colleagues					
Talking with Families					
Conducting Physical Assessments					
Nursing Diagnosis					
Processing Data					
Determining Diagnoses					
Setting Priorities					
Nursing Orders					
Writing Nursing Orders					
Maintaining Individualized Care					
Providing Care					
Giving Direct Care					
Effectively Using Interpersonal Processes					
Quality of Technical Skills					
Quality of Teaching Methods					

	Unacceptable	Acceptable	Distinguished	Not Observed	Not Applicable
Advocating for the Client/Family					
Making Appropriate Referrals					
Coordinating Care					
Delegating Care Appropriately					
Supervising Other Nursing Personnel					
Evaluating Outcome					

Goals for Next Appraisal Period   *Date for Next Appraisal* ____

1. _____

_____

_____

_____

2. _____

_____

_____

_____

3. _____

_____

_____

_____

4. _____

_____

_____

_____

5. _____

_____

_____

Epilogue

For Learners . . . No matter what you do, make it your best.
Leave nothing undone.

Be sensitive to your own way of growing,
And

Have clear goals for yourself.
Be strict in your journey
Toward their fulfillment.

Learn to know and to feel with yourself.
Only then will you be free to know and
To feel with others.

Set high goals and then
Put your mind on reaching them.

In all, only hold on to the positive and
Illuminate it.
Life can then be full of sunshine;
Life can then be successful
At every moment. . . .

Elaine Lynne La Monica

Appendix: Selected Bibliography on Experiential Learning

Benne, K., Bradford, L., Gibb, J., & Lippitt, R. (Eds.). (1975). *Laboratory method of changing and learning: Theory and application.* Palo Alto, CA: Science and Behavior Books.

Brill, N. (1976). *Teamwork: Working together in human services.* Philadelphia: Lippincott.

Burton, A., (Ed.). (1969). *Encounter.* San Francisco: Jossey-Bass.

Corey, G., & Corey, M. (1982). *Groups: Process and practice* (2nd ed.). Monterey, CA: Brooks/Cole.

Dyer, W. (Ed.). (1972). *Modern theory & method in group training.* New York: Van Nostrand Reinhold.

Egan, G. (1970). *Encounter: Group processes for interpersonal growth.* Belmont, CA: Brooks/Cole.

Egan, G. (1973). *Face to face: The small-group experience and interpersonal growth.* Monterey, CA: Brooks/Cole.

Gazda, G., Asbury, F., Balzer, F., Childers, W., Desselle, R., & Walters, R. (1973). *Human relations development: A manual for educators.* Boston: Allyn & Bacon.

Gazda, G., Asbury, F., Balzer, F., Childers, W., & Walters, R. (1977). *Human relations development: A manual for educators.* (2nd ed.). Boston: Allyn & Bacon.

Gazda, G., Asbury, F., Balzer, F., Childers, W., & Walters, R. (1983). *Human relations development: A manual for educators* (3rd ed.). Boston: Allyn & Bacon.

Golembiewski, R., & Blumberg, A. (Eds.). (1970). *Sensitivity training and the laboratory approach: Readings about concepts and applications.* Itasca, IL: Peacock.

Golembiewski, R., & Blumberg, A. (Eds.). (1973). *Sensitivity training and the laboratory approach: Readings about concepts and applications.* (2nd ed.). Itasca, IL: Peacock.

Golembiewski, R. & Blumberg, A. (Eds.). (1977). *Sensitivity training and the laboratory approach: Readings about concepts and applications.* (3rd ed.). Itasca, IL: Peacock.

Goodstein, L., Pfeiffer, J. (Eds.). (1983). *The 1983 annual for facilitators, trainers, and consultants.* San Diego: University Associates.

427

Grove, I. (1976). *Experiences in interpersonal communication*. Englewood Cliffs, NJ: Prentice-Hall.

Harvard Business Reviews on human relations. (1979). New York: Harper & Row.

Johnson, D. (1986). *Reaching out: Interpersonal effectiveness and self-actualization* (3rd ed.). Englewood Cliffs, NJ: Prentice-Hall.

Johnson, D., & Johnson, F. (1987). *Joining together: Group theory & group skills* (3rd ed.). Englewood Cliffs, NJ: Prentice-Hall.

Jones, J., & Pfeiffer, J. (Eds.). (1975). *The 1975 annual handbook for group facilitators*. La Jolla, CA: University Associates.

Jones, J., & Pfeiffer, J. (Eds.). (1977). *The 1977 annual handbook for group facilitators*. La Jolla, CA: University Associates.

Jones, J., & Pfeiffer, J. (Eds.). (1979). *The 1979 annual handbook for group facilitators*. La Jolla, CA: University Associates.

Jones, J., & Pfeiffer, J. (Eds.). (1981). *The 1981 annual handbook for group facilitators*. San Diego: University Associates.

Kolb, D., Rubin, I., & McIntyre, J. (1979). *Organizational psychology: An experiential approach* (3rd ed.). Englewood Cliffs, NJ: Prentice-Hall.

Lieberman, M., Yalom, I., & Miles, M. (1973). *Encounter groups: First facts*. New York: Basic Books.

Luft, J. (1970). *Group processes: An introduction to group dynamics* (2nd ed.). Palo Alto, CA: National Press Books.

Maier, N., Solem, A., & Maier, A. (1975). *The role-play technique: A handbook for management & leadership practice*. La Jolla, CA: University Associates.

Morris, K., & Cinnamon, K. (1974). *A handbook of verbal group exercises*. San Diego: University Associates.

Morris, K., & Cinnamon, K. (1975). *A handbook of non-verbal group exercises*. San Diego: University Associates.

Napier, R., & Gershenfeld, M. (1985). *Groups: Theory & experience* (3rd ed.). Boston: Houghton Mifflin.

O'Banion, T., & O'Connell, A. (1970). *The shared journey: An introduction to encounter*. Englewood Cliffs, NJ: Prentice-Hall

Pfeiffer, J. (Ed.) (1987–88). *The annual series for group facilitators*. San Diego: University Associates.

Pfeiffer, J., & Goodstein, L. (Eds.). (1982–1986). *The annual series for facilitators, trainers, and consultants*. San Diego: University Associates.

Pfeiffer, J. & Jones, J. (Eds.). (1974–85). *A handbook of structured experiences for human relations training* (Vols I–X). La Jolla, CA: University Associates.

Pfeiffer, J. & Jones, J. (Eds.). (1972–81). *The annual series for group facilitators*. La Jolla, CA: University Associates.

Saulnier, L., & Simard, T. (1973). *Personal growth & interpersonal relations*. Englewood Cliffs, NJ: Prentice-Hall.

Schein, E. (1969). *Process consultation: Its role in organization development*. Reading, MA: Addison-Wesley.

Schein, E., & Bennis, W. (1965). *Personal and organizational change through group methods: The laboratory approach*. New York: Wiley.

Author Index

Subject Index